Mixed Affective States: Beyond Current Boundaries

Editors

GABRIELE SANI
ALAN C. SWANN

PSYCHIATRIC CLINICS OF NORTH AMERICA

www.psych.theclinics.com

Consulting Editor
HARSH K. TRIVEDI

March 2020 • Volume 43 • Number 1

ELSEVIER

1600 John F. Kennedy Boulevard • Suite 1800 • Philadelphia, Pennsylvania, 19103-2899

http://www.theclinics.com

PSYCHIATRIC CLINICS OF NORTH AMERICA Volume 43, Number 1
March 2020 ISSN 0193-953X, ISBN-13: 978-0-323-76479-7

Editor: Lauren Boyle
Developmental Editor: Kristen Helm

Psychiatric Clinics of North America (ISSN 0193-953X) is published quarterly by Elsevier Inc., 360 Park Avenue South, New York, NY 10010-1710. Months of issue are March, June, September, and December. Business and Editorial Offices: 1600 John F. Kennedy Blvd., Suite 1800, Philadelphia, PA 19103-2899. Periodicals postage paid at New York, NY and additional mailing offices. Subscription prices are $335.00 per year (US individuals), $734.00 per year (US institutions), $100.00 per year (US students/residents), $406.00 per year (Canadian individuals), $462.00 per year (international individuals), $924.00 per year (Canadian & international institutions), and $220.00 per year (international students/residents), $100.00 per year (Canadian & students/residents). Foreign air speed delivery is included in all *Clinics'* subscription prices. All prices are subject to change without notice. **POSTMASTER: Send address changes to *Psychiatric Clinics of North America*, Elsevier Health Sciences Division, Subscription Customer Service, 3251 Riverport Lane, Maryland Heights, MO 63043. Customer Service: 1-800-654-2452 (US). From outside the United States, call 1-314-447-8871. Fax: 1-314-447-8029. E-mail: journalscustomerservice-usa@elsevier.com (for print support) and journalsonlinesupport-usa@elsevier.com (for online support).**

Reprints. For copies of 100 or more, of articles in this publication, please contact the Commercial Reprints Department, Elsevier Inc., 360 Park Avenue South, New York, New York 10010-1710. Tel.: 212-633-3874, Fax: 212-633-3820, E-mail: reprints@elsevier.com.

Psychiatric Clinics of North America is covered in *MEDLINE/PubMed (Index Medicus), Current Contents/Social and Behavioral Sciences, Social Science Citation Index, Embase/Excerpta Medica,* and PsycINFO.

Printed in the United States of America.

Contributors

CONSULTING EDITOR

HARSH K. TRIVEDI, MD, MBA
President and Chief Executive Officer, Sheppard Pratt Health System, Baltimore, Maryland, USA

EDITORS

GABRIELE SANI, MD
Institute of Psychiatry, Università Cattolica del Sacro Cuore, Department of Psychiatry, Fondazione Policlinico Universitario "Agostino Gemelli" IRCCS, Rome, Italy

ALAN C. SWANN, MD
Professor, Menninger Department of Psychiatry and Behavioral Sciences, Baylor College of Medicine, Staff Psychiatrist, Mental Health Care Line, Michael E. DeBakey VA Medical Center, Houston, Texas, USA

AUTHORS

MONICA AAS, PhD
NORMENT K.G Jebsen Centre for Psychosis Research, Division of Mental Health and Addiction, Institute of Clinical Medicine, University of Oslo, Oslo University Hospital, Oslo, Norway

GLORIA ANGELETTI, MD
Centro Lucio Bini, Azienda Ospedaliera Sant'Andrea, UOC di Psichiatria, NESMOS Department, Sapienza School of Medicine and Psychology, Sant'Andrea University Hospital, Rome, Italy

GERARD ANMELLA, MD
Barcelona Bipolar and Depressive Disorders Program, Hospital Clinic, University of Barcelona, Institute of Neuroscience, IDIBAPS, CIBERSAM, Barcelona, Catalonia, Spain

ROSS J. BALDESSARINI, MD
International Consortium for Research on Mood and Psychotic Disorders, McLean Hospital, Mailman Research Center 3, Belmont, Massachusetts, USA; Department of Psychiatry, Harvard Medical School, Boston, Massachusetts, USA

MARGHERITA BARBUTI, MD
Department of Clinical and Experimental Medicine, University of Pisa, Pisa, Italy

SERGIO A. BARROILHET, MD, PhD
Clínica Psiquiátrica Universitaria, Facultad de Medicina, Universidad de Chile, Santiago, Chile; Department of Psychiatry, Tufts University, School of Medicine, Boston, Massachusetts, USA

EUGENIA CHEN, BS
MD Candidate, Menninger Department of Psychiatry and Behavioral Sciences, Baylor
College of Medicine, Houston, Texas, USA

LAVINIA DE CHIARA, MD
NESMOS Department, Sant'Andrea Hospital, Sapienza University, School of Medicine
and Psychology, Centro Lucio Bini, Rome, Italy

VALERIA DEL VECCHIO, MD, PhD
Department of Psychiatry, University of Campania "Luigi Vanvitelli," Naples, Italy

MARCO DI NICOLA, MD, PhD
Fondazione Policlinico Universitario "A. Gemelli" IRCCS, Università Cattolica del Sacro
Cuore, Rome, Italy

ANDREA FIORILLO, MD, PhD
Department of Psychiatry, University of Campania "Luigi Vanvitelli," Naples, Italy

ALBERTO FORTE, MD
International Consortium for Research on Mood and Psychotic Disorders, McLean
Hospital, Belmont, Massachusetts, USA; Department Neurosciences, Mental Health and
Sensory Organs, Suicide Prevention Center, Sant'Andrea Hospital, Sapienza University of
Rome, Rome, Italy

S. NASSIR GHAEMI, MD, MPH
Department of Psychiatry, Tufts University, School of Medicine, Tufts Medical Center,
Harvard Medical School, Harvard University, Boston, Massachusetts, USA

VINCENZO GIALLONARDO, MD
Department of Psychiatry, University of Campania "Luigi Vanvitelli," Naples, Italy

ANNA GIMENEZ, MD
Barcelona Bipolar and Depressive Disorders Program, Hospital Clinic, University of
Barcelona, Institute of Neuroscience, IDIBAPS, CIBERSAM, Barcelona, Catalonia,
Spain

ADAM GOLDBERG, MD
Child and Adolescent Psychiatry Fellow, Department of Psychiatry and Behavioral
Sciences, McGovern Medical School, The University of Texas Health Science Center at
Houston, Houston, Texas, USA

SUSANA GOMES-DA-COSTA, MD
Barcelona Bipolar and Depressive Disorders Program, Hospital Clinic, University of
Barcelona, Institute of Neuroscience, IDIBAPS, CIBERSAM, Barcelona, Catalonia,
Spain

DELFINA JANIRI, MD
NESMOS Department (Neuroscience, Mental Health, and Sensory Organs), School of
Medicine and Psychology, Sant'Andrea Hospital, Sapienza University, UOC Psichiatria,
Centro Lucio Bini, Rome, Italy; Icahn School of Medicine and Mount Sinai, New York, New
York, USA

LUIGI JANIRI, MD
Fondazione Policlinico Universitario "A. Gemelli" IRCCS, Università Cattolica del Sacro
Cuore, Rome, Italy

GEORGIOS D. KOTZALIDIS, MD, PhD
Centro Lucio Bini, Azienda Ospedaliera Sant'Andrea, UOC di Psichiatria, NESMOS Department, Sapienza School of Medicine and Psychology, Sant'Andrea University Hospital, Rome, Italy

GIORGIO D. KOTZALIDIS, MD, PhD
Neurosciences, Mental Health, and Sensory Organs (NESMOS) Department, Faculty of Medicine and Psychology, Sapienza University, Sant'Andrea University Hospital, UOC Psichiatria, Rome, Italy

ALEXIA EMILIA KOUKOPOULOS, MD, PhD
Azienda Ospedaliera Universitaria Policlinico Umberto I, Sapienza School of Medicine and Dentistry, Centro Lucio Bini, Rome, Italy

SHERIN KURIAN, MD
Research Coordinator, Menninger Department of Psychiatry and Behavioral Sciences, Baylor College of Medicine, Department of Psychiatry, Texas Children's Hospital, Houston, Texas, USA

PIERLUIGI LANZOTTI, MD
Fondazione Policlinico Universitario "A. Gemelli" IRCCS, Università Cattolica del Sacro Cuore, Rome, Italy

DELPHINE LEE, LCSW
Menninger Department of Psychiatry and Behavioral Sciences, Baylor College of Medicine, Houston, Texas, USA

MARIJN LIJFFIJT, PhD
Assistant Professor, Menninger Department of Psychiatry and Behavioral Sciences, Baylor College of Medicine, and the Research Care Line, Michael E. DeBakey VA Medical Center, Houston, Texas, USA

CRISTIAN LLACH, MD
Barcelona Bipolar and Depressive Disorders Program, Hospital Clinic, University of Barcelona, Institute of Neuroscience, IDIBAPS, CIBERSAM, Barcelona, Catalonia, Spain

MARIO LUCIANO, MD, PhD
Department of Psychiatry, University of Campania "Luigi Vanvitelli," Naples, Italy

GIOVANNI MANFREDI, MD, PhD
Centro Lucio Bini, Azienda Ospedaliera Sant'Andrea, UOC di Psichiatria, NESMOS Department, Sapienza School of Medicine and Psychology, Sant'Andrea University Hospital, Rome, Italy

SANJAY J. MATHEW, MD
Michael E. DeBakey VA Medical Center, Menninger Department of Psychiatry and Behavioral Sciences, Baylor College of Medicine, Houston, Texas, USA

LORENZO MAZZARINI, MD, PhD
Neurosciences, Mental Health, and Sensory Organs (NESMOS) Department, Faculty of Medicine and Psychology, Sapienza University, Sant'Andrea University Hospital, UOC Psichiatria, Rome, Italy

PIERPAOLO MEDDA, MD
Psychiatry Unit 2, Azienda Ospedaliero-Universitaria Pisana, Pisa, Italy

LORENZO MOCCIA, MD
Fondazione Policlinico Universitario "A. Gemelli" IRCCS, Università Cattolica del Sacro Cuore, Rome, Italy

MARCO MODICA, MD
Fondazione Policlinico Universitario "A. Gemelli" IRCCS, Università Cattolica del Sacro Cuore, Rome, Italy

DEBBI ANN MORRISSETTE, PhD
Senior Medical Writer, Neuroscience Education Institute, Carlsbad, California, USA

ANDREA MURRU, MD, PhD
Barcelona Bipolar and Depressive Disorders Program, Hospital Clinic, University of Barcelona, Institute of Neuroscience, IDIBAPS, CIBERSAM, Barcelona, Catalonia, Spain

MARTINA NOVI, MD
Department of Clinical and Experimental Medicine, University of Pisa, Pisa, Italy

BRITTANY O'BRIEN, PhD
Michael E. DeBakey VA Medical Center, Menninger Department of Psychiatry and Behavioral Sciences, Baylor College of Medicine, Houston, Texas, USA

ISABELLA PACCHIAROTTI, MD, PhD
Barcelona Bipolar and Depressive Disorders Program, Hospital Clinic, University of Barcelona, Institute of Neuroscience, IDIBAPS, CIBERSAM, Barcelona, Catalonia, Spain

ISABELLA PANACCIONE, MD, PhD
Mental Health Department, ASL Roma 1, Centro Lucio Bini, Rome, Italy

MARIA PEPE, MD
Fondazione Policlinico Universitario "A. Gemelli" IRCCS, Università Cattolica del Sacro Cuore, Rome, Italy

GIULIO PERUGI, MD
Associate Professor, Department of Clinical and Experimental Medicine, University of Pisa, Psychiatry Unit 2, Azienda Ospedaliero-Universitaria Pisana, Pisa, Italy

MAURIZIO POMPILI, MD, PhD
Full Professor and Chair of Psychiatry, Department of Neurosciences, Mental Health and Sensory Organs, Director, Suicide Prevention Center, Director, Sant'Andrea Hospital, Sapienza University of Rome, Rome, Italy

CHIARA RAPINESI, MD
Neurosciences, Mental Health, and Sensory Organs (NESMOS) Department, Faculty of Medicine and Psychology, Sapienza University, Sant'Andrea University Hospital, UOC Psichiatria, Rome, Italy

GAIA SAMPOGNA, MD
Department of Psychiatry, University of Campania "Luigi Vanvitelli," Naples, Italy

GABRIELE SANI, MD
Institute of Psychiatry, Università Cattolica del Sacro Cuore, Department of Psychiatry, Fondazione Policlinico Universitario "Agostino Gemelli" IRCCS, Rome, Italy

JOHANNA SAXENA, BS, BA
Research Coordinator, Menninger Department of Psychiatry and Behavioral Sciences, Baylor College of Medicine, Department of Psychiatry, Texas Children's Hospital, Houston, Texas, USA

KIRTI SAXENA, MD
Associate Professor, Menninger Department of Psychiatry and Behavioral Sciences, Baylor College of Medicine, Department of Psychiatry, Texas Children's Hospital, Houston, Texas, USA

ALESSIO SIMONETTI, MD
Clinical Assistant Professor, Menninger Department of Psychiatry and Behavioral Sciences, Baylor College of Medicine, Houston, Texas, USA; Department of Neurology and Psychiatry, Sapienza University of Rome, Centro Lucio Bini, Rome, Italy

STEPHEN M. STAHL, MD, PhD, DSs (Hon)
Professor, Department of Psychiatry, University of California, San Diego, San Diego, California, USA; Honorary Fellow, University of Cambridge, Cambridge, United Kingdom

ALAN C. SWANN, MD
Professor, Menninger Department of Psychiatry and Behavioral Sciences, Baylor College of Medicine, Staff Psychiatrist, Mental Health Care Line, Michael E. DeBakey VA Medical Center, Houston, Texas, USA

LEONARDO TONDO, MD
International Consortium for Research on Mood and Psychotic Disorders, McLean Hospital, Mailman Research Center 3, Belmont, Massachusetts, USA; Department of Psychiatry, Harvard Medical School, Boston, Massachusetts, USA; Lucio Bini Mood Disorders Center, Cagliari, Italy

BENIAMINO TRIPODI, MD
Department of Clinical and Experimental Medicine, University of Pisa, Pisa, Italy

MARC VALENTÍ, MD, PhD
Barcelona Bipolar and Depressive Disorders Program, Hospital Clinic, University of Barcelona, Institute of Neuroscience, IDIBAPS, CIBERSAM, Barcelona, Catalonia, Spain

GUSTAVO H. VAZQUEZ, MD, PhD, FRCPC
Professor, Department of Psychiatry, Queen's University, Kingston, Ontario, Canada; International Consortium for Research on Mood and Psychotic Disorders, McLean Hospital, Mailman Research Center 3, Belmont, Massachusetts, USA

NORMA VERDOLINI, MD, PhD
Barcelona Bipolar and Depressive Disorders Program, Hospital Clinic, University of Barcelona, Institute of Neuroscience, IDIBAPS, CIBERSAM, Barcelona, Catalonia, Spain

EDUARD VIETA, MD, PhD
Barcelona Bipolar and Depressive Disorders Program, Hospital Clinic, University of Barcelona, Institute of Neuroscience, IDIBAPS, CIBERSAM, Barcelona, Catalonia, Spain

Contents

Mixed states have been discussed for more than 2 millennia. The theoretic conception of the coexistence of presumably opposite symptoms of mood or of different psychic domains is well established, although obscured by the presumed separation between bipolar and depressive disorders. Moreover, the lack of response to treatments and severe psychopathology raise important issues requiring urgent solution. The aim of this article was to review the development of the concept of mixed states from the classic literature to modern nosologic systems and to claim for the need of a new paradigm to address the still-open issues about mixed states.

The construct of mixed states is a robust clinical entity with a high variability of prevalence according to different diagnostic criteria. Despite the changes over the years, current official diagnostic criteria still have poor clinical usefulness. Premorbid characteristics with a potential high clinical importance such as temperament, personality, and emotional reactivity are understudied in patients with mixed states and excluded from the current nosologic systems. The authors provide an overview of current nosography and clinical pictures of mixed states and discuss the role of temperament, personality, and emotional reactivity in mixed states.

Mixed states are frequent clinical pictures in psychiatric practice but are not well described in nosologic systems. Debate exists as to defining mixed states. We review factor and cluster analytical studies and prominent clinical/conceptual models of mixed states. While mania involves standard manic symptoms and depression involves standard depressive symptoms, core additional features of the mixed state are, primarily, psychomotor activation and, secondarily, dysphoria. Those features are more pronounced in mixed mania than in mixed depression but are present in both.

disorders. They are associated with major increases of risk of suicidal behaviors. The authors reviewed the association of suicidal behavior with
mixed features in both major depressive and bipolar disorders, as well
as potentially relevant adverse effects of antidepressant treatment and
use of alternative treatments aimed at minimizing agitation and suicidal
risk.

Pediatric bipolar disorder (PBD) is a severe and chronic illness. The occurrence of mixed symptoms might add further risk of recurrence of treatment
resistance and suicidality. Early recognition and treatment of mixed symptoms might prevent illness progression and development of suicide attempts. This article provides an update on the epidemiology, clinical
profile, and treatment of youth with PBD with mixed states. Mixed states
in PBD are characterized by higher rates of suicide and more chronic
symptoms, and are associated with younger age of onset and greater comorbidity. A careful assessment for mixed states using standardized
criteria is essential.

Mixed states in patients with a perinatal mood episode is seldom encoun-
tered. Lack of appropriate assessment tools could be partly responsible
for this observation. The authors conducted a selective review of studies
dealing with the reporting of mixed symptoms in women during the perinatal period with the intention to quantify the phenomenon. In many in-
stances of reported postpartum depression, either a first onset or an
onset in the context of bipolar disorder, mixed states were identifiable.
However, the strict application of the Diagnostic and Statistical Manual
of Mental Disorders, 5th edition, mixed features specifier to these episodes risks misdiagnosis.

Mixed affective states occur in approximately 40% of patients with mood
disorders and are burdened with a significant rate of comorbidities,
including addictive disorders (AD). The co-occurrence of mixed features
and AD represents a challenge for clinicians because the reciprocal, negative influence of these conditions leads to a worse course of illness, treatment resistance, unfavorable outcome, and higher suicide risk. This article
discusses clinical presentation, possible common pathogenetic pathways,
and treatment options. Further investigations are required to clarify the determinants and the implications of this co-occurrence, and to detect suit-
able approaches in clinical management.

Interest in the coexistence of manic and depressive symptoms fostered hypotheses on neurobiological underpinnings of mixed states. Neurobiological properties of mixed states, however, have not been comprehensively described. The authors searched databases for articles on neurobiological markers related to mixed states. Results showed that mixed states are characterized by elevated central and peripheral monoamine levels, greater alterations in hypothalamic-pituitary-adrenal axis, increased inflammation, and greater circadian rhythms dysfunction than nonmixed forms. Furthermore, the magnitude of pathophysiologic alterations in mixed states exceeds those associated with nonmixed mania or depression and suggest that hyperactivation and hyperarousal are core features of mixed states.

Susceptibility to combined depressive and manic syndromes correlates strongly with arousal-related symptoms including impulsivity, anxiety and agitation. This relationship to a driven, "mixed" activation-depression state, generated by a life-long process, was described in classical times. Course of illness in mixed states includes increased episode frequency, duration, earlier onset, and association with addiction- and trauma/stress-related disorders. Mixed episodes have catecholamine and hypothalamic-pituitary-adrenocortical activity increased beyond nonmixed states of similar symptom severity. These properties resemble behavioral sensitization, where salient, survival-related stimuli (traumatic or rewarding) can generate persistently exaggerated responses with disrupted arousal and reward, with potential for suicide and other severe consequences.

Despite the relatively high prevalence of mixed symptoms and features among patients with mood disorders, the current literature supporting the specific efficacy of second-generation antipsychotics and mood stabilizers for the treatment of mixed symptoms is limited. Several studies have demonstrated that acute affective episodes with mixed symptoms or features tend to respond unsatisfactory to treatments that are usually more effective for the management of other affective phases. There is clearly a need for clinical trials in order to determine the more adequate pharmacologic option for the treatment of individuals suffering from affective episodes with mixed features.

PSYCHIATRIC CLINICS OF NORTH AMERICA

SERIES OF RELATED INTEREST

Child and Adolescent Psychiatric Clinics of North America
https://www.childpsych.theclinics.com/

Neurologic Clinics
https://www.neurologic.theclinics.com/

THE CLINICS ARE AVAILABLE ONLINE!
Access your subscription at:
www.theclinics.com

Preface

Mixed States: Beyond Depression and Mania

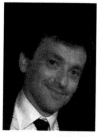
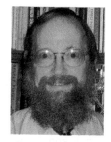

Gabriele Sani, MD   Alan C. Swann, MD
Editors

Mood disorders are usually defined as episode-based, despite evidence that their basis lies in the underlying course of illness. We must characterize the complex structures of mixed episodes, but also look beyond episodes to the characteristics of the underlying illness. In this issue, we examine the history, clinical and diagnostic characteristics, potential mechanisms, and treatment challenges of mixed states.

Our aim is to integrate psychopathology, clinical description, neurobiology, and treatment of mixed states to shed light on this still-apparent clinical paradox. Interpreting the classic clinical description in light of the current knowledge of brain functions can help us to understand the emergence of mixed states from interacting long-term and acute brain mechanisms and to develop strategies for this lifelong challenge.

HISTORY AND CLINICAL IMPACT: RECOGNIZED AND OVERLOOKED SINCE (BEFORE) THE BEGINNING OF PSYCHIATRY

The original descriptions of mood disorders differed from our current diagnostic system. The current model defines affective illnesses as affect-related episodic syndromes. By contrast, the classical description posited a systemic illness defined by its course and typically including aspects of depression, mania, psychosis, and, very importantly, hyperarousal. The constructs of manic and depressive illnesses arose later. Now, as described in this issue, mixed states lead us back toward the classical model, but with observational, scientific, and treatment tools that were unavailable then.

CLINICAL CHARACTERISTICS AND DIAGNOSTIC CHALLENGES OF MIXED SYNDROMES

The articles focusing on clinical characteristics and diagnostic challenges examine mixed states in terms of underlying temperament or personality characteristics and

Psychiatr Clin N Am 43 (2020) xv–xvii
https://doi.org/10.1016/j.psc.2019.11.001
0193-953X/20/© 2019 Published by Elsevier Inc.

their translation into psychopathology. Mixed states challenge the unipolar-bipolar dichotomy. Many individuals exhibit "manic" symptoms only in the context of "depressive" episodes. Despite illness-course and family-history characteristics of "bipolar" disorder, they are often considered "unipolar" because of apparent lack of free-standing manic episodes. Similarly, our current diagnostic system still focuses on "specific" depressive and manic symptoms rather than on symptoms that are more likely to be basic to the underlying illness. This theme, in varying contexts, runs through the articles in this section.

CLINICAL CONTEXTS, COMPLICATIONS, AND CHALLENGES

Mixed states present challenges related to their severe course of illness. Articles in this section address roles of trauma, addictions, and developmental events in mixed states. Regarding course of illness, they address developmental problems, including early-onset and perinatal mixed states. Despite their occurrence at a crucial time (for mother and for offspring) and their high rate of suicide, little attention has been paid to these episodes. Addictions and traumas may both predispose to mixed states and result from them. These challenges may be related to the pathophysiology of recurrent affective disorders and recall classical descriptions linking activation and depression with suicidality and other severe behavioral problems.

MECHANISMS

Understanding mechanisms predisposing to mixed states can facilitate early diagnosis and development of effective treatments. This section addresses neurobiological characteristics of mixed states, going beyond affective symptoms to include underlying hyperarousal. We then discuss long-term sensitization mechanisms, related to neural responses to extremely salient stimuli, and their consequences, which include hyperarousal and fluctuating impulsive behavior.

TREATMENT

Treatment of mixed states must address their complex, shifting symptomatic states and their course of illness. Psychopharmacologic studies of mixed episodes reflect a strength of our current resources: the growing array of symptomatic treatments, and a major problem: the lack of convincing long-term preventive response data. Reported outcomes tend to emphasize manic and/or depressive symptoms over hyperarousal-related symptoms that underlie mixed states. Electroconvulsive treatment is underused but potentially effective in mixed states, regardless of symptomatic characteristics. It is especially valuable for the most severely ill patients, including those with high suicide risk. The review of psychotherapy in mixed states addresses their broader context rather than being limited to syndromal affective symptoms. It describes the challenge of shifting symptoms, emphasizing overarousal, and the preventive/adaptive role of therapy strategies outside of episodes. These challenges are at the heart of mixed states, both as episodes and as the lifetime illness that generates them.

Gabriele Sani, MD
Institute of Psychiatry
Università Cattolica del Sacro Cuore
Largo Francesco Vito 1
00168 Roma, Italy

Department of Psychiatry
Fondazione Policlinico Universitario
"Agostino Gemelli" IRCCS
Roma, Italy

Alan C. Swann, MD
Menninger Department of Psychiatry and
Behavioral Sciences
Baylor College of Medicine
Mental Health Care Line
Michael E. DeBakey Veterans Affairs
Medical Center
Houston, TX, USA

E-mail addresses:
gabriele.sani@unicatt.it (G. Sani)
alan.swann@bcm.edu (A.C. Swann)

History and Clinical Impact: Recognized and Overlooked Since (Before) the Beginning of Psychiatry

Mixed States
Historical Impact and Evolution of the Concept

Check for updates

Gabriele Sani, MD[a,b,1],*, Alan C. Swann, MD[c],*

KEYWORDS

- Bipolar disorder • Differential diagnosis • Manic-depressive illness • Mixed states
- Recurrence

KEY POINTS

- Mixed states challenge our concepts of bipolar disorder, associated with a more severe course of illness, and requiring reconceptualization of our idea of an episode.
- Definitions of mixed states have changed over time, based on the clinical, scientific, and social context.
- The existence and properties of mixed states require a broader concept of bipolar disorder, resembling that of manic-depressive illness, that emphasizes the interaction between lifetime course of illness and properties of individual episodes.

[Mixed states] taught us that our customary grouping into manic and melancholic attacks does not fit the facts, but requires substantial enlargement, if it is to reproduce nature.

—Emil Kraepelin, 1913[1]

INTRODUCTION

Mixed states, broadly defined, are the most frequent clinical manifestations of mood disorders and, perhaps, of all psychopathological alterations. This is consistent with the complex psychopathology of experienced human life and behavior. Each psychic domain lies on continuum from total inhibition to full excitement: depressed and excited mood, retarded and speeded activity, inhibition or acceleration of thinking, emotional hyporeactivity and hyperreactivity, increased or decreased energy, and so on. Dimensionally thinking, it is clear that clinical phenomena are composed of basic underlying constructs at different degrees of inhibition or excitement.

---

[a] Institute of Psychiatry, Università Cattolica del Sacro Cuore, Roma, Italy; [b] Department of Psychiatry, Fondazione Policlinico Universitario "Agostino Gemelli" IRCCS, Roma, Italy; [c] Department of Psychiatry and Behavioral Sciences, Baylor College of Medicine, Michael E. Debakey Veterans Affairs Medical Center, 1977 Butler Boulevard, 4th Floor, Houston, TX 77030, USA
[1] Present address: Institute of Psychiatry, Largo Francesco Vito 1, 00168 Roma, Italy
* Corresponding authors.
E-mail addresses: gabriele.sani@unicatt.it (G.S.); alan.swann@bcm.edu (A.C.S.)

Psychiatr Clin N Am 43 (2020) 1–13
https://doi.org/10.1016/j.psc.2019.10.001
0193-953X/20/© 2019 Elsevier Inc. All rights reserved.

This dimensional view, in fact, runs through more than 2 millennia of clinical descriptions of psychiatric patients. Nevertheless, mixed states have been repeatedly challenged and neglected, and even current nosology does not yet capture the essence of mixed states, leading to inaccurate diagnoses and treatments.

Several reasons underlie the recurrent skepticism and confusion elicited by the concept of mixed states.

First, the term "mixed states," like the term "bipolar disorder," implies that "mania" and "depression," considered as opposites, underlie "bipolar disorder." This is reflected by confusion in nomenclature. Since classic times, the term melancholia was used to describe different forms of mental disorders, many of which could be considered today mixed affective states. In modern times, however, the term melancholia was replaced first by the "endogenous depression" as opposed to "reactive depressive" (according to Meyer's idea of reaction types),[2] followed by "major depression."[3] This unfortunate translation of the classic term melancholia does not convey the dramatic psychic excitation, rage, and fear that were, and are, characteristics of the classic clinical presentation. Although melancholia vividly describes many aspects of mixed states, these states came to be defined in terms of mania rather than as basic expressions of manic-depressive illness.

The relatively recent term "bipolar disorder," replacing "manic-depressive illness," continues this confusion. Kay Redfield Jamison stated: "*I find the word 'bipolar' strangely and powerfully offensive: it seems to me to obscure and minimize the illness it is supposed to represent. The description 'manic-depressive,' on the other hand, seems to capture both the nature and the seriousness of the disease ... splitting mood disorders into bipolar and unipolar categories presupposes a distinction between depression and manic-depressive illness—both clinically and etiologically—that is not always clear, nor supported by science ... it minimizes the importance of mixed manic-and-depressive states, conditions that are common, extremely important clinically, and lie at the heart of many of the critical theoretic issues underlying this particular disease.*"[4]

Finally, the uneasy diagnostic and psychopathological framework of anxiety was combined with the idea of a dichotomy between depression and mania to increase the confusion around the concept of mixed states. From the Latin word anxius, from angĕre ("*to cause pain, choke*"), akin to Ancient Greek ἄγχω (ánkhō, "*to choke*"), anxiety, "*defined as the anticipation of future threat*," has been classically linked to melancholia and, subsequently, to depression.[5] Moreover, the high rate of comorbidity between anxiety and depression[6] and the response of anxiety symptoms to antidepressant treatments,[7] reinforced the hypothesis of this strong connection. Koukopoulos and Koukopoulos[3] stated that there are 2 types of anxiety, one of which is secondary to the depressive state, whereas the other, a strong characteristic of mixed states, appears to be a form of excitation or arousal. This force is so violent that it cannot be anything but excitement in nature and responds well to anti-excitatory agents; correspondingly it is noteworthy that so-called "antidepressant" treatments can be effective for anxiety disorder in people who are not depressed, and response is related to both activated and inhibited components of depression.[7] Anxiety correlates with depression in predominately manic states and with mania in predominately depressive states, so is related to the essence of "mixed" states. A similar situation exists regarding agitation.[8]

The aim of this article was to review the development of the concept of mixed states, exploring depressive and manic symptoms, but emphasizing their combination, through clinical descriptions from the classic literature to modern nosologic systems. In our opinion, the term "mixed states" is likely to become obsolete, as this aspect of manic-depressive illness is recognized as primary, because "mixed states" implies that distinct depressive and manic states are basic to the illness. We will pose the question, based on classic observation, of what drives mixed states, and how this driving force is basic to manic-depressive illness.

FROM ANCIENT CONTRIBUTIONS TO THE EIGHTEENTH CENTURY

The first description of a mixed state was provided by Hippocrates (circa 460–370 BCE) in Disease II: Phrenitis: *something like a thorn seems to be his inward parts and to prick them; loathing attacks the patient, he flees light and people, he loves the dark and he is seized by fear . . . the patient is afraid, he sees terrible things, frightful dreams, and sometimes the dead.*"[9] Aristotle (384–322 BCE) in his Problema XXX described as melancholic Heracles, who in an acute state of madness killed his sons ("*He was changed; his eyes were rolling; he was distraught; his eyeballs were bloodshot and starting from their sockets, and foam was oozing down his bearded cheek. Anon he spoke, laughing the while a madman's laugh...*"[10]), Lysander the Spartan, who "*was now of an altogether harsh disposition, owing to the melancholy which persisted into his old age*"[11] and in which melancholy "*seems to be inextricably associated with violent anger... inextricably confused with the subject's greatness,*"[12] and Ajax, who furiously slaughtered sheep and cattle in the erroneous belief that he was taking his revenge against Agamemnon, Menelaus, and Odysseus.[13] Aretaeus from Cappadocia (first century CE) noted that melancholic individuals are prone "*to sadness and dejection. But additionally, it is possible for them to fly into rage and they spend a lot of their life in madness, doing terrible and humiliating things,*" and observed that mixed states were the most severe form of the illness, were recurrent, and were associated with risk for suicide or violence.[14] Caelius Aurelianus (second or fifth century CE), a prominent representative of the solidist psychiatric trend, provided what could be the first neurobiological hypothesis of mixed states based on brain structures. According to Soranus of Ephesus (second century CE) ("*In the mixed state, looseness and stricture are present in the body at the same time, with each state being more prevalent at different times, or with each being prevalent at the same time, but in different parts of the body*"),[15] Aurelianus described 3 pathologic brain states with corresponding medical and psychiatric symptoms: a tight state, with a diminished diameter of the canalicula; a lax state, with an enlargement of their diameter; and a mixed state with alternation of the 2 conditions. In the lax state, the patients were depressed, asthenic, afraid, sad, lethargic; in the tight states they were anxious, excited, delirious, hallucinated, insomniac; and in the mixed state symptoms from both groups were present.[16]

In the sixth century CE, Alexander of Tralles (circa 525–605 CE), a Byzantine physician, believed that melancholia and mania could present themselves in a cyclical pattern and show mixed characters: "*Mania is nothing else but melancholia in a more intense form.*"[17]

In the following centuries, several interesting contributions on melancholia arrived from the Islamic world. These included texts by Ishaq Ibn Imran (circa 848–906), Raze (Muhammad ibn Zakariya al-Razi, circa 865–925), Avicenna (Abu Ali al-Husayn ibn Abd Allah ibn Sina, 980–1037), and others.[18,19] Among the other major mental disorders, a disease called *ishgh*, a combination of anxiety and depression and characterized by "*assiduous thought of depressive nature,*" was described.

In the first half of the second millennium, European Christian physicians, such as the English John of Gaddesden (circa 1280–1361), the Italian Johannes Manardus (Giovanni Menardo, circa 1462–1536) the Swiss Felix Platter (Platerus, circa 1536–1614), and the Dutch Jason Pratensis (1486–1558) adopted the classic concepts of mania and melancholia, considered to be parts of one disorder by most physicians. This idea was strengthened in the seventeenth century. Thomas Willis (1621–1675), Thomas Sydenham (1624–1689), Giovanni Morgagni (1759–1820), and Vincenzo Chiarugi (1759–1820) reported patients alternating mania and melancholia, clearly highlighting their intimate relationship. The relationship found a nosologic dignity, in which Théophile Bonet (1620–1689) called *maniaco-melancholicus*[20] and Anne-Charles Lorry (1684–1766) called *mania-melancholica.*[21] In our opinion, these terms reflect the integral role of mixed states in manic-depressive illness.

As Koukopoulos and Koukopoulos[3] pointed out, the nosologists of the eighteenth century, such as de Sauvages and Cullen, classified among the melancholias such forms as *melancholia phrontis*, *melancholia moria*, *melancholia sultans*, *melancholia errabunda*, *melancholia silvestris*, *melancholia furens*, and *melancholia enthusiastica*, in which the mixed nature of the disease was evident in the name itself.

Andres Piquer-Arrufat (1711–1772) was a prominent figure in Spanish medicine of the eighteenth century and was the personal physician of King Ferdinand VI (1713–1759). In *Discurso sobre la enfermedad del Rey Nuestro Señor Fernando VI (que dios guarde)* (1759) and *Praxis medica ad usum scholae valentinae* (1764), he described elements of what he called the *affectio melancholico-maniaca*, including mixed manic-depressive states, affective and behavioral instability, and seasonal mood changes. Describing the disease of the King and other patients, he wrote: *"Some who are furious or angry tear their clothes, harm those who serve them or others, and may even harm themselves…. Although these patients are afraid of death, some may kill themselves violently. Whoever considers the afore mentioned characteristics of the melancholic-manic illness and compares them with the King's illness, will find many similarities and will not hesitate to admit that this illness is what His Majesty suffered."*[22]

THE NINETEENTH CENTURY

This neoclassical medical and scientific tradition culminated in the 1800s. Philippe Pinel (1745–1826); Jean-Etienne Dominique Esquirol (1772–1840); Jean Pierre Falret (1794–1870), who provided descriptions of switches between mania and melancholia within mood, ideation, and behavior[23]; Jules Baillarger (1809–1890), who noted that succession of episodes of opposite polarity could occur suddenly, even during sleep, or gradually[24]; Karl-Ludwig Kahlbaum (1828–1899); and Ewald Hecker (1843–1909) essentially founded modern psychiatric thought. This "golden era of psychiatry" was reflected in the evolution of the concept of mixed states.

Johannes Christian August Heinroth (1773–1843), the first professor of psychiatry in Germany (Leipzig), influenced by the Romantics, considered mania and melancholia disorders of mood (Gemüth). In his *Lehrbuch der Stoerungen des Seelenlebens (Textbook of the disorders of the psychic life)* (1818),[25] he recognized 3 "orders" of disorders, according to the change in energy: "exaltation" (*hyperthymias*), "depression" (*asthenias*), and "mixed excitation and depression" (*hyper-asthenias*). Mixed states were divided into "mixed mood disorders" (*animi morbi complicati*), "mixed mental disorders" (*morbi mentis mixti*), and "mixed volition disorders" (*morbi voluntatis mixti*). Many forms of exaltation, manias, and mixed mood states (Ectasis melancholica, Melancholia moria, Melancholica furens, and Melancholia mixta catholica) constituted the main focus of his book.

The Belgian psychiatrist Joseph Guislain (1797–1860) stated that the combination of mania and melancholia was the most frequent presentation of mental illness ("la mélancholie associée à la manie").[26] He provided a clinically meaningful description of the mélancholie-maniaque: "...La figure de l'aliéné, quoique souffrante, est animé; l'oeil est plus mobile, lus expressif, plus étincelant; l'accent est plaintif, mais la voix est forte, sonore; le malade est ausii plu loquace que dans le monopathie mélanchlque... il s'agite, ses mouvements sont prompts.." ("... The figure of the insane, though suffering, is animated; the eye is more mobile, more expressive, more sparkling; the accent is plaintive, but the voice is loud and sonorous; the patient is more loquacious than in melancholy monopathy ... he is agitated, his movements are quick").

Carl Friedrich Flemming (1799–880), the father of the cellular biologist Walther Flemming, developed the concept of mixity across different states. He proposed the diagnosis of "changeable dysthymia" (dysthymia mutabilis), shifting from a depressive (dysthymia atra) to a hypomanic (dysthymia candida) phase or constituted by coexisting elements of both, such as elated melancholia (melancholia hilaris).[27] He considered mixed states the most prevalent forms of mental illness and a diagnostic challenge.[28]

Wilhelm Griesinger (1817–1868), an eminent German psychiatrist, recognized 3 classes of mental disorders: depressive states (psychische Depressionszustände), exaltation states (psychische Exaltationszustände), and weakness states (psychische Schwächezustände). Griesinger described the so-called "mid-forms" (Mittelformen) in which melancholia, from the first class, and mania, from the second class, could occur sequentially or simultaneously.[29] "Melancholia with destructive drives" and "melancholia with long-lasting exaltation of volition" were mid-forms. He had the great intuition that cerebral excitation may underlie psychic pain or depression: "By using the expression 'psychic depressive states' we did not mean to imply that the basic nature of these states is inactivity and weakness and suppression [depression] of the psychic or cerebral processes that underly them. We have much more reason to assume that very intense states of irritation of the brain and excitation of the psychic processes are very often the cause of such states; but the end result of these [psychic and cerebral] states as far as mood is concerned is a state of depression or psychic suffering." Therefore, a physiologically mixed state could appear as "pure" depression on the surface.

Louis-Victor Marcé (1828–1865), student of Baillarger and Moreau de Tours and classmate and close friend of Jules Verne, had a brief, intense, and prolific life. He was a passionate man and a great clinician, who dedicated his life to psychiatry and, overwhelmed by this full life, committed suicide in August 1865. Among Marcé's many important writings, 2 monographs stand out: Traité de la folie des femmes enceintes, des nouvelles accouchées et des nourrices, et considérations médico-légales qui se rattachent à ce sujet (1858) and Traité pratique des maladies mentales (1862). As a deep clinical observer, he described the alternation of recurrent melancholia and mania of limited intensity (resembling modern bipolar II disorder), and the concept of mixed states as the result of combined depressive and excitatory symptoms beyond full-blown mania or depression: "...What is infinitely more common is to see excitation and depression without going into manic or melancholic episodes...I have seen a melancholic episode with profound stupor followed by a period of excitation, characterized only by intellectual overactivity....."[30] Moreover, he was the first to recognize mixed states during the puerperal and post-partum disorders: "...we find in the puerperal state a small number of mixed states that are impossible to classify or to clearly define....."[31] It is noteworthy that this still a neglected issue after 150 years.

EMIL KRAEPELIN AND WILHELM WEYGANDT

Emil Kraepelin (1856–1926) and his pupil Wilhelm Weygandt (1870–1939) systematized mixed states. It is unclear whether Kraepelin originally linked mixed states to manic-depressive illness and then encouraged Weygandt to work on this topic,[3,32] or Weygandt had the original intuition and influenced Kraepelin's conceptualization from the late of 1890s.[33] Kraepelin introduced the concept of mixed states in the fifth edition of his textbook in 1896.[34] Moreover, regarding his first years in Heidelberg (circa 1891), he stated in his "Memoirs": "*Our clinical interest was devoted to the two large groups of dementia praecox and manic-depressive insanity. The classification of the manic stupor was a further step toward understanding the latter group. Some striking observations had let to this new classification, which was first presented in a lecture by Dehio* [Heinrich Dehio, a close collaborator with Kraepelin]. *Subsequently, we discovered other "mixed forms" of mental illness, such as restless depression and mania with lack of thoughts, and gained a better understanding of the inner homogeneity of the whole, large group with its very different forms.*"[35] However, Weygandt's monograph on mixed states "*Über die Mischzustände im circulären Irresein,*"[36] presented in 1898 and published in 1899, apparently influenced Kraepelin's view, leading to the unitary concept of "manic-depressive illness" starting with his 1899 edition. In our opinion, the greatest message of this story is that Kraepelin created one of the best schools of psychiatry that ever existed, assembling the best minds of his times, including Alzheimer, Nissl, Gaupp, and, of course, Weygandt. Their collaborative accomplishments could not have been made by one person alone. Current academicians should keep this in mind.

Kraepelin systematically conceptualized and described mixed states. He considered them the cornerstone of the manic-depressive entity: "*I believe that we can understand these states better, if we assume that they proceed from a mixture of different kinds of fundamental disorders of manic-depressive insanity.*"[1] In conceiving them, Kraepelin started from the excitement or depression of 3 domains of psychic life: intellect (train of thought rather than its contents), mood, and volition, expressed in psychomotor activity. In his dedicated chapter, Kraepelin stated: "*If one follows more closely a considerable number of cases, which belong to the different forms of manic-depressive insanity, one soon observes that numerous transitions exist between the fundamental forms of manic excitement and depression....*"[1] Based on possible combinations of the 3 psychic domains, he eventually described 6 mixed forms; **Table 1** shows the evolution of this formulation. In the fourth edition,[37] he described the manic stupor, and the fifth edition of his textbook (1896) introduced the concept of mixed states.[34] In the sixth edition (1899),[38] he presented manic-depressive insanity and described 5 mixed states: unproductive mania, manic stupor, querulous mania, states of transition, and melancholia with flight of ideas. The seventh edition (1903)[39] introduced depressive agitation and manic inhibition. In the eighth edition (1913),[40] Kraepelin described depressive or anxious mania, excited depression with inhibition of thought, great restlessness, and anxious and despondent mood, mania with poverty of thought, manic stupor, depression with flight of ideas, and inhibited mania. It is important for us to realize that Kraepelin's major contribution lay not in any specific number of basic dimensions or even what they were, as this can be improved (possibly) with advances in neuroscience. The basis of his contribution, which we must build on, was the dimensional structure underlying behavioral phenomena.

Based on longitudinal observations, Kraepelin concluded strongly that mixed states were a basic part of manic-depressive insanity: "*The mixed states here described are*

Table 1
Evolution of Kraepelin's concept of mixed states

Edition IV (1893)	Edition V (1896)	Edition VI (1899)	Edition VII (1903)	Edition VIII (1909–1913)
Manic stupor	1. Manic states with inhibition 2. Depressive states with excitation	1. Unproductive mania 2. Manic stupor 3. Querulous mania 4. Melancholia with flight of ideas 5. Transitional states	1. Furious mania 2. Depressive excitation 3. Unproductive mania 4. Manic stupor 5. Depression with flight of ideas 6. Manic inhibition	1. Depressive or anxious mania 2. Excited depression 3. Mania with poverty of thought 4. Manic stupor 5. Depression with flight of ideas 6. Inhibited mania

Adapted from Marneros A. Origin and development of concepts of bipolar mixed states. J Affect Disord 2001;67(1-3):232; with permission.

with by far the greatest frequency temporary phenomena in the course of the disease … Most frequently we meet with them, as already stated, in the transition periods between the two principal forms of the disease, indeed, only from the history of their development, their transformation from and to the known morbid states, do we derive the justification to interpret them as mixed states of manic-depressive insanity."[1]

Weygandt provided a detailed description of cases with mixed states found among the patients of Clinic in Heidelberg (see Salvatore and colleagues[33] for a full English translation of Weygandt's monograph), stating: *"It is a well-known fact that during both the manic and depressive phases of manic-depressive or circular insanity, transient symptom-free intervals can occur. But even more frequent are periods of hours or days that are characterized by changes in one of the symptoms, so that the illness shows an opposite picture regarding these features compared with the previous course of illness."* According to Kraepelin, Weygandt provided some deep clinical suggestions: *"In mania, euphoric affect and psychomotor excitement are as important as the disturbances in the domain of thought processes. [The latter] are characterized by flight-of-ideas and associations with little conceptual affinity or aim, and thoughts that are connected only on the basis of quick and superficial links or similarities in the sounds of words. In the depressive phase, we find thought-blocking instead of flight of ideas in the domain of associative thinking"* and he highlighted still-persistent diagnostic difficulties: *"…In the [Psychiatric] Clinic of Heidelberg, … fewer than one-third of [manic-depressive] patients have shown no mixed states at all, and over 20% of patients have had one or more episodes in which mixed features predominated. These conditions are well known but are often overlooked due to their brief duration."* He described in detail prototypical clinical pictures of patients with mixed states; although all 6 classic mixed states could be observed, he claimed that *"… for pragmatic rather than speculative reasons, it is useful to consider three particular mixed states that seem to be the most important based on their prevalence and [their potential for a sustained] course":* manic stupor, agitated depression, and unproductive mania (**Table 2**). Only 7.3% of patients had pure recurrent mania or depression!

Weygandt coined the term "agitated depression" (agitierte Depression), although the syndrome was described by Frank Richarz in 1858[41] (melancholia agitans), as acknowledged by Weygandt himself.

Table 2
Prevalence of clinical pictures of patients with manic-depressive insanity observed by Weygandt at the University of Heidelberg Psychiatric Clinic

Clinical Picture	n	%
Pure recurrent mania or depression	11	7.3
Circular manic-depressive	35	23.3
Circular cases with some mixed states	50	33.3
Sustained mixed episodes	22	14.7
Agitated depression	12	8
Manic stupor	11	7.3
Unproductive mania	9	6
Total	150	100

From Salvatore P, Baldessarini RJ, Centorrino F, et al. Weygandt's On the Mixed States of Manic-Depressive Insanity: a translation and commentary on its significance in the evolution of the concept of bipolar disorder. Harv Rev Psychiatry 2002;10(5):255–275; with permission.

THE FALL AND RENAISSANCE OF MIXED STATES

Interest in mixed states waned by the beginning of the twentieth century. Except for Johannes Lange (1898–1938), who described in 1928 *melancholia agitata* as a mixed state,[42] the contemporary great clinicians and researchers expressed their skepticism openly. In 1923, Karl Jaspers (1883–1969) wrote that the issue of mixed states *"did not have any further development, and this was very natural since elements of understanding psychology had been considered as objective components and factors of psychic life."*[43] Specifically, he criticized the division of depression and mania into 3 components (disturbances of thought, mood, and volition), although the concept of mixed states certainly does not require these specific behavioral dimensions. Kurt Schneider (1887–1967) was even more apodictic: *"We do not believe anymore in manic-depressive mixed states."*[44]

This decline in the prominence of mixed states could be related to the focus on clinical detail, unintentionally emphasizing the idea that depression and mania were opposites, losing sight of the classical idea that mixed states had a physiologic basis integral to manic-depressive illness.[45] This produced the notion that mixed states were an oddity rather basic to the illness.

From its inception, the American Diagnostic and Statistical Manual (DSM) system has been uneasy with mixed forms of affective disorders. The first edition (1952)[46] placed mixed features in a peripheral position, together with continuous circular forms, as part of "manic-depressive reaction, other." The second edition (1968),[47] under "Other major affective disorder," stated: "Major affective disorders for which a more specific diagnosis has not been made are included here," such as "mixed manic-depressive illness, in which manic and depressive symptoms appear almost simultaneously." DSM-III (1980)[48] introduced the term "bipolar disorder" instead of manic-depressive illness. "Bipolar disorder, mixed" was defined as "current (or most recent) episode involves the full symptomatic picture of both manic and major depressive episodes, intermixed or rapidly alternating every few days." This definition is substantially preserved, except for the duration criterion of 2 weeks for depressive symptoms, in DSM-III-R, published in 1987.[49] DSM-IV, 1994,[50] and DSM-IV-TR, 2000,[51] narrowed the definition of mixed episodes further, specifically requiring full manic and depressive episodes. This DSM-IV definition proved, with almost 2 decades of experience, to be of little clinical utility because this clinical picture is very rare.

DSM-5[52] introduced the "mixed-features" specifier that can be applied to episodes of major depression, hypomania, or mania. A full mood episode and at least 3 nonoverlapping symptoms of the opposite polarity are required. This revision was found to carry "the limitations of our current categorical systems and polythetic diagnostic criteria"[53] and to have poor clinical utility.[54] Perhaps most important, continuing the overemphasis on "specific" episode types, DSM-5 criteria excluded constructs like anxiety, central to mixed states, for the paradoxic reason that it overlapped depression and mania. Finally, the separation between depression and bipolar disorder made the recognition of mixed sates more difficult. The Viennese School, however, followed Aretaeus and Kraepelin in describing mixed states as "driven" states integral to mood disorders.[55,56]

From the end of the past century, a growing number of psychiatrists[57–65] challenged the official classification of mixed sates, finding it not useful, clinically or therapeutically.[66] This work produced renewed attention to mixed states in the past 2 decades.

Classic clinical-descriptive studies,[67–71] and studies based on careful psychopathological observations,[72–76] specific characteristics, such as suicidality[77,78] and treatment strategies,[79–86] led to alternative diagnostic criteria,[8,87,88] new conceptual models,[89] and specific diagnostic tools,[90,91] including the observation that the extent to which symptoms are mixed may be more important than whether the episode itself was depressive or manic.[8] Nevertheless, response to treatment and long-term outcome in mixed states still remain dramatically unsatisfactory.

SUMMARY

Mixed states have been discussed across the centuries for more than 2 millennia. Moreover, the theoretic conception of the coexistence of presumably opposite symptoms of mood or of different psychic domains is well established, although obscured by the presumed separation between bipolar and depressive disorders. Nevertheless, the lack of response to treatments, severe course of illness, and high risk of suicide raise important issues requiring urgent solution. Three basic issues must be faced: the definition of the most adequate clinical model, especially the nature of mechanisms driving mixed states; the relationship between bipolar and unipolar disorders; and identifying treatments that are at least relatively effective and specific.[92] Answers can come only from neurobiological and epidemiologic studies using valid and clinically based diagnostic criteria. This article discusses modern efforts to achieve these aims.

ACKNOWLEDGMENTS

This work was supported in part by the Program on Mood and Anxiety Disorders, Baylor College of Medicine, and the Michael E. DeBakey VAMC.

DISCLOSURE

The authors declare no conflicts of interest in this article.

REFERENCES

1. Kraepelin E. Manic-depressive illness and paranoia. Edinburgh (Scotland): Livingstone; 1921.
2. Meyer A. Psychobiology. A Science of Man. Springfield, Illinois: 1957.
3. Koukopoulos A, Koukopoulos A. Agitated depression as a mixed state and the problem of melancholia. Psychiatr Clin North Am 1999;22:547–64.

4. Jamison KR. An inquiet mind. New York: Alfred A. Knopf.; 1995.
5. Crocq MA. The history of generalized anxiety disorder as a diagnostic category. Dialogues Clin Neurosci 2017;19:107–16.
6. Katz MM, Bowden CL, Frazer A. Rethinking depression and the actions of antidepressants: uncovering the links between neural and behavioral elements. J Affect Disord 2010;120:16–23.
7. Bighelli I, Castellazzi M, Cipriani A, et al. Antidepressants versus placebo for panic disorder in adults. Cochrane Database Syst Rev 2018;(5):CD010676.
8. Swann AC, Steinberg JL, Lijffijt M, et al. Continuum of depressive and manic mixed states in patients with bipolar disorder: quantitative measurement and clinical features. World Psychiatry 2009;8:166–72.
9. Hippocrates. Affections. Diseases 1. Diseases 2. Translated by Paul Potter. Loeb Classical Library 472. Cambridge (MA): Harvard University Press; 1988.
10. Euripides. Heracles translated by E. P. Coleridge. Available at: http://classics.mit.edu/Euripides/heracles.html. Accessed June 15, 2019.
11. Plutarch, The life of Lysander. Available at: http://penelope.uchicago.edu/Thayer/E/Roman/Texts/Plutarch/Lives/Lysander*.html. Accessed June 15, 2019.
12. Toohey P. Some ancient histories of literary melancholia. III Classical Stud 1990; 15:142–63.
13. Sophocles. Ajax. The Loeb Classical Library. Cambridge (England): Harvard University Press; 1994.
14. Aretaeus. On the causes and symptoms of chronic disease. Boston: Milford House; 1972.
15. Hanson AE, Green MH. Soranus of Ephesus: Methodicorum princeps in Wolfgang Haase and Hildegard Temporini, general editors. [Aufstieg und Niedergang der römischen Welt, Teilband II, Band 37.2]. Berlin: Walter de Gruyter; 1994. p. 968–1075.
16. Aurelianus C. In: Drabkin IE, editor. On acute diseases and on chronic diseases. University of Chicago Press; 1950.
17. Alexander of Tralles. Della melancholia. In: Puschmann T, editor. Alexander von Tralles. Wien (Austria): Wilhelm Braumueller; 1878.
18. Vakili N, Gorji A. Psychiatry and psychology in medieval Persia. J Clin Psychiatry 2006;67:1862–9.
19. Omrani A, Holtzman NS, Akiskal HS, et al. Ibn Imran's 10th century treatise on melancholy. J Affect Disord 2012;10:141, 116–9.
20. Bonet T. Medicina septentrionalis collatitia. [Compendium of medical practice in northern Europe]. Geneva (Swirzerland): Sumptivus Leonardi Choucet and Socij; 1686.
21. Lorry AC. De Melancholia et Morbis Melancholicis. Paris: Lutetia Parisiorum; 1765.
22. Pérez J, Baldessarini RJ, Cruz N, et al. Andrés Piquer-Arrufat (1711-1772): contributions of an eighteenth-century Spanish physician to the concept of manic-depressive illness. Harv Rev Psychiatry 2011;19:68–77.
23. Falret JP. Marche de la folie. Gaz des Hopitaux 24:1851.
24. Baillarger JGF. Note sur un genre de folie dont laccès sont caractérisés par deux périodes régulières, lune de dépression et lautre dexcitation. Bull Acad Impériale Méd Séance 1854.
25. Heinroth JCA. Lehrbuch der Stoerungen des Seelenlebens. Leipzig (Germany): Vogel; 1818.
26. Guislain J. Traité sur les Phrenopathies. Gand (Belgium): Hebbelynck; 1852.

27. Flemming CF. Ueber Classification der Seelenstoerungen. Allg Ztschr Psychiatr 1844;1:97–130.
28. Baldessarini RJ, Pérez J, Salvatore P, et al. History of bipolar manic-depressive disorder. In: Yildiz Y, Ruiz P, Nemeroff C, editors. The bipolar book: history, neurobiology, and treatment. New York: Oxford University Press; 2015. p. 3–19.
29. Griesinger W. Pathologie und Therapie der psychischen Krankheiten. Stuttgart (Germany): Adolf Krabbe Verlag; 1845.
30. Marcé LV. Traité pratique des maladies mentales. Paris: J-B Baillère; 1862.
31. Marcé LV. Traité de la folie des femmes enceintes, des nouvelles accouchées et des nourrices, et considérations médico-légales qui se rattachent à ce sujet. Paris: J-B Baillière et fils; 1858.
32. Marneros A. Origin and development of concepts of bipolar mixed states. J Affect Disord 2001;67:229–40.
33. Salvatore P, Baldessarini RJ, Centorrino F, et al. Weygandt's On the Mixed States of Manic-Depressive Insanity: a translation and commentary on its significance in the evolution of the concept of bipolar disorder. Harv Rev Psychiatry 2002;10: 255–75.
34. Kraepelin E. Psychiatrie. 5th edition. Leipzig (Germany): JA Barth; 1896.
35. Kraepeiln E. Memoirs. In: Hippius H, Peters G, Ploog D, et al, editors. Tanslated by Wooding-Dean C. Berlin: Springer-Verlag; 1987. p. 65.
36. Weygandt W. Ueber die Mischzustaende des manisch-depressiven Irreseins. Muenchen (Germany): Lehmann; 1899.
37. Kraepelin E. Psychiatrie. 4th edition. Leipzig (Germany): JA Barth; 1893.
38. Kraepelin E. Psychiatrie. 6th edition. Leipzig (Germany): JA Barth; 1899.
39. Kraepelin E. Psychiatrie. 7th edition. Leipzig (Germany): JA Barth; 1904.
40. Kraepelin E. Psychiatrie. 8th edition. Leipzig (Germany): JA Barth; 1913.
41. Richarz F. Ueber Wesen und Behandlung der Melancholie mit Aufregung (Melancholia agitans). Allg Ztschr Psychiatr 1858;15:28–65.
42. Lange J. Die endogenen und reaktiven Gemuetserkrankungen und die manischedepressive Konstitution. In: Bumke O, editor. Handbuch der Geisteskrankheiten. Bd. 6, Spezieller Teil 2. Berlin: Springer; 1928.
43. Jaspers K. Allgemeine psychopathologie. 3rd edition. Berlin: Springer; 1923.
44. Schneider K. Klinische psychopathologie. Stuttgart (Germany): Thieme Verlag; 1962.
45. Mathews M. How did pre-twentieth century theories of the aetiology of depression develop? Brighton (England): Priory Lodge Education; 2004.
46. American Psychiatric Association. Diagnostic and statistical manual of mental disorders. 1st edition. Washington, DC: American Psychiatric Association; 1952.
47. American Psychiatric Association. Diagnostic and statistical manual of mental disorders. 2nd edition. Washington, DC: American Psychiatric Association; 1968.
48. American Psychiatric Association. Diagnostic and statistical manual of mental disorders. 3rd edition. Washington, DC: American Psychiatric Association; 1980.
49. American Psychiatric Association. Diagnostic and statistical manual of mental disorders. 3rd edition. Washington, DC: American Psychiatric Association; 1987.
50. American Psychiatric Association. Diagnostic and statistical manual of mental disorders. 4th edition. Washington, DC: American Psychiatric Association; 1994.
51. American Psychiatric Association. Diagnostic and statistical manual of mental disorders. 4th edition-Text Revision. Washington, DC: American Psychiatric Association; 2000.
52. American Psychiatric Association. Diagnostic and statistical manual of mental disorders. 5th edition. Washington, DC: American Psychiatric Association; 2013.

53. Maj M. "Mixed" depression: drawbacks of DSM-5 (and other) polythetic diagnostic criteria. J Clin Psychiatry 2015;76:e381-2.
54. Koukopoulos A, Sani G, Ghaemi SN. Mixed features of depression: why DSM-5 is wrong (and so was DSM-IV). Br J Psychiatry 2013;203:3-5.
55. Janzarik W. Dynamische Grundkonstellationen in endogenen Psychosen. Berlin: Springer; 1959.
56. Berner P, Gabriel E, Katschnig H, et al. Diagnostic criteria for the functional psychoses. 2nd edition. New York: Cambridge University Press; 1993. p. 164.
57. Himmelhoch JM, Coble P, Kupfer DJ, et al. Agitated psychotic depression associated with severe hypo-manic episodes: a rare syndrome. Am J Psychiatry 1976; 133:765-71.
58. Himmelhoch JM, Mulla D, Neil, et al. Incidence and significance of mixed affective states in a bipolar population. Arch Gen Psychiatry 1976;33:1062-6.
59. Akiskal HS, Puzantian VR. Psychotic forms of depression and mania. Psychiatr Clin North Am 1979;2:419-39.
60. Secunda SK, Swann A, Katz AM, et al. Diagnosis and treatment of mixed mania. Am J Psychiatry 1987;144:96-8.
61. Koukopoulos A, Girardi P, Proietti R, et al. Diagnostic and therapeutic considerations on agitated depression understood as a mixed affective state. Minerva Psichiatr 1989;30:283-6.
62. Dell'Osso L, Placidi GF, Nassi R, et al. The manic-depressive mixed state: familial, temperamental and psychopathology characteristics in 108 female inpatients. Eur Arch Psychiatry Clin Neurosci 1991;240:234-9.
63. Swann AC, Secunda SK, Katz MM, et al. Specificity of mixed affective states: clinical comparison of dysphoric mania and agitated depression. J Affect Disord 1993;28:81-9.
64. Bourgeois M, Verdoux H, Mainard CH. Dysphoric mania and mixed states. Encephale 1995;21(Spec No. 6):21-32.
65. Perugi G, Akiskal HS, Micheli C, et al. Clinical subtypes of bipolar mixed states: validating a broader European definition in 143 cases. J Affect Disord 1997;43: 169-80.
66. Koukopoulos A, Sani G. DSM-5 criteria for depression with mixed features: a farewell to mixed depression. Acta Psychiatr Scand 2014;129:4-16.
67. Koukopoulos A, Albert MJ, Sani G, et al. Mixed depressive states: nosologic and therapeutic issues. Int Rev Psychiatry 2005;17:21-37.
68. Koukopoulos A, Sani G, Koukopoulos AE, et al. Melancholia agitata and mixed depression. Acta Psychiatr Scand Suppl 2007;433:50-7.
69. Pacchiarotti I, Mazzarini L, Kotzalidis GD, et al. Mania and depression. Mixed, not stirred. J Affect Disord 2011;133:105-13.
70. Vieta E, Morralla C. Prevalence of mixed mania using 3 definitions. J Affect Disord 2010;125:61-73.
71. Cassidy F. Anxiety as a symptom of mixed mania: implications for DSM-5. Bipolar Disord 2010;12:437-9.
72. Swann AC. Mixed or dysphoric manic states: psychopathology and treatment. J Clin Psychiatry 1995;56(Suppl 3):6-10.
73. Swann AC, Janicak PL, Calabrese JR, et al. Structure of mania: depressive, irritable, and psychotic clusters with different retrospectively-assessed course patterns of illness in randomized clinical trial participants. J Affect Disord 2001;67: 123-32.

74. Koukopoulos A, Sani G, Koukopoulos AE, et al. Endogenous and exogenous cyclicity and temperament in bipolar disorder: review, new data and hypotheses. J Affect Disord 2006;96:165–75.
75. Swann AC, Moeller FG, Steinberg JL, et al. Manic symptoms and impulsivity during bipolar depressive episodes. Bipolar Disord 2007;9:206–12.
76. Perugi G, Angst J, Azorin JM, et al. BRIDGE-II-Mix Study Group. Mixed features in patients with a major depressive episode: the BRIDGE-II-MIX study. J Clin Psychiatry 2015;76(3):e351–8.
77. Popovic D, Vieta E, Azorin JM, et al. Suicide attempts in major depressive episode: evidence from the BRIDGE-II-Mix study. Bipolar Disord 2015;17:795–803.
78. Sani G, Tondo L, Koukopoulos A, et al. Suicide in a large population of former psychiatric inpatients. Psychiatry Clin Neurosci 2011;65:286–95.
79. Swann AC, Bowden CL, Morris D, et al. Depression during mania. Treatment response to lithium or divalproex. Arch Gen Psychiatry 1997;54:37–42.
80. Centorrino F, Fogarty KV, Sani G, et al. Antipsychotic drug use: McLean Hospital, 2002. Hum Psychopharmacol 2005;20:355–8.
81. Centorrino F, Fogarty KV, Cimbolli P, et al. Aripiprazole: initial clinical experience with 142 hospitalized psychiatric patients. J Psychiatr Pract 2005;11:241–7.
82. Bersani FS, Girardi N, Sanna L, et al. Deep transcranial magnetic stimulation for treatment-resistant bipolar depression: a case report of acute and maintenance efficacy. Neurocase 2013;19:451–7.
83. Sani G, Napoletano F, Vöhringer PA, et al. Mixed depression: clinical features and predictors of its onset associated with antidepressant use. Psychother Psychosom 2014;83:213–21.
84. Perugi G, Medda P, Toni C, et al. The role of electroconvulsive therapy (ECT) in bipolar disorder: effectiveness in 522 patients with bipolar depression, mixed-state, mania and catatonic features. Curr Neuropharmacol 2017;15:359–71.
85. Sani G, Fiorillo A. The use of lithium in mixed states. CNS Spectr 2019;28:1–3.
86. Perugi G, De Rossi P, Fagiolini A, et al. Personalized and precision medicine as informants for treatment management of bipolar disorder. Int Clin Psychopharmacol 2019;34:189–205.
87. Swann AC, Lafer B, Perugi G, et al. Bipolar mixed states: an international society for bipolar disorders task force report of symptom structure, course of illness, and diagnosis. Am J Psychiatry 2013;170:31–42.
88. Sani G, Vöhringer PA, Napoletano F, et al. Koukopoulos' diagnostic criteria for mixed depression: a validation study. J Affect Disord 2014;164:14–8.
89. Malhi GS, Irwin L, Hamilton A, et al. Modelling mood disorders: an ACE solution? Bipolar Disord 2018;20(Suppl 2):4–16.
90. Tavormina G, Franza F, Stranieri G, et al. Clinical utilisation and usefullness of the Rating Scale of Mixed States, ("Gt-Msrs"): a multicenter study. Psychiatr Danub 2017;29(Suppl 3):365–7.
91. Sani G, Vöhringer PA, Barroilhet SA, et al. The Koukopoulos Mixed Depression Rating Scale (KMDRS): An International Mood Network (IMN) validation study of a new mixed mood rating scale. J Affect Disord 2018;232:9–16.
92. Swann AC. Mixed features: evolution of the concept, past and current definitions, and future prospects. CNS Spectr 2017;22:161–9.

Clinical Characteristics and Diagnostic Challenges of Mixed Syndromes

Clinical Picture, Temperament, and Personality of Patients with Mixed States

Mario Luciano, MD, PhD[a], Delfina Janiri, MD[b,c],
Andrea Fiorillo, MD, PhD[a], Gabriele Sani, MD[d,e,*]

KEYWORDS

- Agitated/mixed depression • Dysphoric mania • Nosography • Personality
- Temperament • Emotional reactivity

KEY POINTS

- Despite the changes through the different editions, current diagnostic criteria of the official nosologic systems still have poor clinical usefulness.
- Premorbid characteristics with a potential high clinical importance such as temperament, personality, and emotional reactivity are understudied in patients with mixed states and excluded from the current nosologic systems.
- The validation of new diagnostic tools will help clinicians and researchers to better frame the complexity of mixed states.

INTRODUCTION

Mixed states, broadly defined as the simultaneous occurrence of depressive and manic symptoms, are a complex clinical presentation representing a diagnostic and therapeutic challenge for clinicians.[1] Mixed states have heterogeneous clinical pictures, and this partially explains the difficulties in achieving a consensus on their appropriate definition and classification. Mixed states have been scarcely studied in clinical trials, because of the uncertainty in considering them an independent disorder and the difficulties in selecting specific clinical criteria for the recruitment of patients.[2]

[a] Department of Psychiatry, University of Campania "Luigi Vanvitelli", Largo Madonna delle Grazie, Naples 80138, Italy; [b] NESMOS Department (Neuroscience, Mental Health, and Sensory Organs), School of Medicine and Psychology, Sant'Andrea Hospital, Sapienza University, UOC Psichiatria, Via di Grottarossa, 1035-1039, Rome 00189, Italy; [c] Centro Lucio Bini, Rome, Italy; [d] Institute of Psychiatry, Università Cattolica del Sacro Cuore, Roma, Italy; [e] Department of Psychiatry, Fondazione Policlinico Universitario "Agostino Gemelli" IRCCS, Roma, Italy
* Corresponding author. Institute of Psychiatry, Largo Francesco Vito 1, Roma 00168, Italy.
E-mail address: gabriele.sani@unicatt.it

Psychiatr Clin N Am 43 (2020) 15–26
https://doi.org/10.1016/j.psc.2019.10.002
0193-953X/20/© 2019 Elsevier Inc. All rights reserved.

Abbreviations	
DSM	*Diagnostic and Statistical Manual of Mental Disorders*
ICD	*International Classification of Diseases*

Furthermore, the term "mixed states" is not uniformly used in the literature, with a tendency to use the terms "mixed state," mixed mania," "depression during mania," and "dysphoric mania" as synonymous,[3] as well as mixed and agitated depression.[4] Moreover, the clinical picture and course of people with mood disorders is influenced by premorbid characteristics, such as their personality, temperament, and emotional reactivity,[5] and the same seems to happen as far as mixed stares are concerned. Again, no clinical trials have specifically investigated these issues. Nevertheless, the construct of mixed states is a robust clinical entity and, according to the differing definitions provided in different contexts, prevalence rates range from 6% to 28%, if we take into account the narrow definition reported in the *International Classification of Diseases*, 10th edition (ICD)-10, and increase up to 66% when broader definitions are used.[6,7]

In the current nosographic system, mixed states can be conceptualized either as a specific phase of bipolar disorder, as was the case in *Diagnostic and Statistical Manual of Mental Disorders* (DSM)-IV-TR and ICD-10, or as specifiers ("with mixed features") that can be applied to manic, hypomanic, and depressive states (as reported among the diagnostic criteria of the DSM-5). In particular, the latter definition implies that mixed characteristics can be present in each phase of the disorder and that a mood polarity is clearly identifiable. In none of the current systems is the potential diagnostic influence of these premorbid characteristics mentioned. In this article, the authors provide a brief overview of the current nosography and clinical pictures of mixed states. Moreover, we discuss the role of temperament, personality, and emotional reactivity in mixed states.

CURRENT NOSOGRAPHY OF MIXED STATES

The first reports of mixed states can be found already in the work by Hippocrates[8] (460–370 BCE) and Aretaeus of Cappadocia[9] (130 BCE). However, one of the first modern systematization of mixed states has been provided by Kraepelin and Weygandt. In particular, Kraepelin described 6 forms of mixed states:

1. Depressive or anxious mania;
2. Excited or agitated depression;
3. Mania with thought poverty;
4. Manic stupor;
5. Depression with flight of ideas; and
6. Inhibited mania.[10]

Weygandt[11] further systematized the concept of mixed states by describing them as follows: "during manic episodes, the elevated mood suddenly can transform into a deeply depressed one, while otherwise the most vigorous mania persists with its urge of movement and dynamism, its distractibility and irritability, its talkativeness and flight of ideas. However, over the years mixed states were given a substantially lower importance and even their existence was questioned. In 1962, Schneider[12] affirmed that "We no longer believe in manic-depressive mixed states. Anyway, what may look like this is a change or a switch, if it pertains to cyclotymia at all." A revival of clinical and research interest on mixed states has occurred in the past few decades. In fact, since the late 1960s dysphoric mania, a condition characterized by manic symptoms accompanied by prominent depressive symptoms, and agitated or mixed depression (ie, major depression accompanied by symptoms of thought, motor and behavioral overactivation) have been extensively studied.[13]

The concept of mixed states has evolved along the years. The third and fourth edition of the DSM-III[14] and DSM-IV[15] included very stringent criteria for the diagnosis of mixed episodes,[2] requiring the simultaneous presence of full criteria for both a manic and a major depressive episode (except the 2-week duration), nearly every day for at least 1 week. The episode must be associated with marked impairment in functioning, psychosis, or hospitalization and not owing to the direct physiologic effects of a substance or a general medical condition. The DSM-IV clinical characterization of mixed episodes has been criticized as being inconsistent with clinical and research evidence. In fact, the majority of patients present some, but not all, symptoms of the opposite polarity, which are insufficient to be diagnosed as "mixed affective episodes."[16] Therefore, the majority of patients with mixed symptoms were excluded by that definition, and labeled as bipolar disorder, unspecified.[1]

The definition of mixed episodes provided by the ICD-10 (World Health Organization, 1992)[17] has subtle differences from that of the DSM-IV-TR.[18] The ICD-10 requires either a mixture or a rapidly alternating pattern (ie, within a few hours) of prominent manic and depressive symptoms for at least 2 weeks. The 2 sets of symptoms must be "both prominent for the greater part of the current episode of illness." Additionally, patients must have had at least 1 previous, well-defined hypomanic, manic, depressive, or mixed affective episode. The differences between the DSM-IV-TR and the ICD-10 criteria, such as the duration of symptoms (1 week vs 2 weeks), the cyclicity or the rapid alteration, and the exclusion that the first bipolar episode should have a mixed presentation in the ICD-10, present diagnostic challenges for clinicians. The ICD-10 definition of mixed states is less restrictive than that proposed by the DSM-IV, also acknowledging the existence of mixed depression and mixed mania.[19]

To overcome the limits of DSM-IV classification of mixed episodes, DSM-5 removed the category of mixed episodes and introduced the specifier "with mixed features" to the diagnosis of both mania/hypomania and major depression.[20] In the manic pole, contropolar mixed specifiers include dysphoria or depressed mood, loss of interest and pleasure, psychomotor retardation, fatigue or loss of energy, feelings of worthlessness or excessive or inappropriate guilt and thoughts of death, recurrent suicidal ideation, or a suicide attempt or a specific plan for committing suicide. In the depression pole, mixed specifiers include elevated mood, inflated self-esteem or grandiosity, decreased need for sleep, increased goal-directed activities, increased engagement in potentially risky behaviors, pressure of speech and flight of ideas, or the subjective experience that thoughts are racing. The threshold for adopting these specifiers was set to 3 contropolar symptoms. However, despite the significant changes made, the list of manic symptoms included in these specifiers has been widely criticized.[21] In fact, the list includes manic symptoms, such as elevated mood and grandiosity, that are rarely reported by patients with depression with mixed features, whereas other symptoms, such as irritability, psychomotor agitation, and distractibility—which are more frequently reported—have been excluded.[13] Moreover, the specifier "with mixed features" can be applied also to patients suffering from (unipolar) major depressive disorder who present hypomanic or manic symptoms.[22] This issue has raised the critique that, according to the DSM-5, the presence of 3 manic symptoms in patients with a major depressive episode is classified as a unipolar depression, whereas the development of a fourth manic symptom in the same patient determines that the episode is classified as bipolar.[16]

Following this debate, the World Health Organization decided not to remove the mixed episode from the eleventh revision of their chapter on mental and behavioral disorders.[23] According to the ICD-11, recently released by the World Health Organization, a mixed episode is characterized by (1) the presence of prominent manic or depressive symptoms that occur simultaneously or alternate very rapidly and (2) a significant impairment in personal, family, social, educational, occupational, or other important area of functioning.[24] The ICD-11 also specify that, when a depressive episode is predominant, contropolar symptoms should include irritability, racing or crowded thoughts, increased talkativeness, and psychomotor agitation. Dysphoric mood, expressed beliefs of worthlessness or hopelessness, and suicidal ideation are depressive symptoms that should be present when manic symptoms are predominant. Overall, the ICD-11 definition of mixed states seems to be much more consistent with both classical descriptions and recent research evidences.

CLINICAL DESCRIPTIONS OF MIXED STATES

Mixed episodes are associated with more severe forms of bipolar disorder, along with a worse course of illness and higher rates of comorbid conditions.[25,26] The onset of bipolar disorders with mixed episodes is earlier compared with "pure" bipolar disorder, with shorter symptom-free periods and longer time to resolution compared with depressive or manic episodes.[27–29]

Compared with patients with bipolar disorder without mixed episodes, those with mixed episodes usually experience more severe levels of psychopathology, more episodes per year, a worse long-term outcome and higher comorbidity rates.[30] In fact, more often people with mixed episodes present co-occurring anxiety disorders,[31] borderline personality disorder,[32] and alcohol and substance abuse.[33] Furthermore, patients with mixed episodes are considered to be at a particularly high risk for suicide, regardless the specific constellation of symptoms or predominant polarity.[34,35] Individuals with history of mixed episodes have more suicide attempts than those with pure affective episodes (31% vs 13%).[36]

There is a general agreement that in clinical practice mixed states can present with 2 main clusters of symptoms according to their mood polarity: one characterized by depressive symptoms intruding into a manic states (also called manic dysphoria),[37] and a second with manic features in patients with predominantly depressed mood.[2] Manic episodes with mixed features present more often with greater emotional lability and irritability, less euphoria, prolonged emotional instability, reduced involvement in pleasant activities, and less decreased need of sleep. Dysphoric mood, anxiety, excessive guilt, and suicidal symptoms are also common.[1] When a predominant depressed mood is present, mixed episodes occur with irritability, emotional liability, increased cognitive activity (ie, tachypsychia and distractibility), and psychomotor hyperactivity (ie, restlessness, impulsivity, and increased talkativeness).[38]

Psychomotor agitation is prominent in mixed states, independent of mood polarity, and includes 2 basic disturbances: painful inner tension and increased, poorly regulated goal-directed activity.[31] Painful inner tension is at the base of non–goal-directed motor activity and is often prominent in depressive episodes, whereas increased and poorly regulated goal-directed activity is often associated with irritability and impatience, mainly prominent in manic episodes. In mixed episodes, both aspects of agitation are present.

From a therapeutic viewpoint, patients with mixed episodes are difficult to treat, because these patients are generally poor responders. Lithium and other mood stabilizers are classically considered less effective in these patients,[39] although there are important reasons for still considering them a valid therapeutic option.[40] Antidepressants should be avoided because of exacerbation of manic symptoms and increased risk of suicidality.[2,7,34] Atypical antipsychotics[41,42] as well as nonpharmacologic treatments, such as electroconvulsive therapy[43] and transcranial magnetic stimulation[44] have been used. More studies are needed on the most appropriate treatment strategy in patients with mixed episodes.

TEMPERAMENT AND MIXED STATES

Temperament has been defined as a temporally stable biological "core" of personality and it refers to an individual's activity level, rhythms, moods and related cognitions.[45] Akiskal and colleagues[46] classified affective temperaments in 5 major subtypes, that is, hyperthymic, cyclothymic, dysthymic (depressive), anxious, and irritable, suggesting that temperaments are largely heritable and represent subclinical spectrum variants of the major affective disorders.[45] Premorbid affective temperament types have an important role in the clinical evolution of mood episodes, including the direction of affective polarity. Various studies specifically focused on the relationship between temperament and episode polarity, highlight that when temperaments are "congruent" with the affective episode, the resultant episode is often of the same sign (ie, euphoric mania in patients with hyperthymic temperament). Conversely, when the affective episode occurs in a temper of opposite polarity, the resulting clinical picture is characterized by mixed features (ie, mixed depression in patients with hyperthymic temperament). In 1992, for the first time, Akiskal[47] suggested that acute mixed manic (bipolar I) states might arise from a depressive temperamental base, whereas more protracted nonpsychotic depressive mixed states might arise from a cyclothymic-bipolar II and/or hyperthymic temperamental base. In this context, 2 subsequent studies, the Pisa–San Diego study[48] and the EPIMAN[49] study, can be considered as the 2 milestones in evaluating the impact of temperament on mixed states.

The Pisa–San Diego study explored the clinical, temperamental, and familial characteristics of 143 mixed state patients compared with a group of 118 patients who met DSM-III-R criteria for mania. The authors emphasized that the phenomenology of mixed states is more than the mere overlap of opposite affective symptoms; it rather represents an expansive–excited phase intruding into a depressive temperament and a melancholic episode intruding into a hyperthymic temperament. They found mania arising from a hyperthymic background, and mixed state from both depressive or hyperthymic temperaments. They also applied a mixed threshold of temperamental traits (ie, a patient meeting few criteria for traits of both types) and found that the mixed state group had higher rates than the manic group for these mixed temperamental traits, suggesting that when traits of the 2 temperaments coexisted, they represented a mixed-irritable form. Therefore, they hypothesized that this mixed-irritable temperament could impart dysphoric features to a manic episode.

The EPIMAN study by Akiskal and colleagues[49] characterized the clinical and temperamental features of 104 manic patients during hospitalization. Mixed mania was defined, according to McElroy's criteria,[50] as presenting with 2 depressive symptoms superimposed on mania and it was found in 37% of the sample. The EPIMAN study validated the significantly higher rate of hyperthymic temperament in classical mania compared with the significantly higher rate of depressive temperament in the mixed manic form. Akiskal and colleagues found a female over-representation in mixed mania. They linked this to the higher rates of hyperthymic temperament in men, which could be protective against depressive symptom development during a manic episode. In the EPIMAN study, irritable and cyclothymic temperaments have been related to mixed mania as well.

More recently, Röttig and colleagues[51] further supported Akiskal's original assumption of significantly higher scores of depressive, irritable, and cyclothymic temperaments in patients with prior mixed episodes compared with patients without. This finding underlines the importance of assessing temperament in the clinical evaluation of patients with affective disorders, particularly considering the greater affective instability and fluctuation that can occur in mood episodes and temperaments of opposite polarity.[5] Further studies with larger sample sizes are needed to expand these observations.

PERSONALITY AND MIXED STATES

Although temperament identifies temporally stable and biologically defined characteristics, personality, a broader phenotype, refers to acquired characterological determinants and interpersonal operations.[45] Although there is evidence that patients with mixed manic episodes may differ from patients with pure manic or depressive episodes concerning their temperament, few studies have investigated the relationship between mixed states and personological traits. Brieger and colleagues[52] assessed 16 patients with a mixed manic episode and 26 patients with a pure manic episode with the NEO-5-factor inventory of personality disorders. They found no difference between patients with mixed mania and patients with pure mania concerning their personality features. Röttig and colleagues[51] confirmed this observation in a larger sample size but also found significantly higher rates of personality disorders in patients with prior mixed episodes compared with those without. In a large, 2811-patient sample with a major depressive episode, Perugi and colleagues[53] provided evidence of high prevalence of borderline personality disorder in patients with depression presenting with mixed features. Mixed features were defined according to the DSM-5. The authors suggested that the irritable, aggressive, and impulsive behaviors present in borderline personality disorder may overlap in the clinical picture of mixed mood features. Similar considerations apply for affective instability, which is a key feature in borderline personality disorder and has generally been attributed to marked mood reactivity in interpersonal contexts. Interestingly, the authors suggested alternative explanations to the affective instability in those patients, surmising that it is possible for interpersonal problems to trigger emotional reactions, or conversely, the patient's unstable mixed mood can cause an excessive interpersonal sensitivity.[53]

EMOTIONAL REACTIVITY AND MIXED STATES

In the Pisa–San Diego study, Perugi and colleagues[48] operationalized new mixed state criteria, which were in part based on the concept of emotional instability. Mixed states were defined as a state of sustained (at least 2 weeks) emotional instability, and labile or hypersyntonic emotional resonance was proposed as one of the diagnostic criteria. This formulation emphasized the dynamic dimension of psychic life derived from an intimate mixture of the individual's drive and emotions. The authors proposed that, in a mixed state, the affective oscillations would be the result of instability in this dynamic dimension. In the BRIDGE study,[53] emotional lability was confirmed as a core feature of mixed states.

Henry and colleagues[54] assessed 139 patients with Bipolar I with a dimensional scale defining emotions not as a function of their tonality (eg, euphoria, irritability, sadness, and anxiety), but as quantitative dimensions defined by the intensity of emotional reactivity. Accordingly, emotional hyper-reactivity implies that all emotions can be felt with an unusual intensity. The authors found that bipolar disorder patients in a mixed state were characterized by high emotional hyper-reactivity and suggested this dimensional approach as the most appropriate to describe mixed states. Accordingly, mixed states could directly pertain to biological excitatory processes underlying emotion dysregulation in bipolar disorders.[55–57] They also found higher risk of suicide attempts in patients with emotional hyper-reactivity associated with depressive mood. This finding is in line with the high suicidal risk reported in mixed states and agitated depression.[4,48,49,58]

Intriguingly, a recent study found high emotional hyper-reactivity/affective lability in bipolar patients reporting childhood trauma.[59] Childhood trauma is strongly associated with both bipolar disorder type I and type II[60] and worsening of the clinical course of the illness (ie, increased suicide risk)[61] and could well bear specific neurobiological links with emotional reactivity in patients.[62–64] No studies to date have investigated the relationship between childhood trauma and mixed states in bipolar disorders. This investigation could potentially help to clarify the link between mixed states and emotional instability/reactivity.

DIAGNOSTIC TOOLS

Diagnostic tools reflect definitional issues in the diagnostic approach to mixed states. The current nosography of mixed states, identifying both depression and mania with mixed features, can be assessed through the Structured Clinical Interview for DSM-5.[65] Given the application of DSM-5 criteria for mixed depression carry poor clinical usefulness,[21,66] alternative diagnostic criteria and, hence, diagnostic are needed. Research Diagnostic Criteria[67] and the Koukopoulos criteria[68] for mixed depression with and without psychomotor agitation, have been proposed (**Table 1**).

The criteria for mixed depression were recently operationalized, and the first rating scale specifically designed to assess mixed symptoms cross-sectionally, that is, the Koukopoulos Mixed Depression Rating Scale, was validated.[69]

As discussed, the assessment of temperament could be crucial in the evaluation of mixed states. Temperament should always be assessed in patients with affective

Table 1
Proposed diagnostic criteria for mixed depression with (agitated depression) and without (mixed depression) psychomotor agitation

Agitated Depression Research Diagnostic Criteria Criteria[67]	Mixed Depression (Koukopoulos' Criteria)[68]
Major depression with at least 2 manifestations of psychomotor agitation (not mere subjective anxiety) present for several days: 1. Pacing 2. Hand wringing 3. Unable to sit still 4. Pulling or rubbing on hair, skin, clothing, or other objects 5. Outbursts of complaining or shouting 6. Talking on and on or "can't seem to stop talking"	Major depression with at least 3 of the following: 1. Inner tension/agitation 2. Racing or crowded thoughts 3. Irritability or unprovoked feeling of rage 4. Dramatic description of suffering or frequent spells of weeping 5. Talkativeness 6. Absence of signs of retardation 7. Mood lability and marked emotional reactivity 8. Early insomnia

disorders in everyday clinical practice. Considering previous studies on temperament and mixed states[49,51] the most reliable instrument in assessing temperament seems to be the Temperament Evaluation of Memphis, Pisa, Paris and San Diego-Autoquestionnaire version. Its constituent subscales and items were formulated on the basis of the diagnostic criteria for affective temperaments (cyclothymic, dysthymic, irritable, hyperthymic, and anxious), originally developed by Akiskal and his collaborators.[46] Assessing personality traits could be useful also for patients at risk for developing mixed symptoms. Nevertheless, insufficient and inconsistent data do not allow to identify which is the best assessment of personality. However, previous studies have specifically suggested considering mood episodes with mixed symptoms in patients with borderline personality disorder. Of consequence, we believe that emotional reactivity should be investigated in patients with affective disorders at risk for mixed states. Brancati and colleagues[70] very recently proposed and validated a new tool for the evaluation of emotional reactivity, the Reactivity, Intensity, Polarity and Stability questionnaire. This scale assesses emotional dysregulation and identifies 5 subscales, namely, affective instability, emotional impulsivity, and negative and positive emotionality, and it could be a promising instrument to better characterize patients with mixed states.

SUMMARY

Mixed states are a complex clinical entity, characterized by severe psychopathology and course of illness, a high risk of suicide, and unfavorable response to usual treatments. Moreover, diagnosis is not easy because of the various clinical presentations. Current official diagnostic criteria, based only on the presence and the count of manic or depressive symptoms, did not show enough clinical usefulness. A different approach needs to be used. The assessment of premorbid characteristics, such as temperament, personality and emotional reactivity, may be useful to detect mixed states earlier and understand better their complexity, and to develop personalized,[71] and hopefully effective, treatment strategies.

ACKNOWLEDGMENTS

The authors acknowledge the valuable collaboration of Matthew Brown.

DISCLOSURE

The authors declare that there are no conflicts of interest in this article.

REFERENCES

1. Solé E, Garriga M, Valentí M, et al. Mixed features in bipolar disorder. CNS Spectr 2017;22:134–40.
2. Castle DJ. Bipolar mixed states: still mixed up? Curr Opin Psychiatry 2014;27: 38–42.
3. Dilsaver SC, Chen YR, Shoaib AM, et al. Phenomenology of mania: evidence for distinct depressed, dysphoric, and euphoric presentations. Am J Psychiatry 1999;156:426–30.
4. Koukopoulos A, Sani G, Koukopoulos AE, et al. Melancholia agitata and mixed depression. Acta Psychiatr Scand 2007;115:50–7.
5. Koukopoulos A, Sani G, Koukopoulos AE, et al. Endogenous and exogenous cyclicity and temperament in bipolar disorder: review, new data and hypotheses. J Affect Disord 2006;96:165–75.

6. Azorin JM, Kaladjian A, Adida M, et al. Self-assessment and characteristics of mixed depression in the French national EPIDEP study. J Affect Disord 2012; 143:109–17.
7. Sani G, Napoletano F, Vöhringer PA, et al. Mixed depression: clinical features and predictors of its onset associated with antidepressant use. Psychother Psychosom 2014;83:213–21.
8. Hippocrates. Affections. Diseases 1. Diseases 2. Translated by Paul Potter. Loeb Classical Library 472. Cambridge (MA): Harvard University Press; 1988.
9. Aretaeus. On the causes and symptoms of chronic disease. Boston: Milford House; 1972.
10. Kraepelin E. Manic-depressive illness and paranoia. Edinburgh (United Kingdom): Livingstone; 1921.
11. Weygandt W. Ueber die Mischzustaende des manisch-depressiven Irreseins. Lehmann: Muenchen; 1899.
12. Schneider K. Klinische psychopathologie. Stuttgart (Germany): Thieme Verlag; 1962.
13. Maj M. "Mixed" depression: drawbacks of DSM-5 (and other) polythetic diagnostic criteria. J Clin Psychiatry 2015;76:e381–2.
14. American Psychiatric Association. Diagnostic and statistical manual of mental disorders. 3rd edition. Washington, DC: American Psychiatric Association; 1980.
15. American Psychiatric Association. Diagnostic and statistical manual of mental disorders. 4th edition. Washington, DC: American Psychiatric Association; 1994.
16. Malhi GS, Fritz K, Elangovan P, et al. Mixed states: modelling and management. CNS Drugs 2019;33:301–13.
17. World Health Organization. ICD-10: international statistical classification of diseases and related health problems: tenth revision. 2nd edition. Geneve: World Health Organization; 2004.
18. American Psychiatric Association. Diagnostic and statistical manual of mental disorders. 4th edition. Washington, DC: American Psychiatric Association; 2000.
19. Maj M. Development and validation of the current concept of major depression. Psychopathology 2012;45:135–46.
20. American Psychiatric Association. Diagnostic and statistical manual of mental disorders. 5th edition. Washington, DC: American Psychiatric Association; 2013.
21. Koukopoulos A, Sani G. DSM-5 criteria for depression with mixed features: a farewell to mixed depression. Acta Psychiatr Scand 2014;129:4–16.
22. Kaltenboeck A, Winkler D, Kasper S. Bipolar and related disorders in DSM-5 and ICD-10. CNS Spectr 2016;21:318–23.
23. World Health Organization. ICD-11: international statistical classification of diseases and related health problems: eleventh revision. Geneve: World Health Organization; 2018.
24. Reed GM, Sharan P, Rebello TJ, et al. The ICD-11 developmental field study of reliability of diagnoses of high-burden mental disorders: results among adult patients in mental health settings of 13 countries. World Psychiatry 2018;17:174–86.
25. Cassidy F, Carroll BJ. The clinical epidemiology of pure and mixed manic episodes. Bipolar Disord 2001;3:35–40.
26. Dell'Osso B, Dobrea C, Cremaschi L, et al. Italian bipolar II vs. I patients have better individual functioning, in spite of overall similar illness severity. CNS Spectr 2016;24:1–8.
27. Shim IH, Woo YS, Bahk WM. Prevalence rates and clinical implications of bipolar disorder "with mixed features" as defined by DSM-5. J Affect Disord 2015;173: 120–5.

28. Baldessarini RJ, Bolzani L, Cruz N, et al. Onset-age of bipolar disorders at six international sites. J Affect Disord 2010;121:143–6.
29. Undurraga J, Baldessarini RJ, Valenti M, et al. Suicidal risk factors in bipolar I and II disorder patients. J Clin Psychiatry 2012;73:778–82.
30. Fagiolini A, Coluccia A, Maina G, et al. Diagnosis, epidemiology and management of mixed states in bipolar disorder. CNS Drugs 2015;29:725–40.
31. Swann AC, Lafer B, Perugi G, et al. Bipolar mixed states: an international society for bipolar disorders task force report of symptom structure, course of illness, and diagnosis. Am J Psychiatry 2013;170:31–42.
32. Fagiolini A, Forgione R, Maccari M, et al. Prevalence, chronicity, burden and borders of bipolar disorder. J Affect Disord 2013;148:161–9.
33. Strakowski SM, Faedda GL, Tohen M, et al. Possible affective-state dependence of the Tridimensional Personality Questionnaire in first-episode psychosis. Psychiatry Res 1992;41:215–26.
34. Sani G, Tondo L, Koukopoulos A, et al. Suicide in a large population of former psychiatric inpatients. Psychiatry Clin Neurosci 2011;65:286–95.
35. Persons JE, Coryell WH, Solomon DA, et al. Mixed state and suicide: is the effect of mixed state on suicidal behavior more than the sum of its parts? Bipolar Disord 2018;20:35–41.
36. González-Pinto A, Barbeito S, Alonso M, et al. Poor long-term prognosis in mixed bipolar patients: 10-year outcomes in the Vitoria prospective naturalistic study in Spain. J Clin Psychiatry 2011;72:671–6.
37. Berk M, Dodd S, Malhi GS. 'Bipolar missed states': the diagnosis and clinical salience of bipolar mixed states. Aust N Z J Psychiatry 2005;39:215–21.
38. Pacchiarotti I, Nivoli AM, Mazzarini L, et al. The symptom structure of bipolar acute episodes: in search for the mixing link. J Affect Disord 2013;149:56–66.
39. Krüger S, Trevor Young L, Bräunig P. Pharmacotherapy of bipolar mixed states. Bipolar Disord 2005;7:205–15.
40. Sani G, Fiorillo A. The use of lithium in mixed states. CNS Spectr 2019;28:1–3.
41. Centorrino F, Fogarty KV, Sani G, et al. Antipsychotic drug use: McLean Hospital, 2002. Hum Psychopharmacol 2005;20:355–8.
42. Centorrino F, Fogarty KV, Cimbolli P, et al. Aripiprazole: initial clinical experience with 142 hospitalized psychiatric patients. J Psychiatr Pract 2005;11:241–7.
43. Perugi G, Medda P, Toni C, et al. The role of electroconvulsive therapy (ECT) in bipolar disorder: effectiveness in 522 patients with bipolar depression, mixed-state, mania and catatonic features. Curr Neuropharmacol 2017;15:359–71.
44. Bersani FS, Girardi N, Sanna L, et al. Deep transcranial magnetic stimulation for treatment-resistant bipolar depression: a case report of acute and maintenance efficacy. Neurocase 2013;19:451–7.
45. Von Zerssen D, Akiskal HS. Personality factors in affective disorders: historical developments and current issues with special reference to the concepts of temperament and character. J Affect Disord 1998;51:1–5.
46. Akiskal HS, Akiskal KK, Haykal RF, et al. TEMPS-A: progress towards validation of a self-rated clinical version of the temperament evaluation of the Memphis, Pisa, Paris, and San Diego Autoquestionnaire. J Affect Disord 2005;85:3–16.
47. Akiskal HS. The distinctive mixed states of bipolar I, II, and III. Clin Neuropharmacol 1992;15(Suppl 1):632A–3A.
48. Perugi G, Akiskal HS, Micheli C, et al. Clinical subtypes of bipolar mixed states. J Affect Disord 1997;43:169–80.

49. Akiskal HS, Hantouche EG, Bourgeois ML, et al. Gender, temperament, and the clinical picture in dysphoric mixed mania: findings from a French national study (EPIMAN). J Affect Disord 1998;50:175–86.

50. McElroy SL, Keck PE, Pope HG, et al. Clinical and research implications of the diagnosis of dysphoric or mixed mania or hypomania. Am J Psychiatry 1992; 149:1633–44.

51. Röttig D, Röttig S, Brieger P, et al. Temperament and personality in bipolar I patients with and without mixed episodes. J Affect Disord 2007;104:97–102.

52. Brieger P, Ehrt U, Roettig S, et al. Personality features of patients with mixed and pure manic episodes. Acta Psychiatr Scand 2002;106:179–82.

53. Perugi G, Angst J, Azorin JM, et al. Relationships between mixed features and borderline personality disorder in 2811 patients with major depressive episode. Acta Psychiatr Scand 2016;133:133–43.

54. Henry C, M'Baïlara K, Desage A, et al. Towards a reconceptualization of mixed states, based on an emotional-reactivity dimensional model. J Affect Disord 2007;101:35–41.

55. Kotzalidis GD, Rapinesi C, Savoja V, et al. Neurobiological Evidence for the Primacy of Mania Hypothesis. Curr Neuropharmacol 2017;15:339–52.

56. Janiri D, Di Nicola M, Martinotti G, et al. Who's the leader, mania or depression? Predominant polarity and alcohol/polysubstance use in bipolar disorders. Curr Neuropharmacol 2017;15(3):409–16.

57. Janiri D, Ambrosi E, Danese E, et al. Bipolar disorders. In: Spalletta G, Piras F, Gili T, editors. Brain morphometry. New York: Springer; 2018. p. 339–83.

58. Rapinesi C, Kotzalidis GD, Scatena P, et al. Alcohol and suicidality: could deep transcranial magnetic stimulation (DTMS) be a possible treatment? Psychiatr Danub 2014;26:281–4.

59. Aas M, Henry C, Bellivier F, et al. Affective lability mediates the association between childhood trauma and suicide attempts, mixed episodes and co-morbid anxiety disorders in bipolar disorders. Psychol Med 2017;47:902–12.

60. Janiri D, Sani G, Danese E, et al. Childhood traumatic experiences of patients with bipolar disorder type I and type II. J Affect Disord 2014;175:92–7.

61. Janiri D, Rossi P De, Kotzalidis GD, et al. Psychopathological characteristics and adverse childhood events are differentially associated with suicidal ideation and suicidal acts in mood disorders. Eur Psychiatry 2018;53:31–6.

62. Janiri D, Sani G, De Rossi P, et al. Hippocampal subfield volumes and childhood trauma in bipolar disorders. J Affect Disord 2019;253:35–43.

63. Janiri D, Sani G, De Rossi P, et al. Amygdala and hippocampus volumes are differently affected by childhood trauma in patients with bipolar disorders and healthy controls. Bipolar Disord 2017;19(5):353–62.

64. Del Casale A, Kotzalidis GD, Rapinesi C, et al. Neural functional correlates of empathic face processing. Neurosci Lett 2017;655:68–75.

65. First M, Williams J, Karg R, et al. Structured clinical interview for DSM-5 (SCID-5 for DSM-5). Am Psychiatr Assoc 2015.

66. Koukopoulos A, Sani G, Ghaemi SN. Mixed features of depression: why DSM-5 is wrong (and so was DSM-IV). Br J Psychiatry 2013;203:3–5.

67. Spitzer RL, Endicott J, Robins E. Research diagnostic criteria: rationale and reliability. Arch Gen Psychiatry 1978;35(6):773–82.

68. Sani G, Vöhringer PA, Napoletano F, et al. Koukopoulos' diagnostic criteria for mixed depression: a validation study. J Affect Disord 2014;164:14–8.

69. Sani G, Vöhringer PA, Barroilhet SA, et al. The Koukopoulos Mixed Depression Rating Scale (KMDRS): an International Mood Network (IMN) validation study of a new mixed mood rating scale. J Affect Disord 2018;232:9–16.
70. Brancati GE, Barbuti M, Pallucchini A, et al. Reactivity, intensity, polarity and stability questionnaire (RIPoSt-40) assessing emotional dysregulation: development, reliability and validity. J Affect Disord 2019;257:187–94.
71. Perugi G, De Rossi P, Fagiolini A, et al. Personalized and precision medicine as informants for treatment management of bipolar disorder. Int Clin Psychopharmacol 2019;34:189–205.

Psychopathology of Mixed States

Sergio A. Barroilhet, MD, PhD[a,b,*], S. Nassir Ghaemi, MD, MPH[b,c]

KEYWORDS

- Mixed states • Psychopathology • Factor structure • Conceptual models
- Mixed depression • Mixed mania

KEY POINTS

- Mixed states are not only a mixture of depressive and manic symptoms, but reflect manic and depressive symptoms combined with the core feature of psychomotor activation.
- Psychomotor activation is the core feature of mixed states, independent of polarity.
- Dysphoria (irritability/hostility) is the next most important feature of mixed states.
- Kraepelin and Koukopoulos provide conceptual models that fit the empirical data regarding mixed states well and are useful clinically.

INTRODUCTION

Mixed states pose a problem for the concept of bipolar illness. The term, *bipolar*, implies that mood varies between 2 opposite poles, mania and depression. Mixed states have been seen as transitional, and uncommon, phases between depression and mania.[1,2] Kraepelin, who emphasized course of illness rather than polarity of mood states in the diagnosis of manic-depressive insanity (MDI), argued that most mood episodes were neither depressive nor manic, but both at the same time, ie, mixed.[3] He did not emphasize polarity (depression vs mania) because he considered pure polarity (pure mania or pure depression) as infrequent, whereas mixed states were common. Influenced by Kraepelin's opponents in the Wernicke-Kleist-Leonhard school, the *Diagnostic and Statistical Manual of*

[a] Clínica Psiquiátrica Universitaria, Facultad Medicina Universidad de Chile, Santiago, Chile; [b] Department of Psychiatry, Tufts University, School of Medicine, Tufts Medical Center, Pratt Building, 3rd Floor, 800 Washington Street, Box 1007, Boston, MA 02111, USA; [c] Department of Psychiatry, Harvard Medical School, Harvard University, Boston, MA, USA
* Corresponding author. Clínica Psiquiatrica Universitaria, Av. La Paz 1003, Recoleta, Santiago, Chile.
E-mail address: sbarroilhet@hcuch.cl

Psychiatr Clin N Am 43 (2020) 27–46
https://doi.org/10.1016/j.psc.2019.10.003
0193-953X/20/© 2019 Elsevier Inc. All rights reserved.

Mental Disorders (Third Edition) (*DSM-III*) changed the emphasis of diagnosis of MDI from course of illness to polarity and replaced the MDI diagnosis with 2 offshoots: bipolar disorder and the newly invented major depressive disorder (MDD). Mixed states were legislated out of existence, being defined as simultaneous full manic and depressive episodes, a rare occurrence. Common mixed state symptoms like irritability or agitation became nosologically irrelevant. After 4 decades, the *Diagnostic and Statistical Manual of Mental Disorders* (Fifth Edition) (*DSM-5*) introduced a mixed features specifier to MDD but still denied any diagnostic validity to core mixed features of psychomotor agitation and dysphoria.[4,5]

Despite this anti-Kraepelinian *Diagnostic and Statistical Manual of Mental Disorders* (*DSM*) ideology, the research literature in the past few decades has contradicted the Leonhardian viewpoint, finding that coexistence of manic and depressive symptoms is the rule more than the exception.[6,7] Mood states with mixed symptoms may be the most common presentation of bipolar illness[8] and also common in unipolar depression.[9–11] These studies challenge the current *DSM* nosology and suggest a need for further attention to the psychopathology of mixed states.

A prominent approach to the psychopathology of mixed states is through 2 methods: factor analysis and cluster analysis. In factor analysis, clinical symptoms are analyzed into underlying components. In cluster analysis, clinical symptoms are combined to identify homogenous patient subgroups.[12] A complementary approach is based on systematic clinical observation, producing hypotheses to test with factor and cluster analytical methods.

This article summarizes factor and cluster analytical studies of the psychopathology of mixed states and relates those results to clinical models of mixed states.

METHODS

This article updates a prior review of factor and cluster analytical studies conducted by the 2013 International Society for Bipolar Disorders Task Force on mixed states (**Tables 1** and **2**).[13] Searches were done in PubMed from 1998 to 2019 using combinations of relevant terms, "mixed, "mania", "hypomania" "subtype", "factor structure", "factor analysis", and "cluster analysis", to explore structural analysis and cluster classification studies that included patients with mania and mixed mania. Likewise, for patients with depression and mixed depression, several searches were done in PubMed from 1998 to 2019 using combinations of relevant terms, "mixed depression", '"mixed depressive state", "depressive mixed state", "mixed depressive syndrome", "subtype", "factor structure", "factor analysis", and "cluster analysis." Additional bibliographic cross-referencing was conducted. Data on frequency of symptomatic domains were added as complementary information when found.

RESULTS

The results of this review are presented in 2 parts. The first summarizes factor and cluster analysis studies of empirical data on the psychopathology of mixed states. The second summarizes proposed clinical/conceptual models of mixed states. This discussion attempts to integrate the empirical factor analysis literature with proposed clinical/conceptual models.

Table 1
Symptomatic structure of pure and mixed manic episodes

Study	Sample	Measures	Factor Structure	Notes
Cassidy et al,[30] 1998	204 manic 33 mixed *DSM-III-R*	Rating scale derived by authors	Dysphoric mood,[a,b] psychomotor acceleration, psychosis, increased hedonia, irritable-aggression	Time of assessment: 2–5 d of admission Measure included mania depression, and psychosis items (20 items) Medication: as appropriate during inpatient stay Results did not change when removing mixed patients
Dilsaver & Shoaib,[24] 1999	48 manic 57 mixed RDC and *DSM-III-R*	SADS	Depressive state, sleep disturbance, manic state, and irritability-paranoia	Time of assessment: "before starting treatment"
Akiskal et al,[22] 2001	104 manic *DSM-IV*	MVAS-BP	Expansiveness Activation Psychomotor acceleration Anxiety depression Social desinhibition Sleep Anger	Based on ≥2 concurrent depressive symptoms 64.5% had pure mania and 35.5 had depressive mixed mania
Kumar et al,[38] 2001	100 manic ICD-10-DCR	SMS	Mania (psychomotor acceleration) Psychosis Irritability-aggression	Outpatients Patients with mixed mania were excluded Substance abuse excluded
Perugi et al,[23] 2001	153 manic *DSM-III-R*	CPRS	Depressive Irritable-agitated Euphoric-grandiose Accelerated-sleepless Paranoid-anxious	Time of assessment: within 7 d of admission Medication: as appropriate during inpatient stay Substance abuse excluded
Rossi et al,[19] 2001	124 manic *DSM-III-R*	BRMaS BRMeS	Activation-euphoric Depression Psychomotor retardation Hostility-destructiveness sleep disturbance	Time of assessment: within 3 d of admission

(continued on next page)

Table 1
(continued)

Study	Sample	Measures	Factor Structure	Notes
Swann et al,[31] 2001	162 manic or mixed RDC and *DSM-III-R*	SADS ADRS	Impulsivity, anxious pessimism,[b] hyperactivity, distressed appearance, hostility, psychosis	Inpatients, screened during washout of medication; 50% were delusional
Sato et al,[25] 2002	518 manic 58 mixed *DSM-IV*	SADS (37 symptoms)	Depressive mood, irritable aggression, insomnia, depressive inhibition, pure mania, lability/agitation, psychosis	Time of assessment: 1–5 d of admission Medication: as appropriate during inpatient stay
González-Pinto et al,[26] 2003, and González-Pinto et al,[15] 2004	78 manic 25 mixed SCID-I	YMRS HAM-D-21	Depression,[b] dysphoria, hedonism, psychosis, activation	Time of assessment: first day after admission Medication: patients on medication when assessed Substance abuse excluded
Akiskal et al,[18] 2003	104 manic *DSM-IV*	MSRS HAM-D-17	Disinhibition Hostility Deficit (lack of self-care) Psychosis Elation Depression Sexuality	Inpatients Sample: Consecutive admissions without selection
Harvey et al,[14] 2008	363 manic 71 mixed SCID-I	HAM-D-21 MRS (SADS)	Manic: energy/activity, lack of insight, depression, racing thoughts, and reduced sleep Mixed: 5-factor solution differed to energy/activity, judgment, elation, depression/thinking, and reduced sleep	Inpatients Substance abuse excluded
Picardi et al,[37] 2008	88 manic *ICD-10*	BPRS	Mania Disorganization Positive symptoms Dysphoria	Time of assessment: within 3 d of admission Sample: subsample of acute manic hospitalized patients, from a national multicenter sample in Italy

Study	Sample	Scale	Symptoms/Factors	Comments
Gupta et al,[20] 2009	225 manic ICD-10-DCR	SMS	Psychosis, irritability/aggression, dysphoria,[a] accelerated thought stream, hedonia, hyperactivity	Sample: excluded patients if they had received a diagnosis of mixed affective disorder
Hanwella and de Silva,[36] 2011	131 manic ICD-10	YMRS	Irritable mania, elated mania, psychotic mania	Time of assessment: within 24 h of admission. Inpatients
Swann et al,[16] 2013	1535 manic 644 mixed DSM-IV	MADRS YMRS	Depression, mania, sleep disturbance, judgment/impulsivity, irritability/hostility	Time of assessment: before randomization. Sample: patients pooled from 6 RCT with aripiprazole. Medication: no meds or in washout. Substance abuse excluded (<3 mo)
Perugi et al,[27] 2013	202 mixed DSM-IV	HAM-D-18 YMRS	Depression, agitation/irritability/aggression, psychosis. Anxiety, sleep disorder, anxiety/language-thought disorder, motor retardation/somatic symptoms/guilt	Time of assessment: first week of admission. Sample: resistant inpatient derived for trial of ECT; 70% psychosis. Factor analysis: considered 9 non-redundant items of YMRS, and 12 items of HAM-D-18
Perugi et al,[28] 2014	202 mixed DSM-IV	BPRS	Psychotic-positive symptoms, mania, disorientation–unusual motor behavior, depression. Negative symptoms and anxiety	Time of assessment: first week of admission. Sample: resistant inpatient derived for trial of ECT; 70% psychosis
Filgueiras et al,[21] 2014	117 manic DSM-IV	SADS-C	Depression, suicide, insomnia, mania, psychosis, anxiety	Time of assessment: first week of admission
Güçlü et al,[17] 2015	96 manic SCID-I	YMRS MADRS SAPS	Increased, psychomotor activity, dysphoria,[a] psychosis	Time of assessment: within 3 d of admission. Sample: only males. High prevalence of alcohol and marijuana use
Shah et al,[29] 2017	50 manic or mixed ICD-10 RDC	YMRS BPRS	Pure mania, dysphoric mania,[a] hostile mania, delirious mania	Unmedicated

Abbreviations: ADRS, Affective Disorder Rating Scale; BPRS, Brief Psychiatric Rating Scale; BRMaS, Bech–Rafaelsen Mania Scale; BRMeS, Bech–Rafaelsen Melancholia Scale; CPRS, Comprehensive Psychopathological Rating Scale; *DSM-III-R, Diagnostic and Statistical Manual of Mental Disorders* (Third Edition Revised); ECT, Electro-convulsive Therapy; HAM-D-21, Hamilton Depression Rating Scale, 21 items; HAM-D-18, Hamilton Depression Rating Scale, 18 items; HAM-D-17, Hamilton Depression Rating Scale, 17 items; *ICD-10, International Classification of Diseases, Tenth Revision*; ICD-10-DCR, International Classification of Diseases, Tenth Revision, Diagnostic Criteria for Research; MADRS, Montgomery–Åsberg Depression Rating Scale; MRS, Mania Rating Scale; MSRS, Beigel-Murphy Manic-State Rating Scale; MVAS-BP, Multiple Visual Analogue Scales of Bipolarity; RDC, Research Diagnostic Criteria; SADS, Schedule for Affective Disorders and Schizophrenia; SADS-C, Schedule for Affective Disorders and Schizophrenia (Changed); SAPS, Scale for the Assessment of Positive Symptoms; SCID-I, Structured Clinical Interview for *DSM-IV* Axis I Disorders; SMS, Scale for Manic States; YMRS, Young Mania Rating Scale.

  a Dysphoria used as a synonym of depressive.
  b Biphasic distribution.

Table 2
Symptomatic structure of depressive and mixed depressive episodes

Study	Sample	Measures	Factor Structure	Notes
Benazzi & Akiskal,[48] 2005	348 BP II MDE 254 UP MDE SCID	HIG	Psychomotor activation Irritability–mental activation	Depressed outpatients Excluded patients with substance abuse, borderline personality, or significant medical illness Unmedicated
Biondi et al,[51] 2005	380 UP MDE 143 UP MDE DSM-IV	Author-derived scale MMPI-2	Depression Anxiety Activation	Depressed outpatients Measure assessed a broad range of behavior, beyond conventional mood symptoms Excluded: bipolar unmedicated
Sato et al,[52] 2005	863 UP MDE 25 BP II MDE 70 BP I MDE ICD-10	AMDP system	Typical vegetative symptoms Depressive retardation/loss of feeling, hypomanic syndrome, anxiety, psychosis, depressive mood/hopelessness	Depressive inpatients Medicated before admission Measured 43 symptoms of the AMDP
Benazzi,[49] 2008	441 BP II MDE 289 UP MDE 275 remitted BP II SCID	SCID (modified) HIG	Irritable mental overactivity Elevated mood, motor overactivity	Depressed outpatients Excluded patients with SUS, BPD, or significant medical illness Unmedicated
Frye et al,[50] 2009	172 BP I or II MDE SCID	YMRS	Motor/verbal activation Thought content/insight Aggressiveness Appearance	Moderate severity of depression

Abbreviations: AMDP, Association for Methodology and Documentation in Psychiatry; BP II, Bipolar Disorder, type II; HIG, hypomania interview guide; *ICD-10, International Classification of Diseases, Tenth Revision;* MDE, Major Depressive Episode; MMPI-2, Minnesota Multiphasic Personality Inventory; SCID, Structured Clinical Interview for *DSM-IV;* UP, Unipolar; YMRS, Young Mania Rating Scale.

Part I: Factor and Cluster Analysis Studies of the Empirical Psychopathology of Mixed States

Factor analysis studies: pure and mixed mania

All manic episodes, whether pure or mixed, shared a similar multidimensional structure according to factor analysis (see **Table 1**). The 3 main components were manic, depressive, and non–mood-related symptoms (ie, psychomotor activation, dysphoria, psychosis, and anxiety).

Depression Contrary to common belief, pure mania was associated with an underlying depressive factor in most studies,[14–31] mainly depressed mood, guilt, and suicidality.[13,32] Depressive symptoms can be found in 12.8% to 29% of pure manic patients[15,32] and may rise to 30% to 40%, depending on the methodology.[33] This may be due to a lack of specificity of *DSM* and *International Classification of Diseases* (*ICD*) diagnostic criteria,[30] which are insufficient to rule out mixed mania, and, because of the low frequency of pure forms, as Kraepelin predicted. Using the mixed features specifier in *DSM-5*, incidence of depressive symptoms in patients with mania/hypomania rises to 24% to 34%.[34,35]

Dysphoria A dysphoria (irritability/hostility) factor presented as a consistent independent factor across most studies,[16,18–20,22–27,29–31,36–38] although sometimes it covaried with other symptoms like lack of insight[14,23,25,26] or increased motor activity.[17,19,21,23,27] This factor often is more frequent in mixed than pure mania,[8] though not in all studies.[15] It includes irritability, subjective and overt anger, uncooperativeness, impatience, suspiciousness, hostility, and aggression, and is present in 22.7% to 72% of manic patients.[32,39]

Psychomotor activation This factor showed a variable pattern, sometimes covarying with manic elation symptoms (ie, euphoria, increased self-esteem, and grandiosity)[16,17,19,21,22,24,28,31,37] or dysphoria,[13,17,23,27,36] and sometimes presenting as an independent factor.[14,18,20,26,30,38] Common symptoms were racing thoughts, distractibility, pressured speech, intrusiveness and increased contacts with other people, hyperactivity, and increased goal-directed activities. Sometimes a separate factor was expressed in the opposite dimension, with retarded or inhibited thought and inhibited drive and motor activities,[19,25,27] all of which were independent of depressive mood,[25] pointing to an inhibited mania subtype, as described by Kraepelin.

Anxiety The anxiety component of mania includes inner tension, somatic symptoms, worry, indecisiveness, and panic symptoms. It correlates with severity of depressive symptoms and in most studies loads in the depressive factor.[15,16,20,24,25,31] In some studies with more severely ill patients, it is present as an individual factor,[21,27] while also overlapping with other factors of language/thoughts or motor/agitation.[27] Hence, anxiety may be a marker of severity of mixed states, with a strong correlation with depression scores in manic subjects.[40] Although many studies do not measure anxiety directly, it appears that anxiety is present in 17% to 32% of manic patients.[32]

Psychosis In most studies, psychosis presented as an independent factor of mania,[17–21,25–28,31,32,36–38] characterized by hallucinations, delusions, paranoia (hypervigilance and suspiciousness), lack of insight, impaired self-care, and bizarre or disorganized behavior. Psychotic symptoms can be found in up to 70% of severely ill manic patients[27] and can present with equal frequency in pure and mixed mania,[25,32] being more common in the manic than in the depressive pole.[13,27] It has been conceptualized as a marker of severity in pure and mixed manic patients.[13,36,41]

In contrast to abnormal thought content, abnormalities of thought process had no consistent role in manic states. In some studies, thoughts process loaded mainly with psychomotor symptoms,[26,30] whereas in other studies, it loaded with affective components of mania (euphoria, increased self-esteem, and grandiosity)[25,36] or even as an independent factor.[14,20]

Sleep disturbance Sleep symptoms loaded independently from mania or depression factors,[14,16,19,21,22,24,25] perhaps because patients experience insomnia in different ways; for example, some patients with manic insomnia lack insight into their decreased need for sleep and do not see it as a problem, whereas other insomniac patients without decreased need for sleep experience it as a subjectively painful state.[21]

Subtypes of pure and mixed mania
A majority of cluster studies demonstrated 4 consistent clusters of manic subtypes: euphoric, dysphoric, depressive, and psychotic manic states. A fifth possible group is mixed hypomania.

Euphoric mania Euphoric mania entails elevated mood, increased self-esteem or grandiosity, and increased energy and activity,[16,24,31] with little or no irritability/hostility,[16] anxiety, or psychosis.[24,31] Sleep disturbance may be present or not.[16] The main characteristic is the relative (although not complete) absence of depressive symptoms.[16,24]

Dysphoric mania In this subtype, classical manic symptoms are present with lower scores in manic hyperactivity.[24,31] There are high levels of distress and hostility[31] and high scores for depressed state, anxiety, and irritability/paranoia, compared with pure manic patients,[16,24] and more treatment refusal compared with other mixed or pure manic patients.[23] A severely ill subgroup demonstrates high anxiety (panic attacks), higher hyperactivity, and psychotic symptoms,[27] resembling Kraepelin's depressive-anxious mania.

Depressive mania In this subtype, the clinical picture of depressive mania tends to meet *DSM-5* criteria for mixed states. There is high psychomotor activation, with variable degrees of irritability and paranoia.[16] Depression is characteristically prominent.[16,17,24,25] Patients are prone to have a negative evaluation of self, have self-reproach, feel discouragement, suffer from psychic and somatic anxiety,[31] and experience emotional lability/agitation, which may increase suicidality.[17,25,42] Some patients show psychomotor inhibition with retarded thoughts and inhibited drive, along with emotional lability/agitation,[25] resembling Kraepelin's "excited depression," where depressive-anxious mood and thought inhibition are combined with agitation and restlessness.[27]

Depressive mania and dysphoric mania are different.[31,42] The latter has milder depressive symptoms and the former has more suicidality. These differences can be linked to baseline temperaments, depressive and irritable, respectively.[42] Some investigators see dysphoric mania as an intermediate state in a continuum between pure euphoric mania and depressive mania.[24] Bimodal distribution of the depressive factor in some studies support this view.[16,26,30,31]

Psychotic mania In this subtype, there is psychomotor activation along with psychotic features, ranging from impairment of judgment and insight[16] to overt delusions.[31]

Besides manic symptoms, such patients present little or no irritability/hostility (except in patients with substance abuse[17]) or depressive symptoms.[16,25,30,31] There is low frequency of rapid cycling[23,31,43] but more chronic residual manic and psychotic symptoms.[27]

Mixed hypomania The clinical picture of mixed hypomania has been little studied, with no factor analysis studies to date. The most frequent symptom is irritability, with or without depressive symptoms, the latter being more frequent among women.[44,45] Crowded thoughts may be more frequent compared with pure mania or depression.[46] Psychotic symptoms are not common. *DSM-5*–defined MDD with mixed features captures a clinical picture that is equivalent to mixed hypomania, not mixed depression.[4]

Factor analysis studies: pure and mixed depression
Manic symptoms are frequent in depressive episodes, whether unipolar or bipolar (see **Table 2**). Concurrent manic symptoms are present in 38.1% to 47% of cases of unipolar depression[9,10] and in 68.8% of cases of bipolar depression.[6] The specific manic symptoms that occur during depressive episodes are similar in both unipolar and bipolar depression, especially psychomotor agitation and racing/crowded thoughts.[4,6] Pure depression versus mixed depression is best distinguished by manic symptoms of irritability, language/thought disorder, rate and amount of speech, and increased psychomotor activity/energy.[47]

Table 2 summarizes factor analysis studies on this topic. A limiting factor was that no studies used both depressive and manic symptom scales in current depressive episodes. In general, psychomotor activation and dysphoria appear as the main underlying factors, explaining a major part of the variance.[48–50]

Psychomotor activation
Psychomotor activation was the strongest and most consistent factor present in mixed depression, whether unipolar or bipolar. In unipolar depression, it was present in 20% to 27% of cases and loaded on a factor characterized by motor overactivation[51] and agitation,[48,49] along with talkativeness,[48,49] acceleration of ideas, impulsiveness, and unstable mood.[51] It covaried with irritability and aggressiveness (dysphoria). In bipolar depression, the activation factor had the same symptomatic profile but with higher amount of increased energy and overactivation of thought process (racing thoughts and flight of ideas).[50] This factor included standard *DSM* manic symptoms except euphoria, increased self-esteem, or grandiosity.[48,49,52] Baseline psychomotor activation (racing thoughts, talkativeness, and increased activities) was related to antidepressant-induced mania.[50] As seen in factor analysis studies of mania and mixed mania, however, a separate factor expressed the opposite extreme of the dimension, with retarded and inhibited thinking, loss of emotion, perplexity, inhibited drive, social withdrawal, and objective retardation.[52]

Dysphoria Dysphoria also was present consistently in mixed depression, both unipolar and bipolar, with 40% to 73.3% prevalence[6,39] (vs 15%–17.5% in pure depression[39,53,54]). It is characterized by irritability[48,49] and increased risky activities.[48] Associated features that covaried with it were racing/crowded thoughts, distractibility, and psychomotor activation.[48,49] In unipolar depression, a composite factor included intolerance toward social rules, impulsiveness, sensitivity, and aggressiveness, but overtly disruptive aggressive behavior loaded in this factor only in bipolar depression.[50] Standard manic and psychotic symptoms were covariates of the dysphoria factor in unipolar depression.[51]

Psychosis Psychotic symptoms were present in up to 30.0% of subjects with unipolar and bipolar mixed depression,[9] including paranoia (vigilance, sensitivity, litigiousness, distrust, and suspicion), along with delusions of poverty, guilt, reference, and hypochondria[52] as well as lack of insight.[50] Psychosis covaried with psychomotor activation.[51]

Anxiety In unipolar mixed depression, the anxiety factor comprised apprehension, fear, preoccupation, and somatization,[51] along with somatic inner restlessness, complaints, somatic anxiety, and panic attacks.[52] Anxiety scores correlated strongly with manic scores.[40]

Phenomenology of depressive features in mixed depression The experience of the core depressive state in mixed depression was similar in both unipolar and bipolar types. It included sadness, demoralization, apathy, hopelessness, feeling of inadequacy, and suicidal ideation.[51,52] There also was a somatic factor comprising initial insomnia, interrupted sleep, shortened sleep, early waking, decreased appetite, tiredness, loss of vitality, and decreased sexual interest.[52] The latter study also identified a factor that included psychomotor inhibition with motor retardation, inhibited affectivity and drive, retarded thinking, and social withdrawal.[52]

Subtypes of pure and mixed depression
Available studies suggest 2 main clusters of depressive subtypes: an activated/hyperreactive cluster and a retarded/hyporeactive cluster.

Activated/hyperreactive mixed depression This subtype is characterized by psychomotor agitation, irritability, emotional lability, distractibility, and mood reactivity.[55] In bipolar depression, there is increased psychomotor activation with many plans and activities[56]; increased speech,[57] racing thoughts, and distractibility[56]; suicidal ideation; and psychotic symptoms.[57] This subtype of depression presents with emotional hyperreactivity, marked emotional lability,[56] somatic symptoms like appetite disturbance,[57] and enhanced sensory perception.[56] Psychomotor activation can lead to agitation[57] and suicide attempts.[56] A characteristic of this subtype is higher intensity and frequency of emotions like irritability, anger, panic, anxiety, and exaltation,[56,57] which previously have been labeled in the psychiatric literature with other terms, such as agitated depression or irritable-hostile depression.

Retarded/hyporeactive pure depression This other main subtype of depression, is characterized centrally by psychomotor retardation.[55] In bipolar depression, it is characterized by reduced energy[56,57] and more inhibition in thoughts process and motor activities[56] and loss of motivation,[56,57] diminished interests, reduced social engagement,[57] indecision,[56] and impaired concentration and memory.[57] In the affective domain, this subtype is characterized by anhedonia along with feelings of worthlessness, helplessness and hopelessness, depressed mood, anxiety, and guilt,[57] with notable affective flattening,[56,57] emotional hyporeactivity, sensorial numbness,[56] and sleep disturbances.[57] This clinical picture resembles classic melancholic depression.[58]

Threshold for diagnosis of mixed states
In contrast to *DSM-III* through *DSM-5*, there is no scientific rationale at all for the *DSM* requirement of 3 or 4 manic symptoms as the threshold for mixed episodes or mixed modifier definitions. Instead, the reviewed literature consistently and strongly supports a cutoff of 2 or 3 symptoms of the opposite polarity during a depressive or manic/hypomanic episode.[9,10,15,32] This threshold correlates with

diagnostic validators of differing course of illness, prognosis, comorbidities, and treatment response.

Part II: Clinical/Conceptual Models of Mixed States

Kraepelin/Weygandt model

Kraepelin acknowledged that mixed states were propelled by a mechanism similar to hyperarousal and emphasized the importance of course, distinguishing a transitional and an autonomous form. Following Weygandt, Kraepelin held that mixed states resulted from the combination of 3 independent domains—mood, thought, and volition—on an excitation-inhibition continuum. Different combinations of these domains constituted different subtypes of MDI. Accordingly, he described 8 mood states, 2 pure (pure mania and pure depression) and 6 mixed: depression with flight of ideas, exited or agitated depression, depressive/anxious mania, inhibited mania, mania with poverty of thoughts, and manic stupor.[59]

The most prevalent mixed states were depressive/anxious mania, excited or agitated depression, and depression with flight of ideas.[13] The first subtype was characterized by increased thought production and speed manifested externally in logorrhea and pressured speech, along with restlessness, high anxiety, and increased activities. Psychomotor excitation was prominent, and delusions of guilt, persecution and hypochondriac delusions were common. The second subtype was similar to the latter but with inhibition of thought. The third subtype consisted of depressive mood and inhibition of motor activity, including speech, but with abnormal thought processes. Patients could even become mute and rigid.[60]

Malhi and colleagues[12] proposed a revised formulation of the Kraepelin/Weygandt model, the activity-cognition-emotion (ACE) model. These 3 dimensions interact with each other. One can be primary but combine with other dimensions for secondary symptoms. Mixed states result from overactivation of one dimension along with inhibition of another. Dimensions can shift in occurrence and severity over time, accounting for myriad mixed state presentations.

Mentzos/Berner model

The Greek-German psychiatrist Stavros Mentzos defined mood states on 2 domains: boost (the underlying force behind the psychic process) and mood (the predominant affective tone that colored thoughts and conscienceless).[5,61] Pure forms would result from concordant boost and mood, whereas mixed states resulted from contradictory or quickly changing boost and mood.[5,59] Based on this structure, Berner explained mixed states as the "persistent presence of a drive state contradictory to the mood state and/or the emotional resonance."[62] Mixed states were classified in stable and unstable (ie, rapid cycling) forms and included diurnal variations and sleep disturbances as key aspects.[63] This group proposed a dysphoric dimension (morose, tense, and irritated mood) as a third field in mood disorders, distinguishable from mixed states[64] that also may mix with depression and mania.[65] Other investigators have proposed that the dysphoric syndrome (inner tension, irritability, aggressive behavior, and hostility) is the core marker of mixed states.[39]

Akiskal model

Akiskal proposed that mixed states were the result of interaction of a mood episode with a temperament in the opposite polarity, such as a depressive episode in a person with hyperthymic or cyclothymic temperament.[66,67] Likewise, pure depressive episodes occur when an episode aligns with temperamental predisposition (such as, euphoric mania in a person with hyperthymic temperament) or occurs in someone with no affective temperament at all (a depressive episode in a person with a normal personality).[23,42,62] Empirical data to support this view include evidence that affective temperaments are more frequent in mixed than pure depressive or manic episodes.[68]

Koukopoulos model

Koukopoulos advocated for the Kraepelin and Akiskal models but saw depression as the effect of manic states, not an independent phenomenon. He followed Griesenger in the view that excitatory brain processes (producing mania) are the cause of inhibitory brain processes (producing depression).[69] The "primacy of mania"[70] hypothesis put forward by Koukopoulos holds that depressive symptoms in mixed states are caused by manic processes.[71] Furthermore, even pure depressive episodes are caused by prior manic episodes or symptoms (such as manic temperaments). His metaphor for this theory was that "mania is the fire, depression is the ash."

This theory explains why mixed states occur, not as an accident or coincidence but because they are the outcome of depressive symptoms fueled by mania. Therefore, because mania causes depression, it is mania that has to be prevented or treated directly, not depression.[71]

Clinically, Koukopoulos sees mixed depression as the presence of a depressive episode with psychomotor excitation, manifested as psychomotor agitation and/or marked rage. *DSM* manic symptoms may or may not be present.[4] As noted, his view is consistent with Akiskal's emphasis on affective temperaments, specifically those with manic features, that is, cyclothymic, hyperthymic, and irritable temperaments.

The following quotation from Koukopoulos and colleagues brings out his meaning: "When a sad or stressful event provokes a depressive reaction, or a seasonal or endogenous depression occurs in such a person, the psychic reaction is intense and exacerbates the depression itself. In turn, the emotional reaction heightens and unleashes this energy, which produces manic symptoms, such as restlessness and racing thoughts, while it also triggers anxiety and aggravates the depressive psychic pain. This tight interweaving of manic traits and depressive states of agitated depression makes it an authentic mixed state."[60]

DISCUSSION

A summary of the factor/cluster analytical studies reviewed is as follows: Besides mood-related factors of depression and mania, the core additional features of the mixed state are psychomotor activation and secondarily, in some subtypes, dysphoria. Those central features are more pronounced in mixed mania than in mixed depression but are present nonetheless in both mood states. These central features of mixed states are independent of illness polarity (ie, are similar in both unipolar and bipolar illness). Anxiety and psychosis reflect severity of the mixed state in both mania and depression and are not core features. Psychomotor inhibition, although sometimes present in some mixed states (ie, depressive mania) mainly is present in pure depression.

In classification studies, 4 main subtypes of manic states—euphoric, dysphoric, depressive, and psychotic—and 2 main subtypes of depressive states—activated/hyperreactive mixed depression and retarded/hyporeactive pure depression—were identified (**Fig. 1**).

Clinical/conceptual models acknowledge the multidimensionality of mood disorders and the myriad of possible presentations. Weygandt and Kraepelin saw mixed states as a combination of contradictory forces from 3 dimensions: mood, thought, and volition (recently reformulated in the ACE model as affect, emotion, and

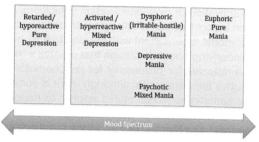

Fig. 1. Subtypes of mood states supported by cluster analysis studies. Note: the 6 subtypes of mood states supported by cluster analysis studies are individualized, and myriad intermediate forms may have not yet been captured given the lack of psychopathologic nuance of current instruments and limitations of studies.

cognition). Metzos and Berner underscored that an underlying alteration (drive or boost) at a physiologic level, contradictory to mood or emotional resonance, was the basis of mixed states. Akiskal held that mixed states were the result of mood episodes interacting with affective temperaments of the opposite pole. Koukopoulos highlighted the importance psychomotor excitation (with clinical presentation as rage and lability) as the crucial process causing subsequent depressive symptoms.

Importance of Psychomotor Activation

Frequently, psychomotor overactivation is interpreted in terms of *agitation* or *excitation*. Agitation to many clinicians implies observable physical activity, although it need not do so, because the concept of *psychic agitation*, without motor changes, also has existed for many years. Another term that is used confusedly is *psychomotor*. This term means either psychological or motor changes, not both psychological and motor changes. In other words, motor abnormalities are not necessary for the presence of psychomotor disturbance.

One approach to clarifying any confusion in terms is to prefer the term, *activation*, as Scott and colleagues[72] have proposed: as "a multilevel construct emerging from underlying physiologic change... measurable in objectively observed behavior (motor activity) and the related subjective experience of the overt behavior (energy)." Activation also broadly comprehends other less observable phenomena like fine motor movements, reaction times, and speech articulation and production[73] and is tightly related to thought production and flow[46,74] and to feelings, emotions, and volitions.[75,76] An apt metaphor may be voltage, the push that causes the charge to move in a functional system.

Correlation of Empirical Factor/Cluster Analytical Studies with Clinical/Conceptual Models

The empirical results, described previously, with emphasis on core features of psychomotor activation and dysphoria, are consistent with the clinical/conceptual models provided.

The Kraepelin/Weygandt model is consistent with the notion that psychomotor activation would drive affectivity (intensity, reactivity, and stability), thoughts or cognitions (speed, shifts, and quantity), and volition (impulsivity, intensity, and endurance or shifts of behavior). For each symptom domain, this psychomotor activation may demonstrate in over-activation or over-deactivation (inhibition), presenting as mixed states when activation in some domains coincide with deactivation in other domains.

The Metzos/Berner model is consistent with the idea that a physiologic psychomotor activation is the underlying boost or voltage that creates a mixed state. The Akiskal model provides a rationale for propensity for psychomotor activation as being related to manic affective temperaments, although there is some evidence opposed to this view because sometimes mixed states appear to happen without affective temperaments.

The Koukopoulos model, like Metzos/Berner, views psychomotor excitation as primary and causative not only of mixed states but also depressive states. The Koukopoulos model not only fits the empirical factor analytical data but also is the only model that provides a conceptual rationale for those data, namely that manic states and depressive states go together, because the former cause the latter. This "primacy of mania" claim can be rephrased as the "primacy of psychomotor overactivation" if the core of mania is defined as psychomotor overactivation, as is shown to be the case in the factor analytical studies. This concept, that the central feature of mania is psychomotor overactivation and that the central feature of depression is psychomotor inhibition, also has been a central idea of classical European psychopathology, dating to Pinel and Kraepelin in the eighteenth and nineteenth centuries and forward to Binswanger, Jaspers, Schneider, and Kuhn in the twentieth century.[73,77] The concept of melancholia specifically was characterized by psychomotor inhibition as its central feature in this classical literature.[58] The Koukopoulos model is consistent with all the other models described as well, because underlying biology (Metzos/Berner) and/or temperament may predispose to manic symptoms (Akiskal). Of the 3 Kraepelinian domains, the Koukopoulos model emphasizes volition as primary (elevated activity).

In sum, all the models fit these empirical data somewhat, but the Kraepelin/Weygandt and Koukopoulos models seem to fit those data best, and integrate that evidence well into clinical experience and the traditional psychopathology literature.

Differential Diagnosis with Borderline Personality and Neurotic Depression

It often is stated that mixed states resemble borderline personality, due to mood instability. It also is important to distinguish mixed depression from other kinds of depression that are unrelated to manic-depressive illness. The most important depressive presentation that was not seen as part of manic-depressive illness used to be called *neurotic depression*. This concept has been legislated away by *DSM-III* and folded into the *DSM* concept of major depressive disorder.[78] **Table 3** provides some distinguishing features between mixed states of bipolar and unipolar depression, versus neurotic depression and borderline personality.[60,79]

The key clinical distinction is that psychomotor activation is primary and central to mixed states of MDI but absent in neurotic depression and more variable in borderline personality (sometimes present, sometimes not, and typically secondary to life events, unlike mixed states, where it can be spontaneous). Furthermore, there are other diagnostic differences of importance in genetics, course, and prognosis between MDI, neurotic depression and borderline personality, which must be taken into account, as described in **Table 3**.

Clinical Consequences

This review suggests some important clinical consequences. First, mixed states are not the result of opposing symptoms of only depression and mania but rather a

Table 3
Differential diagnosis of mixed states versus borderline personality/neurotic depression

Anxious Syndrome	Neurotic Depression	Mixed States
Psychomotor activation	• Secondary to life stressors and less present at baseline	• Primary, present at baseline, and not only with life stressors
Thought content and process	• Depressive, obsessive, or anxious ruminations with worry-based content • Analytical pattern of thinking that is constantly present or repetitive	• Racing thoughts, flight of ideas, and, more specifically, crowded thoughts
Arousal and tension	• Very emotionally reactive to painful life experiences • Feelings of apprehension, fearfulness, or impending doom • Feelings of worthlessness, pessimism	• Inner tension, restlessness • Overwhelming despair and sense of lack of power to do things
Genetics and course	• Absent manic-depressive genetics and chronic course • Extremely reactive to life events and stressors	• Strong manic-depressive genetics and episodic course • Sometimes reactive to life events and stressors but sometimes spontaneous

Dysphoric Syndrome	Borderline Personality	Mixed States
Hyperarousal	• Secondary to emotional tension • Hyper-reactivity triggered by interpersonal stressors	• Primary: somatic tension • Hyper-reactivity triggered from the somatic realm: very sensitive to noise, light, touch
Hostility	• Anger combined with fear • Experience of fragility • Attention oriented to the environment • Behavior oriented to receiving attention and help	• Rage combined with despair; no fear • Attention oriented inward, not to the external environment • Behavior oriented to end visceral discomfort and extreme tension
Suicidality	• Secondary: very reactive to interpersonal triggers • Parasuicidal behavior, with self-cutting and other self-harm • High frequency of low-lethality attempts	• Primary: less reactive to interpersonal triggers • Little to no parasuicidal behavior • High risk of impulsive suicidality with high-lethality attempts
Genetics and course	• Absent manic-depressive genetics and chronic course • Extremely reactive to life events and stressors	• Strong manic-depressive genetics and episodic course • Sometimes reactive to life events and stressors but sometimes spontaneous

combination of psychomotor activation and dysphoria with standard depressive or manic symptoms. Second, the *DSM*-based unipolar-bipolar ideology is questionable because mixed states are so frequent, and thus polarity is not a good basis for diagnosis.[80] Other depressive presentations, like neurotic depression and borderline personality, can be distinguished from mixed states based on the role of psychomotor activation as well as other clinical features (like genetics and course of illness). Third, mixed states involving dimensional domains of affect, thought, and volition argue against *DSM*-based overly categorical approaches to diagnosis. Fourth, this review puts into doubt the conventional psychopharmacological treatment of mood conditions, with antidepressants for unipolar depression and mood stabilizers and antipsychotics for bipolar illness. Instead, because mixed states occur in both unipolar and bipolar illnesses, their treatments may be similar, with less emphasis on traditional antidepressants and more emphasis on treating psychomotor disturbance with lithium, some anticonvulsants, and dopamine-blocking agents.

DISCLOSURE

S.A. Barroilhet has no disclosures to report and no commercial or financial conflicts of interest. S.N. Ghaemi is currently employed at Novartis Institutes for Biomedical Research in Cambridge, Massachusetts.

REFERENCES

1. Schneider K, Sánchez-Pascual A. Psicopatología Clínica. Madrid: Fundación Archivos de Neurobiología; 1997.
2. Goodwin FK, Jamison KR. Manic-depressive illness: bipolar disorders and recurrent depression, vol. 1. New York: Oxford University Press; 2007.
3. Angst J, Marneros A. Bipolarity from ancient to modern times: conception, birth and rebirth. J Affect Disord 2001;67(1–3):3–19.
4. Koukopoulos A, Sani G. DSM-5 criteria for depression with mixed features: a farewell to mixed depression. Acta Psychiatr Scand 2014;129(1):4–16.
5. Tortorella A, Albert U, Nivoli AMA, et al. Mixed states: still a modern psychopathological syndrome? J Psychopathol 2015;21(4):332–40.
6. Goldberg JF, Perlis RH, Bowden CL, et al. Manic symptoms during depressive episodes in 1,380 patients with bipolar disorder: findings from the STEP-BD. Am J Psychiatry 2009;166(2):173–81.
7. Grunze H, Vieta E, Goodwin GM, et al. The World Federation of Societies of Biological Psychiatry (WFSBP) guidelines for the biological treatment of bipolar disorders: acute and long-term treatment of mixed states in bipolar disorder. World J Biol Psychiatry 2018;19(1):2–58.
8. Solé E, Garriga M, Valentí M, et al. Mixed features in bipolar disorder. CNS Spectr 2017;22(2):134–40.
9. Perlis RH, Uher R, Ostacher M, et al. Association between bipolar spectrum features and treatment outcomes in outpatients with major depressive disorder. Arch Gen Psychiatry 2011;68(4):351–60.
10. Angst J, Azorin JM, Bowden CL, et al. Prevalence and characteristics of undiagnosed bipolar disorders in patients with a major depressive episode: the BRIDGE study. Arch Gen Psychiatry 2011;68(8):791–8.
11. Nusslock R, Frank E. Subthreshold bipolarity: diagnostic issues and challenges. Bipolar Disord 2011;13(7–8):587–603.
12. Malhi GS, Irwin L, Hamilton A, et al. Modelling mood disorders: an ACE solution? Bipolar Disord 2018;20(S2):4–16.
13. Swann AC, Lafer B, Perugi G, et al. Bipolar mixed states: an international society for bipolar disorders task force report of symptom structure, course of illness, and diagnosis. Am J Psychiatry 2013;170(1):31–42.

14. Harvey PD, Endicott JM, Loebel AD. The factor structure of clinical symptoms in mixed and manic episodes prior to and after antipsychotic treatment. Bipolar Disord 2008;10(8):900–6.
15. González-Pinto A, Aldama A, Pinto AG, et al. Dimensions of mania: differences between mixed and pure episodes. Eur Psychiatry 2004;19(5):307–10.
16. Swann AC, Suppes T, Ostacher MJ, et al. Multivariate analysis of bipolar mania: retrospectively assessed structure of bipolar I manic and mixed episodes in randomized clinical trial participants. J Affect Disord 2013;144(1–2):59–64.
17. Güclü O, Şenormancı Ö, Aydın E, et al. Phenomenological subtypes of mania and their relationships with substance use disorders. J Affect Disord 2015;174: 569–73.
18. Akiskal HS, Azorin JM, Hantouche EG. Proposed multidimensional structure of mania: beyond the euphoric-dysphoric dichotomy. J Affect Disord 2003; 73(1–2):7–18.
19. Rossi A, Daneluzzo E, Arduini L, et al. A factor analysis of signs and symptoms of the manic episode with Bech–Rafaelsen Mania and Melancholia Scales. J Affect Disord 2001;64(2–3):267–70.
20. Gupta SC, Sinha VK, Praharaj SK, et al. Factor structure of manic symptoms. Aust N Z J Psychiatry 2009;43(12):1141–6.
21. Filgueiras A, Nunes ALS, Silveira LAS, et al. Latent structure of the symptomatology of hospitalized patients with bipolar mania. Eur Psychiatry 2014;29(7): 431–6.
22. Akiskal HS, Hantouche EG, Bourgeois ML, et al. Toward a refined phenomenology of mania: combining clinician-assessment and self-report in the French EPIMAN study. J Affect Disord 2001;67(1):89–96.
23. Perugi G, Maremmani I, Toni C, et al. The contrasting influence of depressive and hyperthymic temperaments on psychometrically derived manic subtypes. Psychiatry Res 2001;101(3):249–58.
24. Dilsaver SC, Shoaib AM. Phenomenology of mania: evidence for distinct depressed, dysphoric, and euphoric presentations. Am J Psychiatry 1999; 156(3):426–30.
25. Sato T, Bottlender R, Kleindienst N, et al. Syndromes and phenomenological subtypes underlying acute mania: a factor analytic study of 576 manic patients. Am J Psychiatry 2002;159(6):968–74.
26. González-Pinto A, Ballesteros J, Aldama A, et al. Principal components of mania. J Affect Disord 2003;76(1):95–102.
27. Perugi G, Medda P, Reis J, et al. Clinical subtypes of severe bipolar mixed states. J Affect Disord 2013;151(3):1076–82.
28. Perugi G, Medda P, Swann AC, et al. Phenomenological subtypes of severe bipolar mixed states: a factor analytic study. Compr Psychiatry 2014;55(4):799–806.
29. Shah S, Aich TK, Subedi S. A factor analytical study report on mania from Nepal. Indian J Psychiatry 2017;59(2):196–201.
30. Cassidy F, Forest K, Murry E, et al. A factor analysis of the signs and symptoms of mania. Arch Gen Psychiatry 1998;55(1):27–32.
31. Swann AC, Janicak PL, Calabrese JR, et al. Structure of mania: depressive, irritable, and psychotic clusters with different retrospectively-assessed course patterns of illness in randomized clinical trial participants. J Affect Disord 2001; 67(1–3):123–32.
32. Cassidy F, Murry E, Forest K, et al. Signs and symptoms of mania in pure and mixed episodes. J Affect Disord 1998;50(2):187–201.

33. Suppes T, Eberhard J, Lemming O, et al. Anxiety, irritability, and agitation as indicators of bipolar mania with depressive symptoms: a post hoc analysis of two clinical trials. Int J Bipolar Disord 2017;5(1):36.

34. Shim IH, Woo YS, Bahk W-M. Prevalence rates and clinical implications of bipolar disorder "with mixed features" as defined by DSM-5. J Affect Disord 2015;173: 120–5.

35. McIntyre RS, Tohen M, Berk M, et al. DSM-5 mixed specifier for manic episodes: evaluating the effect of depressive features on severity and treatment outcome using asenapine clinical trial data. J Affect Disord 2013;150(2):378–83.

36. Hanwella R, de Silva VA. Signs and symptoms of acute mania: a factor analysis. BMC Psychiatry 2011;11(1):137.

37. Picardi A, Battisti F, de Girolamo G, et al. Symptom structure of acute mania: a factor study of the 24-item Brief Psychiatric Rating Scale in a national sample of patients hospitalized for a manic episode. J Affect Disord 2008;108(1):183–9.

38. Kumar R, Sinha BNP, Chakrabarti N, et al. Phenomenology of Mania - A factor analysis approach. Indian J Psychiatry 2001;43(1):46–51.

39. Bertschy G, Gervasoni N, Favre S, et al. Frequency of dysphoria and mixed states. Psychopathology 2008;41(3):187–93.

40. Swann AC, Steinberg JL, Lijffijt M, et al. Continuum of depressive and manic mixed states in patients with bipolar disorder: quantitative measurement and clinical features. World Psychiatry 2009;8(3):166–72.

41. Canuso CM, Bossie CA, Zhu Y, et al. Psychotic symptoms in patients with bipolar mania. J Affect Disord 2008;111(2–3):164–9.

42. Akiskal HS, Hantouche EG, Bourgeois ML, et al. Gender, temperament, and the clinical picture in dysphoric mixed mania: findings from a French national study (EPIMAN). J Affect Disord 1998;50(2–3):175–86.

43. Haro JM, van Os J, Vieta E, et al. Evidence for three distinct classes of 'typical', 'psychotic' and 'dual' mania: results from the EMBLEM study. Acta Psychiatr Scand 2006;113(2):112–20.

44. Benazzi F. Delineation of the clinical picture of Dysphoric/Mixed Hypomania. Prog Neuropsychopharmacol Biol Psychiatry 2007;31(4):944–51.

45. Suppes T, Mintz J, McElroy SL, et al. Mixed hypomania in 908 patients with bipolar disorder evaluated prospectively in the Stanley Foundation Bipolar Treatment Network: a sex-specific phenomenon. Arch Gen Psychiatry 2005;62(10): 1089–96.

46. Weiner L, Ossola P, Causin J-B, et al. Racing thoughts revisited: a key dimension of activation in bipolar disorder. J Affect Disord 2019;255:69–76.

47. Miller S, Suppes T, Mintz J, et al. Mixed depression in bipolar disorder: prevalence rate and clinical correlates during naturalistic follow-up in the stanley bipolar network. Am J Psychiatry 2016;173(10):1015–23.

48. Benazzi F, Akiskal H. Irritable-hostile depression: further validation as a bipolar depressive mixed state. J Affect Disord 2005;84(2):197–207.

49. Benazzi F. A tetrachoric factor analysis validation of mixed depression. Prog Neuropsychopharmacol Biol Psychiatry 2008;32(1):186–92.

50. Frye MA, Helleman G, McElroy SL, et al. Correlates of treatment-emergent mania associated with antidepressant treatment in bipolar depression. Am J Psychiatry 2009;166(2):164–72.

51. Biondi M, Picardi A, Pasquini M, et al. Dimensional psychopathology of depression: detection of an 'activation' dimension in unipolar depressed outpatients. J Affect Disord 2005;84(2):133–9.

52. Sato T, Bottlender R, Kleindienst N, et al. Irritable psychomotor elation in depressed inpatients: a factor validation of mixed depression. J Affect Disord 2005;84(2–3):187–96.

53. Sato T, Bottlender R, Schröter A, et al. Frequency of manic symptoms during a depressive episode and unipolar 'depressive mixed state' as bipolar spectrum. Acta Psychiatr Scand 2003;107(4):268–74.

54. Maj M, Pirozzi R, Magliano L, et al. Agitated "unipolar" major depression: prevalence, phenomenology, and outcome. J Clin Psychiatry 2006;67(5):712–9.

55. Brancati GE, Vieta E, Azorin J-M, et al. The role of overlapping excitatory symptoms in major depression: are they relevant for the diagnosis of mixed state? J Psychiatr Res 2019;115:151–7.

56. Henry C, M'Baïlara K, Poinsot R, et al. Evidence for two types of bipolar depression using a dimensional approach. Psychother Psychosom 2007;76(6):325–31.

57. Chang JS, Ahn YM, Yu HY, et al. Exploring clinical characteristics of bipolar depression: internal structure of the bipolar depression rating scale. Aust N Z J Psychiatry 2009;43(9):830–7.

58. Parker G. Defining melancholia: the primacy of psychomotor disturbance. Acta Psychiatr Scand Suppl 2007;(433):21–30.

59. Marneros A. Origin and development of concepts of bipolar mixed states. J Affect Disord 2001;67(1):229–40.

60. Koukopoulos A, Sani G, Albert MJ, et al. Agitated depression: spontaneous and induced. In: Marneros A, Goodwin F, editors. Bipolar disorders: mixed states, rapid-cycling, and atypical forms. 1st edition. New York: Cambridge University Press; 2005. p. 157–86.

61. Maina G, Bertetto N, Boccolini FD, et al. The concept of mixed state in bipolar disorder: from Kraepelin to DSM-5. J Psychopathol 2013;19:287–95.

62. Perugi G, Akiskal HS. Emerging concepts of mixed states: a longitudinal perspective. In: Marneros A, Goodwin FK, editors. Bipolar disorders: mixed states, rapid-cycling, and atypical forms. 1st edition. New York: Cambridge University Press; 2005. p. 45–60.

63. Berner P, Gabriel E, Katschnig H, et al. Diagnostic criteria for schizophrenic and affective psychoses. Washington: World Psychiatric Press; 1983.

64. Berner P, Musalek M, Walter H. Psychopathological concepts of dysphoria. Psychopathology 1987;20(2):93–100.

65. Dayer A, Aubry JM, Roth L, et al. A theoretical reappraisal of mixed states: dysphoria as a third dimension. Bipolar Disord 2000;2(4):316–24.

66. Akiskal HS. The distinctive mixed states of bipolar I, II, and III. Clin Neuropharmacol 1992;15(Suppl 1 Pt A):632A–3A.

67. Akiskal HS, Pinto O. The evolving bipolar spectrum: prototypes I, II, III, and IV. Psychiatr Clin North Am 1999;22(3):517–34.

68. Iasevoli F, Valchera A, Di Giovambattista E, et al. Affective temperaments are associated with specific clusters of symptoms and psychopathology: a cross-sectional study on bipolar disorder inpatients in acute manic, mixed, or depressive relapse. J Affect Disord 2013;151(2):540–50.

69. Marneros A, Goodwin FK. Bipolar disorders: mixed states, rapid-cycling, and atypical forms. 1st edition. New York: Cambridge University Press; 2005.

70. Koukopoulos A, Ghaemi SN. The primacy of mania: a reconsideration of mood disorders. Eur Psychiatry 2009;24(2):125–34.

71. Ghaemi SN, Vohringer PA. Athanasios koukopoulos' psychiatry: the primacy of mania and the limits of antidepressants. Curr Neuropharmacol 2017;15(3):402–8.

72. Scott J, Murray G, Henry C, et al. Activation in bipolar disorders: a systematic review. JAMA Psychiatry 2017;74(2):189.
73. Sobin C, Sackeim HA. Psychomotor symptoms of depression. Am J Psychiatry 1997;154(1):4–17.
74. Carrol BJ. Psychopathology and neurobiology of manic-depressive disorders. In: Carrol BJ, Barrett JE, editors. Psychopathology and the brain. New York: Raven Press; 1991. p. 265–85.
75. Capponi R. Psicopatología y Semiología Psiquiátrica. Santiago, Chile: Editorial Universitaria; 1987.
76. Koukopoulos A, Koukopoulos A. Agitated depression as a mixed state and the problem of melancholia. Psychiatr Clin North Am 1999;22(3):547–64.
77. Day RK. Psychomotor agitation: poorly defined and badly measured. J Affect Disord 1999;55(2-3):89–98.
78. Ghaemi SN, Vohringer PA, Vergne DE. The varieties of depressive experience: diagnosing mood disorders. Psychiatr Clin North Am 2012;35(1):73–86.
79. Risco L, Herane A. Estados mixtos. In: Trastornos bipolares. 2nd edition. Santiago (Chile): Mediterráneo; 2006. p. 151–64.
80. Malhi GS, Berk M, Morris G, et al. Mixed mood: the not so united states? Bipolar Disord 2017;19(4):242–5.

Diagnosis, Clinical Features, and Therapeutic Implications of Agitated Depression

Gaia Sampogna, MD*, Valeria Del Vecchio, MD, PhD,
Vincenzo Giallonardo, MD, Mario Luciano, MD, PhD,
Andrea Fiorillo, MD, PhD

KEYWORDS

- Agitated "unipolar" depression • Mixed states • Suicide • Psychomotor agitation
- Treatments

KEY POINTS

- Depression is a complex disorder with multiple symptomatic clusters, including affective, cognitive, and physical dimensions, with a heterogeneous clinical presentation.
- Agitated "unipolar" depression is a distinct affective syndrome conceptualized as lying on the continuum of the bipolar disorder spectrum or as a distinct unipolar depression. This difference has obvious therapeutic and prognostic implications.
- The clinical picture of agitated "unipolar" depression is characterized by low mood, diminished interest in activities, and psychomotor excitation, whereas melancholic depression is characterized by retarded psychomotor functioning and anhedonia.
- Agitated "unipolar" depression requires a personalized management and treatment plan, which should include mood stabilizers, atypical antipsychotics, and benzodiazepines. The use of antidepressants is controversial.

INTRODUCTION

Depression is a complex, severe mental disorder with multiple symptomatologic dimensions, including affective, cognitive, and physical symptoms.[1,2] In the last decade, a significant increase in the incidence of the disorder of almost 20% has been observed.[3,4] In 2015, depressive disorders were the greatest contributor to nonfatal health loss. The average lifetime prevalence of major depressive disorder (MDD) is estimated to be 14.6% in high-income countries.[5] Moreover, MDD represents the leading cause of disability worldwide,[6] accounting for 2.5% of global Disability

Department of Psychiatry, University of Campania "Luigi Vanvitelli", Largo Madonna delle Grazie, Naples 80138, Italy
* Corresponding author.
E-mail address: gaia.sampogna@gmail.com

Psychiatr Clin N Am 43 (2020) 47–57
https://doi.org/10.1016/j.psc.2019.10.011
0193-953X/20/© 2019 Elsevier Inc. All rights reserved.

Adjusted Life Years lost, especially in women. Depression has been traditionally described as a clinical state characterized by low mood, reduced levels of energy, and reduction in motor and physic activity, with disturbances in motivation, reward, and arousal.[7] Some patients with major depression present activation as a product of inner tension and anxiety, which is defined as "psychic pain," a type of activation completely different from the goal-oriented one present during a manic episode. Therefore, the clinical presentation of major depressive disorder can be very heterogeneous, with some patients presenting features of psychomotor excitation together with sad mood and diminished interest in activities. Patients with agitated depression are characterized by a depressed and anxious mood with inner, psychic agitation, whereas psychomotor agitation could even not be present.[8] This clinical condition has been neglected in recent years, and it does not appear as a full clinical diagnosis in modern classification systems. However, more recently, there has been a renewed clinical and research interest toward this syndrome, which is a "difficult to treat" subtype of depression, often refractory to antidepressant treatments.

Along the years, agitated "unipolar" depression has been conceptualized as a mixed affective state[9] or as a type of major depressive episode associated with subsyndromal symptoms of mania.[10] Historically, Kraepelin[11] and Weygandt[12] defined "excited depression," in which symptoms of excitement and inhibition were present in the same episode, which was developed from the concept of *melancholia agitata*. More recently, Akiskal and colleagues[13] underlined that agitated depression is a distinct affective syndrome characterized by intraepisode noneuphoric hypomanic symptoms and a family history of bipolar disorder, lying on a continuum of the bipolar disorder spectrum.

THE PROBLEM OF CLASSIFICATION OF AGITATED "UNIPOLAR" DEPRESSION

In the modern classification systems, the diagnosis of agitated depression is unclear and misleading. In 1978, with the approval of Research Diagnostic Criteria, agitated depression was considered a subtype of depressive episode, which could be present either during a major depressive disorder or during a bipolar disorder.[10] In the third edition of the Diagnostic and Statistical Manual for Mental Disorders (DSM-III),[14] the category of MDD included several depressive states, such as melancholic depression (with psychomotor retardation and anhedonia) and agitated depression. However, this categorization has not been acknowledged in the subsequent versions of the DSM and in the International Classification of Diseases (ICD). In the DSM-IV, a diagnosis of mixed episode could be formulated as a combination of a full manic episode with a major depressive episode at the same time in the course of bipolar disorders. However, this condition was very rare in ordinary clinical practice,[15] and it has not been used routinely by clinicians worldwide. The DSM-5 has included the specifier "with mixed features" in both the chapters on depressive and bipolar disorders.[16] The main advantage of the introduction of this specifier is that it can be applied to both groups of patients, increasing the clinical utility of those diagnoses. In fact, this change has given to clinicians the possibility to capture the most common subthreshold presentations of mixed states; however, some limitations still persist.[17,18] The "mixed features" specifier is defined by the presence of at least 3 hypomanic signs or symptoms during a depressive episode in the context of major depressive disorder or bipolar disorder or by more than 3 depressive features present during a (hypo)manic episode in bipolar disorder. According to the DSM-5, in order to reach the symptoms' criteria threshold for mixed features, agitation, distractibility, impulsivity, and sleep-loss should not be considered, because these symptoms are nonspecific and already listed among the symptoms of both depressive and (hypo)manic episodes.[19,20] More in detail, the definition provided in the DSM-5 focuses on the presence of nonoverlapping manic symptoms during a major depressive episode. However, the exclusion of these features has been highly criticized, because it limits the identification of many mixed affective states.[21–23] Other investigators have argued that nonspecific and common symptoms shall not be excluded if robust scientific evidence confirm that they have enough sensitivity for making the diagnosis.[24–26] This controversy underlines the limitations of the current categorial diagnostic systems, in which the identification of clear boundaries between pure mania and pure depression, as well as between unipolar and bipolar disorders, is not possible.[27–30] These clinical conditions lay on a continuum and probably a prototypical approach, as described in the seminal works by Kraepelin[11] and Weygandt,[31] is needed, considering the clinical presentation of the syndrome as a whole and not just its individual symptoms.[32–34]

In contrast to the DSM-5, the 11th revision of the International Classification of Disorders released by the World Health Organization[35,36] categorizes mixed episodes as characterized by the presence of persistent, prominent, and rapidly alternating manic/hypomanic and depressive symptoms in a single episode lasting for at least 2 weeks. Moreover, the ICD-11 provides additional details on the contrapolar symptoms and episode-qualifiers.[37–39] The decision to keep the definition of mixed episodes similar to that of the ICD-10 is due to the fact that this approach was validated by several studies. Guidance is provided regarding the typical contrapolar symptoms observed when manic or depressive symptoms predominate.

Recently, using the criteria developed by Koukopoulos and colleagues,[9] an alternative model for classifying depressive mixed states has been proposed, focusing on the presence of psychic agitation, marked irritability, and marked mood lability, with or without other excitatory symptoms.[24,40] Koukopoulos' perspective is broad, including not only DSM-based manic symptoms but also psychic excitation.[9,41] Sani and colleagues[8] have provided a definition of mixed depression using diagnostic validators such as the presence of psychic agitation, marked irritability, and mood reactivity, with an absence of psychomotor retardation, thus further confirming the validity of these criteria. This concept of mixed depression is in line with the Kraepelinian nosology, in which a central role is given to psychic agitation, accompanied or not by motor agitation. According to this model, psychic pain, suicidal ideas, anxiety, agitation, and other symptoms, which are the core features of mixed depression, are due to an excitatory process.[9]

WHAT IS AGITATED "UNIPOLAR" DEPRESSION?

The original definitions of agitated "unipolar" depression described an affective state in which mood and ideation were in the negative polarity and activity in the opposite polarity.[11] It has also been called "excited depression" or "depression with excitatory symptoms," pointing out the presence of symptoms of excitement (ie, restlessness, talkativeness, flight of ideas, irritability) together with a depressed mood within the same affective episode.

Koukopoulos and Koukopoulos[9] proposed that agitated depression should be considered as a mixed affective state, laying on the bipolar disorder spectrum. Akiskal and colleagues[13] in a clinical sample of 254 "unipolar" patients found a strong association between agitated depression and depressive mixed state, as regards the presence of distractibility, racing/crowded thoughts, irritable mood, talkativeness, and risky behaviors in both definitions. They concluded that bipolar features can be found also in "unipolar" depressed patients and that agitated major depression can be considered as part of the bipolar spectrum, defining what we call a depressive mixed state.[42]

This conceptualization is in line with the classical definitions proposed by German psychopathologists, who included agitated depression among mixed states. "Activated depression," "agitated depression," and "depression with mixed features" would represent three overlapping clinical categories.[13] Compared with nonagitated depressed patients, during a depressive episode, patients with agitated depression present several bipolar features, including distractibility, racing/crowded thoughts, irritability, talkativeness, and risky behaviors (all classified as hypomanic symptoms).[13]

Several clinical studies have been conducted in order to describe the clinical features of agitated "unipolar" depression. In a sample of day-care patients, Perugi and colleagues[43] found that patients with agitated depression have irritable mood, pressured speech, flight of ideas, psychotic symptoms, and psychomotor agitation. Other studies[44,45] carried out in clinical samples confirmed that agitated depression is a more severe variant of bipolar depression, whose most common manic symptoms are irritability, greater talkativeness, distractibility, and racing thoughts.

Agitated depression is quite common in outpatient settings,[13] but patients with these clinical characteristics can be found also in other settings, such as primary care, tertiary care, outpatient, and inpatient units, further supporting the idea that agitated depression is a common clinical presentation.

In agitated depression, psychomotor agitation is not a sufficient symptom for characterizing this subtype of affective disorder,[13] whereas the main feature is the combination of low mood with many hypomanic symptoms.

Two subtypes of mixed depression have been proposed recently[46]: the classic agitated depression, characterized by anxiety and restlessness with motor agitation, and a second type, mainly characterized by inner psychic tension, racing and crowded thoughts, mood lability, and talkativeness, without motor agitation.[9,46] Koukopoulos identified several independent predictors of the mixed depressive state, such as premorbid temperament, course of illness, family history, worsening of the clinical status with antidepressants, and improvement with sedatives.[46] In both forms, patients can present suicidal ideation and psychotic features. Many sociodemographic and lifetime clinical features are associated with the presence of agitated depression, such as female gender,[47] more lifetime mixed episodes,[22] and the presence of suicide attempts.[48] Also, some characteristics of the index episode are associated with a higher risk of developing agitated features, such as distractibility, increased talkativeness, longer duration of the episode,[49] suicidal ideation,[50] and suicidal behavior[51] (Box 1).

Agitated depression occurs in 7% to 60% of patients with major depressive disorder. In a recent study by Serra and colleagues,[51] agitated depression was present in 32% of patients, with a slightly higher prevalence in patients with bipolar II disorder (BD-II) (36.8%) compared with patients with BD-I (30.3%). However, in this study the lifetime diagnosis was not a significant predictor of the presence of agitated depression, even after controlling for other clinical and sociodemographic characteristics. The investigators argued that the different prevalence rates found between the two disorders could be due to the heterogeneity of the definition of depression with mixed features.[50] Patients with agitated depression have a poorer prognosis compared with patients with a nonagitated depression, given the inadequate response to antidepressants in the former group.[13,52]

Box 1
Main clinical features of agitated depression

- Dysphoric mood
- Emotional lability
- Psychic and/or motor agitation
- Talkativeness, crowded and/or racing thoughts
- Rumination
- Initial or middle insomnia
- Impulsive suicidal attempts
- Verbal outbursts

The mixed depressive syndrome is not a transitory condition, but it can persist for several weeks or months. The clinical picture is characterized by dysphoric mood, emotional lability, psychic and/or motor agitation, talkativeness, crowded and/or racing thoughts, rumination, and initial or middle insomnia. Impulsive suicidal attempts are also frequent. The most frequently reported complaints by family members include patients' irritability, verbal outbursts, physical aggression, and hypersexuality.[46]

However, according to Swann,[7] agitation can be considered a dimensional part of the core depressive syndrome. Therefore, agitated depression should not necessarily be considered a mixed state, laying on the bipolar spectrum disorder. In particular, agitation can be considered a cross-cutting symptom of both bipolar and depressive disorders, with two different types of agitation: the former characterized by inner tension, which is most typical of depressive states, corresponding to "psychic pain"; and the latter characterized by disinhibited goal-oriented behavior, which is more frequent in manic episodes.

SUICIDALITY IN AGITATED DEPRESSION

Suicidal behaviors are due to the interaction between biological, psychosocial, and sociocultural factors. People suffering from agitated depression are at high risk of suicide, especially for the presence of racing thoughts and general restlessness. Because of flight of ideas and high levels of impulsivity, patients can take life-threatening decisions and risky behaviors. Other elements concurring to the high suicidal risk include the rapid cycling course, the predominant depressive polarity, the high levels of anxiety, the use of substances, and the presence of hopelessness and insomnia.[53–57]

Akiskal and colleagues[13] identified the presence of suicidal ideation as an independent predictive factor of having agitated depression, whereas other previous studies found a robust association between psychomotor agitation and suicidal ideation.[58–61]

More recently, Popovic and colleagues[62] found that depressed patients with impulsivity, risky behaviors, reckless driving or promiscuity, psychomotor agitation (such as pacing around a room, wringing one's hands or pulling off clothing and putting it back on, and other similar actions) have a 50% higher risk of attempting suicide compared with depressed patients without these behaviors. Therefore, the early identification of risky behaviors, psychomotor agitation, and impulsivity in patients with a major depressive episode may be crucial to reduce the risk of suicide and to develop appropriate suicide prevention plans.

Another important issue in suicidal patients with agitated depression is the role of antidepressant medications.[62] Patients taking antidepressants who become suicidal are usually in an activated state, characterized by increased energy before mood improvement. This phase, which has been defined as "activation syndrome," is characterized by agitation, irritability, impulsivity, and hostility. These symptoms represent the most common (hypo)manic symptoms occurring during a major depressive episode.[51,63] Therefore, it may be that those "unipolar" depressed patients treated with antidepressants have a paradoxic (or poor) response to antidepressants, resulting in increased suicidal behaviors.

THERAPEUTIC IMPLICATIONS

Agitated depression is a severe clinical condition that requires a specific management and treatment plan. The main challenge is represented by its adequate identification and appropriate diagnosis.[50,64] In case of patients with treatment-resistant depression, who failed to respond to treatment with 4 or 5 sequential trials of antidepressants over a period of years, a diagnosis of agitated depression should always be considered.[65] Moreover, many patients with this disorder—even if they are on a long-term pharmacologic management—do not remit and report a worsening of symptoms, mainly an exacerbation of irritability, sleep disturbances, restlessness, anxiety, or dysphoric mood for a year or more. Moreover, when psychomotor symptoms are present during a depressive episode and are misdiagnosed, there is the risk to prescribe inappropriate pharmacologic or psychological treatments. The concept of agitated depression proposes that the origin of psychic pain, suicidal ideas, anxiety, agitation, and other symptoms is an excitatory process, instead of a depressive one.

An accurate description of the clinical features of agitated "unipolar" depression is essential for successful treatment, because these patients need different treatments compared with those with a nonagitated depression.

One of the main challenges for psychiatrists in managing agitated depression is the lack of specific clinical guidelines.[66] In fact, available guidelines provide clinical recommendations for the treatment of unipolar depression, bipolar depression, and bipolar mania, whereas the authors found only one guideline specifically focusing on patients with a major depressive episode with mixed features.[67] Therefore, clinicians manage agitated depression following the guidelines for the treatment of major depressive disorder or bipolar disorder. The authors believe that this approach should be revised, because agitated depression represents a clinical condition with specific features and different prognostic implications compared with nonagitated depression.

In fact, the use of antidepressants in this condition is still controversial, because many studies found that these drugs can induce hypomanic symptoms.[68] In particular, patients with bipolar I disorder with a current mixed depression episode have a higher risk of mood switching when they take antidepressants compared with patients with BD-I without a mixed depression.[12,69] Therefore, an antidepressant monotherapy is not recommended in patients with mixed depression of any type (unipolar, BP II, or BP I), given the potential role of these drugs to increase psychomotor agitation,[70] whereas mood stabilizers or antipsychotics may reduce agitation and associated hypomanic symptoms.[9,65,68]

Although no drugs are currently approved by the Food and Drug Administration and European Medicines Agency for the treatment of agitated depression, antipsychotics and benzodiazepines have been used successfully for the treatment of this clinical condition. In particular, second-generation antipsychotics, such as asenapine, lurasidone, olanzapine, quetiapine and ziprasidone, have been tested for the treatment of depression with mixed features. Also, aripiprazole and cariprazine have shown some efficacy in improving both manic and depressive symptoms.[64]

Mood stabilizers can be used in patients with agitated depression in order to prevent mood swings and angry outbursts. However, except lamotrigine, no other mood stabilizer is approved for use in any kind of depression (unipolar, mixed, bipolar). As regards lithium, it is well known that it has antisuicidal, antiaggression, anticycling, and antimanic effects, and therefore it should be considered, whenever possible, as an effective augmentation strategy in these patients.[71,72] Benzodiazepines may be used as additional short-term medications and their beneficial effects confirm the excitatory nature of agitated depression.[73]

SUMMARY

Agitated "unipolar" depression represents a potentially dangerous clinical entity, given the high associated risk of suicide. It is extremely relevant for clinicians, mental health professionals, patients, carers, and all mental health stakeholders to adequately identify, diagnose, and treat it. This clinical condition has been neglected for many years, and therefore, there is still an open and ongoing debate about the correct classification of this disorder. In particular, it should be clarified whether this condition belongs to the group of depressive disorders or to the group of bipolar disorders. However, although already Kraepelin identified this state more than a century ago, during the evolution of modern psychiatry, the importance of mixed states has been inconstantly recognized by psychiatrists. Infact, the concept of a continuum between manic and depressive states has not been incorporated into the modern psychiatric diagnostic systems. With the approval of the DSM-5, the introduction of the specifier "with mixed features" has broadened the diagnosis of major depression, although this definition is still not adequate to capture the complexity of this clinical syndrome.

In conclusion, agitated "unipolar" depression is a severe psychiatric condition, too often misdiagnosed, which needs to be adequately addressed by researchers and identified and treated by clinicians.[74,75] In particular, considering the high levels of suicidal ideation and suicidal behaviors in these patients, it is also a public health priority to promote a correct identification and clinical management of these patients.

ACKNOWLEDGMENTS

The authors would like to acknowledge Carmela Palummo, Benedetta Pocai, Luca Steardo Jr, Arcangelo Di Cerbo, and Francesca Zinno, all from the Department of Psychiatry of the University of Campania "L. Vanvitelli", Naples, Italy.

DISCLOSURE

The authors have nothing to disclose.

REFERENCES

1. Fiorillo A, Carpiniello B, De Giorgi S, et al. Assessment and management of cognitive and psychosocial dysfunctions in patients with major depressive disorder: a clinical review. Front Psychiatry 2018;9:493.
2. McIntyre RS, Cha DS, Soczynska JK, et al. Cognitive deficits and functional outcomes in major depressive disorder: determinants, substrates, and treatment interventions. Depress Anxiety 2013;30:515–27.

3. Reynolds CF RD, Patel V. Screening for depression: the global mental health context. World Psychiatry 2017;16:316–7.
4. Ormel J, Cuijpers P, Jorm AF, et al. Prevention of depression will only succeed when it is structurally embedded and targets big determinants. World Psychiatry 2019;18:111–2.
5. Kessler RC, Bromet EJ. The epidemiology of depression across cultures. Annu Rev Public Health 2013;34:119–38.
6. World Health Organization. Depression and other common mental disorders: global health estimates. 2017. Available at: http://apps.who.int/iris/bitstream/10665/254610/1/WHO-MSD-MER-2017.2-eng.pdf. Accessed November 25, 2019.
7. Swann AC. Activated depression: mixed bipolar disorder or agitated unipolar depression? Curr Psychiatry Rep 2013;15(8):376.
8. Sani G, Vöhringer PA, Napoletano F, et al. Koukopoulos' diagnostic criteria for mixed depression: a validation study. J Affect Disord 2014;164:14–8.
9. Koukopoulos A, Koukopoulos A. Agitated depression as a mixed state and the problem of melancholia. Psychiatr Clin North Am 1999;22:547–64.
10. Spitzer RL, Endicott J, Robins E. Research diagnostic criteria for a selected group of functional disorders. 3rd edition. New York: New York State Psychiatric Institute Biometrics Inst; 1978.
11. Kraepelin E. Manic-depressive insanity and paranoia. Edinburgh (Scotland): E & S Livingstone; 1921.
12. Benazzi F. Agitated depression: a valid depression subtype? Prog Neuropsychopharmacol Biol Psychiatry 2004;28:1279–85.
13. Akiskal HS, Benazzi F, Perugi G, et al. Agitated "unipolar" depression reconceptualized as a depressive mixed state: implications for the antidepressant-suicide controversy. J Affect Disord 2005;85:245–58.
14. American Psychiatric Association. Diagnostical and statistical manual of mental disorders (DSM-III). DSM–III. 3rd edition. Washington, DC: American Psychiatric Association; 1980.
15. First MB, Rebello TJ, Keeley JW, et al. Do mental health professionals use diagnostic classifications the way we think they do? A global survey. World Psychiatry 2018;17:187–95.
16. Benazzi F. Depressive mixed states: unipolar and bipolar II. Eur Arch Psychiatry Clin Neurosci 2000;250:249–53.
17. American Psychiatric Association. Diagnostic and statistical manual of mental disorders. 5th edition. Washington, DC: American Psychiatric Association; 2013.
18. Luciano M, Sampogna G, Del Vecchio V, et al. Critical evaluation of current diagnostic classification systems in psychiatry: the case of DSM-5. Riv Psichiatr 2016;51:116–21.
19. Pingani L, Luciano M, Sampogna G, et al. The crisis in psychiatry: a public health perspective. Int Rev Psychiatry 2014;26:530–4.
20. Malhi GS, Byrow Y, Outhred T, et al. Exclusion of overlapping symptoms in DSM-5 mixed features specifier: heuristic diagnostic and treatment implications. CNS Spectr 2017;22:126–33.
21. Zimmerman M. Measures of the DSM-5 mixed-features specifier of major depressive disorder. CNS Spectr 2017;22:196–202.
22. Perugi G, Angst J, Azorin J-M, et al. Mixed features in patients with a major depressive episode: the BRIDGE-IIMIX study. J Clin Psychiatry 2015;76:e351–8.
23. Tondo L, Vázquez GH, Pinna M, et al. Characteristics of depressive and bipolar disorder patients with mixed features. Acta Psychiatr Scand 2018;138:243–52.

24. Brancati GE, Vieta E, Azorin JM, et al. The role of overlapping excitatory symptoms in major depression: are they relevant for the diagnosis of mixed state? J Psychiatr Res 2019;115:151–7.

25. Koukopoulos A, Sani G, Ghaemi SN. Why DSM-5 is wrong (and so was DSM-IV). Br J Psychiatry 2013;203:3–5.

26. Malhi GS, Lampe L, Coulston CM, et al. Mixed state discrimination: a DSM problem that won't go away? J Affect Disord 2014;158:8–10.

27. Lahey BB, Krueger RF, Rathouz PJ, et al. Validity and utility of the general factor of psychopathology. World Psychiatry 2017;16:142–4.

28. Maj M. Why the clinical utility of diagnostic categories in psychiatry is intrinsically limited and how we can use new approaches to complement them. World Psychiatry 2018;17:121–2.

29. Fulford KWM, Handa A. Categorical and/or continuous? Learning from vascular surgery. World Psychiatry 2018;17:304–5.

30. Jablensky A. The dialectic of quantity and quality in psychopathology. World Psychiatry 2018;17:300–1.

31. Ghaemi SN. After the failure of DSM: clinical research on psychiatric diagnosis. World Psychiatry 2018;17:301–2.

32. Weygandt W. Uber die mischzustande des manisch-depressiven irreseins. Munchen (Germany): Verlag von S.F. Lechmann; 1899.

33. Borsboom D, Robinaugh DJ, Rhemtulla M, et al, Psychosystems Group. Robustness and replicability of psychopathology networks. World Psychiatry 2018;17: 143–4.

34. Kendler KS. Classification of psychopathology: conceptual and historical background. World Psychiatry 2018;17:241–2.

35. Schultze-Lutter F, Theodoridou A. The concept of basic symptoms: its scientific and clinical relevance. World Psychiatry 2017;16:104–5.

36. Reed GM, Keeley JW, Rebello TJ, et al. Clinical utility of ICD-11 diagnostic guidelines for high-burden mental disorders: results from mental health settings in 13 countries. World Psychiatry 2018;17:306–31.

37. Luciano M, Sampogna G, Del Vecchio V, et al. The Italian ICD-11 field trial: inter-rater reliability in the use of diagnostic guidelines for schizophrenia and related disorders. Riv Psichiatr 2019;54:109–14.

38. Chakrabarti S. Mood disorders in the international classification of Diseases-11: Similarities and differences with the diagnostic and statistical manual of mental Disorders 5 and the international classification of Diseases-10. Indian J Social Psychiatry 2018;34:17–22.

39. Perugi G. ICD-11 mixed episode: nothing new despite the evidence. Bipolar Disord 2019;21:376–7.

40. Koukopoulos A, Sani G, Koukopoulos AE, et al. Melancholia agitata and mixed depression. Acta Psychiatr Scand 2007;115:50–7.

41. Koukopoulos A, Sani G. DSM-5 criteria for depression with mixed features: a farewell to mixed depression. Acta Psychiatr Scand 2014;129:4–16.

42. Koukopoulos A, Sani G, Koukopoulos AE, et al. Endogenous and exogenous cyclicity and temperament in bipolar disorder: review, new data and hypotheses. J Affect Disord 2006;96:165–75.

43. Akiskal HS, Benazzi F. Family history validation of the bipolar nature of depressive mixed states. J Affect Disord 2003;73:113–22.

44. Perugi G, Akiskal HS, Micheli C, et al. Clinical characterization of depressive mixed state in bipolar-I patients: Pisa-San Diego collaboration. J Affect Disord 2001;67:105–14.

45. Maj M, Pirozzi R, Magliano L, et al. Agitated depression in bipolar I disorder: prevalence, phenomenology, and outcome. Am J Psychiatry 2003;160:2134–40.
46. Maj M, Pirozzi R, Magliano L, et al. Agitated "unipolar" major depression: prevalence, phenomenology, and outcome. J Clin Psychiatry 2006;67:712–9.
47. Faedda GL, Marangoni C, Reginaldi D. Depressive mixed states: a reappraisal of Koukopoulos' criteria. J Affect Disord 2015;176:18–23.
48. Benazzi F, Helmi S, Bland L. Agitated depression: Unipolar? Bipolar? or Both? Ann Clin Psychiatry 2002;14:97-104.
49. Rihmer A, Gonda X, Balazs J, et al. The importance of depressive mixed states in suicidal behaviour. Neuropsychopharmacol Hung 2008;10:45–9.
50. Vázquez GH, Lolich M, Cabrera C, et al. Mixed symptoms in major depressive and bipolar disorders: A systematic review. J Affect Disord 2018;225:756–60.
51. Serra F, Gordon-Smith K, Perry A, et al. Agitated depression in bipolar disorder. Bipolar Disord 2019;21(6):547–55.
52. Takeshima M, Oka T. Association between the so-called "activation syndrome" and bipolar II disorder, a related disorder, and bipolar suggestive features in outpatients with depression. J Affect Disord 2013;151:196–202.
53. Maj M. "Mixed" depression: drawbacks of DSM-5 (and other) polythetic diagnostic criteria. J Clin Psychiatry 2015;76:e381–2.
54. Batty GD, Gale CR, Tanji F, et al. Personality traits and risk of suicide mortality: findings from a multi-cohort study in the general population. World Psychiatry 2018;17:371–2.
55. Oquendo MA, Bernanke JA. Suicide risk assessment: tools and challenges. World Psychiatry 2017;16:28–9.
56. Pietrzak RH, Pitts BL, Harpaz-Rotem I, et al. Factors protecting against the development of suicidal ideation in military veterans. World Psychiatry 2017;16:326–7.
57. Erbuto D, Innamorati M, Lamis DA, et al. Mediators in the association between affective temperaments and suicide risk among psychiatric inpatients. Psychiatry 2018;81:240–57.
58. Fico G, Caivano V, Zinno F, et al. Affective temperaments and clinical course of bipolar disorder: an exploratory study of differences among patients with and without a history of violent suicide attempts. Medicina 2019;55:390.
59. Sato T, Bottlender R, Schröter A, et al. Frequency of manic symptoms during a depressive episode and unipolar 'depressive mixed state' as bipolar spectrum. Acta Psychiatr Scand 2003;107:268–74.
60. Fisher K, Houtsma C, Assavedo BL, et al. Agitation as a moderator of the relationship between insomnia and current suicidal ideation in the military. Arch Suicide Res 2017;21:531–43.
61. Stange JP, Kleiman EM, Sylvia LG, et al. Specific mood symptoms confer risk for subsequent suicidal ideation in bipolar disorder with and without suicide attempt history: multi-wave data from STEP-BD. Depress Anxiety 2016;33:464–72.
62. Popovic D, Vieta E, Azorin JM, et al. Suicide attempts in major depressive episode: evidence from the BRIDGE-II-Mix study. Bipolar Disord 2015;17:795–803.
63. Courtet P, Lopez-Castroman J. Antidepressants and suicide risk in depression. World Psychiatry 2017;16:317–8.
64. Caligiuri MP, Gentili V, Eberson S, et al. A quantitative neuromotor predictor of antidepressant non-response in patients with major depression. J Affect Disord 2003;77:135–41.
65. Stahl SM, Morrissette DA, Faedda G, et al. Guidelines for the recognition and management of mixed depression. CNS Spectr 2017;22:203–19.

66. Steinert T. Chance of response to an antidepressant: what should we say to the patient? World Psychiatry 2018;17:114–5.
67. Bak M, Weltens I, Bervoets C, et al. The pharmacological management of agitated and aggressive behaviour: a systematic review and meta-analysis. Eur Psychiatry 2019;57:78–100.
68. University of South Florida, College of Behavioural & Community Sciences. Florida best practice psychotherapeutic medication guidelines for adults. Florida Medicaid Drug Therapy Management Program for Behavioral Health. University of South Florida; 2015.
69. Ghaemi SN, Hsu DJ, Soldani F, et al. Antidepressants in bipolar disorder: the case for caution. Bipolar Disord 2003;5:421–33.
70. Bottlender R, Sato T, Kleindienst N, et al. Mixed depressive features predict maniform switch during treatment of depression in bipolar I disorder. J Affect Disord 2004;78:149–52.
71. Akiskal HS, Pinto O. The evolving bipolar spectrum. Prototypes I, II, III, and IV. Psychiatr Clin North Am 1999;22:517–34.
72. Alda M. Who are excellent lithium responders and why do they matter? World Psychiatry 2017;16:319–20.
73. Sani G, Fiorillo A. The use of lithium in mixed states. CNS Spectr 2019;28:1–3.
74. Dell'Osso B, Albert U, Atti AR, et al. Bridging the gap between education and appropriate use of benzodiazepines in psychiatric clinical practice. Neuropsychiatr Dis Treat 2015;11:1885–909.
75. Kessing LV, Bukh JD. The clinical relevance of qualitatively distinct subtypes of depression. World Psychiatry 2017;16:318–9.

Mixed Features in Depression

The Unmet Needs of Diagnostic and Statistical Manual of Mental Disorders Fifth Edition

Isabella Pacchiarotti, MD, PhD[a], Giorgio D. Kotzalidis, MD, PhD[b],
Andrea Murru, MD, PhD[a], Lorenzo Mazzarini, MD, PhD[b],
Chiara Rapinesi, MD[b], Marc Valentí, MD, PhD[a],
Gerard Anmella, MD[a], Susana Gomes-da-Costa, MD[a],
Anna Gimenez, MD[a], Cristian Llach, MD[a], Giulio Perugi, MD[c],
Eduard Vieta, MD, PhD[a],*, Norma Verdolini, MD, PhD[a]

KEYWORDS

- Major depressive disorder • Bipolar disorder • DSM-5 • Mixed features specifier
- Nonoverlapping symptoms • Overlapping symptoms

KEY POINTS

- The identification of mixed features during a major depressive episode is important due to the worse course and treatment issues associated with this condition.
- Diagnostic and Statistical Manual of Mental Disorders Fifth Edition mixed features specifier criteria are controversial, because it includes typical manic symptoms, whereas it excludes overlapping excitatory symptoms that are frequently reported in mixed depression.
- Psychomotor agitation, mood lability, and aggressiveness are the new proposed criteria based on the results of the Bipolar Disorders: Improving Diagnosis, Guidance and Education-II-Mix study.
- Several clinical and course indicators of bipolarity were found to be associated with the presence of mixed characteristics, mainly overlapping excitatory symptoms, during a major depressive episode.

---

[a] Barcelona Bipolar and Depressive Disorders Program, Hospital Clinic, University of Barcelona, Institute of Neuroscience, IDIBAPS, CIBERSAM, 170 Villarroel st, 12-0, Barcelona, Catalonia 08036, Spain; [b] Neurosciences, Mental Health, and Sensory Organs (NESMOS) Department, Faculty of Medicine and Psychology, Sapienza University, Sant'Andrea University Hospital, UOC Psichiatria, Via di Grottarossa 1035-1039, Rome 00189, Italy; [c] Department of Clinical and Experimental Medicine, University of Pisa, Via Roma 67, Pisa 56100, Italy
* Corresponding author. Bipolar Disorders Unit, Institute of Neuroscience, IDIBAPS, CIBERSAM, Hospital Clínic de Barcelona, c/Villarroel, 170, 12-0, Barcelona 08036, Spain.
E-mail address: EVIETA@clinic.cat

Psychiatr Clin N Am 43 (2020) 59–68
https://doi.org/10.1016/j.psc.2019.10.006
0193-953X/20/© 2019 Elsevier Inc. All rights reserved.

INTRODUCTION

The identification of mixed features in bipolar disorder (BD) and major depressive disorder (MDD) is an open challenge in psychiatry, because an accurate diagnosis is a prerequisite for the initiation of adequate therapeutic approaches.[1–4] Although the importance of mixed states was increasingly recognized in the last decades, the Kraepelinian concept of a continuum between manic and depressive states was not incorporated into major psychiatric diagnostic systems such as the Diagnostic and Statistical Manual of Mental Disorders Third Edition (DSM-III), DSM-III-R, DSM-IV, DSM-IV-TR,[5–8] and the International Classification of Diseases, Tenth Edition.[9] Substantial changes to the diagnosis of BD mixed state were made in the DSM-5.

The DSM-IV–defined categorical approach of diagnosing mixed states (ie, a period of 1 week when the criteria are met for both a manic episode and a major depressive episode [MDE] nearly every day) has been replaced in DSM-5 by the dimensional mixed features specifier (MFS).[10] Despite the introduction of the MFS, substantial controversy still remains as to whether the definition proposed reflects the empirical evidence.[11,12]

MAJOR DEPRESSIVE EPISODE WITH MIXED FEATURES

The importance of promptly recognizing the presence of mixed characteristics during an MDE is mostly due to clinical variables associated with greater severity, namely the higher number of episodes[13]; the lower response or switch with antidepressants (ADs)[14]; the high prevalence of psychiatric comorbidities such as anxiety, substance use,[13] and borderline personality disorder[15]; the increased risk of suicide[16]; worse psychosocial functioning; and quality of life.[17]

In DSM-5, a depressive episode with MFS would apply if the criteria for an MDE are met along with 3 or more of the following nonoverlapping symptoms: elevated/expansive mood, inflated self-esteem, talkativeness, flight of ideas, increased energy, goal-directed activity, decreased need for sleep, and excessive involvement in activities that have high potential for adverse consequences.[10]

Major concerns still exist for the DSM-5 specifier particularly due to the exclusion of overlapping symptoms, such as distractibility, irritability, and psychomotor agitation. As a consequence, different classifications have been developed, such as the research-based diagnostic criteria for mixed depression (RBDC) that are defined by the presence of an MDE plus 3 out of 14 hypomanic symptoms. The included hypomanic symptoms differ between the 2 classifications: the DSM-5 includes the symptom "decreased need for sleep" that is not included in the RBDC. The RBDC includes overlapping symptoms between episodes of opposite poles and other symptoms such as aggression and affective lability that are not considered in the rubric of mixed symptoms in the DSM-5.

In 2015, a large multicenter study, the Bipolar Disorders: Improving Diagnosis, Guidance and Education (BRIDGE)-II-Mix study, was conducted in order to estimate the frequency of depressive mixed features during an MDE, considering not only the DSM-5 criteria but also the RBDC criteria. The latter identified 4 times more patients with MDE as having mixed features and yielded statistically more robust associations with several illness characteristics of BD than did DSM-5 criteria, such as family history of mania; lifetime suicide attempts; duration of the current episode greater than 1 month; atypical features; early onset history of AD-induced mania/hypomania; and lifetime comorbidity with anxiety, alcohol, and substance use disorders, attention-deficit/hyperactivity disorder, and borderline personality disorder.[18]

A recent cluster analysis of the same study identified an algorithm of predictive symptoms of mixed depression and supported the predominant role for overlapping "manic" symptoms in defining mixed depressive states, namely irritability, psychomotor agitation, and distractibility, together with other excitatory features shared with mania and atypical features, such as emotional lability, mood reactivity, absence of reduced appetite, and absence of psychomotor retardation, rather than by nonoverlapping manic symptoms.[19]

WHY DSM-5 DOES NOT FIT WITH REAL MIXED DEPRESSION?

Several aspects of the clinical presentation of MDE with MFS commonly seen in clinical practice unfortunately seem not to be reflected by the diagnostic DSM-5 criteria for mixed features. Particularly, it is quite infrequent to observe euphoria and grandiosity as mixed features in the context of an MDE both in bipolar and unipolar depression. Indeed, findings from the BRIDGE-II-Mix study highlighted that euphoria and grandiosity were rare mixed features (4.6% and 3.7%, respectively) among the entire sample.[18] Similarly, Sato and colleagues[20] found that in their sample euphoria and grandiosity ranged from 1% to 4% and stated that euphoria and grandiosity were too uncommon to be used for the selection of patients with depressive mixed states. Maj and colleagues[21] reported that no depressive patients, either agitated or nonagitated, presented elevated mood, inflated self-esteem, or grandiosity. Results from the Systematic Treatment Enhancement Program for Bipolar Disorder, including data of 1380 bipolar depressed patients, found that in those patients presenting subsyndromal mania or a full mixed episode the specific manic symptoms with the highest frequency did not include either elation or grandiosity.[22] These findings suggest that the "real-world" depressive patients with mixed features may have characteristics of hypo/manic behavior but they lack expansiveness typical of euphoria and grandiosity.[12]

With the aim of avoiding overdiagnosis, DSM-5 MFS has excluded the overlapping "manic" symptoms, leaving many patients with mixed depression undiagnosed.[12] Many investigators have claimed how overlapping symptoms, such as anxiety, psychomotor agitation, mood lability, irritability, and distractibility, are the most frequently observed in mixed patients and may actually represent the core features of mixed depression.[12,23,24] In the BRIDGE-II-Mix study including 2811 unipolar or bipolar depressed patients, the most frequent manic/hypomanic symptoms according to the RBDC mixed criteria were irritable mood (32.6%), emotional/mood lability (29.8%), distractibility (24.4%), psychomotor agitation (16.1%), impulsivity (14.5%), aggression (14.2%), racing thoughts (11.8%), and pressure to keep talking (11.4%).[18] Interestingly, in a recent cluster analysis of the BRIDGE-II-Mix study, although nonoverlapping DSM-5 mixed symptoms were more represented among the group of depressive patients with mixed features, the symptoms that better predicted the mixed cluster were irritable mood, emotional/mood lability, psychomotor agitation, distractibility mood reactivity, absence of reduced appetite, and absence of psychomotor retardation, pointing out that none of these correspond to DSM-5 MFS criteria.[19]

Noteworthy, most of the overlapping symptoms have been found to be associated with clinical and course variables related to a bipolar diathesis such as BD diagnosis, family history of hypomania, atypical features, early age of onset, history of switch with ADs, suicide attempts, comorbidity with alcohol and substances disorders, attention deficit hyperactivity disorder (ADHD) and borderline personality disorder, probably indicating a better "affinity" of these features to the bipolar spectrum.[18] Similarly, Malhi and colleagues[23] found that the so-called DIP symptoms, including distractibility, irritability, and psychomotor agitation, were fundamental to define mixed depression and all 3 were key features in indicating a clinical course that suggests a bipolar spectrum disorder.

This leads to another important issue: the capability of the DSM-5 to capture the real accurate diagnosis of mixed presentations. In fact, overlapping criteria have been excluded by DSM-5 because they were thought to be nonspecific.[23] As a consequence, the choice of a more "specific" approach has been made at the expenses of the "sensitivity" of the classification.[25,26] In fact, DSM-5 MFS presented a 100% specificity but only 5.1% sensitivity,[27] as also highlighted in the recent cluster analysis of the BRIDGE-II-Mix group.[19] This means that up to 95% of patients presenting with mixed features according to the DSM-5 are wrongly diagnosed as having "pure" affective episodes with huge clinical and therapeutic implications.[25,27]

The speculative wish to avoid "overlapping" symptoms, such as psychomotor agitation, irritability, and mood lability, the most common features of mixed depression across the literature, is very restrictive, allowing the diagnosis of mixed depression only in 1 out of 4 cases.[18] Certainly, these symptoms may be nonspecific but to exclude them entirely may be not justified, in the absence of any evidence that the remaining criteria are sufficiently sensitive.[28]

THE CLINICAL RELEVANCE OF MIXED SYMPTOMS NOT INCLUDED IN DSM-5 CRITERIA: RESULTS FROM BRIDGE-II-MIX STUDY
Psychomotor Agitation

DSM-5 criteria for MFS currently exclude psychomotor agitation, making it diagnostically irrelevant because it represents one of the symptoms defining the B criterion of an MDE in DSM-5. Conversely, the concept of agitation and psychomotor excitement has been consistently proposed as the key point of mixed depression across the literature. Actually, Koukopoulos and colleagues,[12,16] based on their clinical experience, considered the classic "agitated depression" the most dramatic clinical picture of depressive mixed states, being psychomotor agitation, when present, a fairly distinctive symptom to make the diagnosis of mixed depression. Moreover, in a pooled post hoc analysis of both the BRIDGE and the BRIDGE-II-Mix studies, psychomotor agitation was closely related to bipolarity and was found to characterize an especially difficult-to-treat subgroup of patients, requiring a more complex regimen of pharmacologic treatment.[29]

Affective Lability

The psychopathologic construct of affective lability assumed a central role both as a traitlike clinical feature in mixed episodes[30] and as one of the 3 most frequent state features in mixed depression, together with agitation and irritability.[12] Traditionally, affective lability in a depressive mixed episode was considered as a risk factor of shifting between MDD and BD[31,32] and was found to be strongly associated with atypical depression, in which the core symptom is mood reactivity,[10] that has been typically related to bipolar depression.[32]

In a post hoc analysis of the BRIDGE-II-Mix study,[33] more than a half of the patients reporting affective lability were diagnosed with a DSM-5 MDE with mixed features. Several findings from this study seem to support that the presence of affective lability during an MDE was associated with mixicity, particularly with a more severe clinical condition, such as the severity of cooccurring hypo/manic symptoms during an MDE. Furthermore, mood reactivity was the variable most significantly associated with affective lability, and vice versa, leading the investigators to review their results in the light of a unique continuum between mood states, concluding that the intertwined association between affective lability and mood reactivity might bridge the gap between mixed and atypical depression.[33] Consistently, affective lability and mood reactivity are 2 of the 7 clinical features proved to be the best predictors of membership of the mixed cluster in the cluster analysis of the BRIDGE-II-Mix study.[19]

Aggressiveness

Aggressiveness is not currently considered as a DSM diagnostic criterion of MFS in either bipolar or unipolar depressive episodes despite its prevalence being around 15% in an MDE, according to RBDC mixed criteria.[18] In a post hoc analysis of the BRIDGE-II-Mix study[34] focused on this behavioral construct, the most relevant clinical variable associated with aggressiveness was the presence of a DSM-5 MDE with mixed features. Several findings from this study supported its association with bipolarity per se, independently from comorbid disorders such as borderline personality disorder and substance abuse, for example, the higher frequency of BD diagnosis in depressed patients with aggressiveness, whereas a diagnosis of unipolar depression was negatively correlated with aggressive behaviors. Moreover, MDE patients with aggressiveness showed higher rates of family history for BD as well as younger age at the first depressive episode. Taken together, these results might have important implications in terms of the reconsideration of aggressiveness for diagnostic criteria for the MFS.

The proposed mixed features are shown in **Fig. 1**.

CLINICAL INDICATORS OF "MIXICITY" THAT SUGGEST A BIPOLAR DIATHESIS

Interestingly, the RBDC criteria, but not DSM-5 criteria, for MFS were found to be associated with several indicators of bipolarity, as mentioned earlier.[18]

Since the publication of the BRIDGE-II-Mix study, several post hoc analyses found that different clinical variables related to a bipolar diathesis were more likely associated with the presence of mixed features during a bipolar or unipolar MDE (**Fig. 2**).

Suicidality

The presence of suicidality was the focus of a post hoc analysis by Popovic and colleagues,[35] which found that depressed patients with a previous history of suicide attempts presented distinct clinical features that suggest a bipolar diathesis, such as a first-degree family history of BD, psychotic and atypical features, more (hypo)manic switches with AD, and higher rates of treatment resistance. Moreover, suicidal

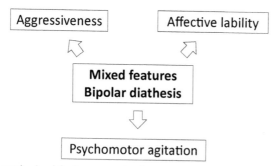

Fig. 1. New proposed mixed features: results from BRIDGE-II-Mix study.

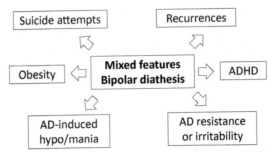

Fig. 2. Clinical and course features that suggest BD: results from BRIDGE-II-Mix study.

behavior was associated with RBDC mixed features, particularly risky behavior, psychomotor agitation, and impulsivity.

Antidepressant-Induced Hypomania

The emergence of new hypo/manialike responses to AD treatment in patients diagnosed as having a major depressive disorder (MDD-AIHM) has been assessed by Barbuti and colleagues.[36] The investigators compared patients in the MDD-AIHM group with those suffering from MDD or BD without a history of AD-induced hypo/mania and found that in the MDD-AIHM group, familiarity for BD and rates of atypical features and comorbid psychiatric disorders were similar to that of patients with BD and significantly more frequent compared with the MDD group. MDD-AIHM patients presented clinical course variables associated with BD, such as more than 3 affective episodes and higher rates of treatment resistance. The frequency of MDE with MFS was similar in patients of the MDD-AIHM and BD groups and significantly higher in both groups than in the MDD group. This led the investigators to claim the need for the DSM-5 inclusion of patients with MDD with AIHM within the rubric of BD.

Treatment Resistance or Worsening of Depression Associated with Antidepressant

Another recent analysis from the BRIDGE-II-Mix group was aimed at exploring the possible association between different inadequate patterns of response to ADs and bipolarity in unipolar depressive patients.[37]

Patients with or without a history of resistance to AD treatment and with or without a previous AD-induced irritability and mood lability have been compared. Those with AD treatment resistance showed higher rates of psychotic features, history of suicide attempts, emotional lability and impulsivity as mixed features, comorbid borderline personality disorder, and polypharmacologic treatment.

Patients presenting previous affective lability and irritability following AD treatment showed significantly higher rates of first-degree family history for BD, previous treatment-resistant depression, atypical features, psychiatric comorbidities, lifetime suicide attempts, and lower age at first psychiatric symptoms. Among mixed features, distractibility, impulsivity, and hypersexuality were significantly associated with worsening of depression with AD. The investigators concluded that in unipolar depressed patients, a lifetime history of resistance and/or irritability/mood lability in response to ADs was associated with the presence of mixed features and a possible underlying bipolar diathesis.

Higher Rates of Depressive Recurrences

The presence of mixed features frequency was assessed comparing unipolar depressive patients with high versus low recurrences rates.[38] Patients with higher recurrences presented more hypomanic symptoms during current MDE, resulting in higher rates of mixed depression according to both DSM-5 and RBDC criteria. Moreover, they presented clinical indicators of bipolarity such as earlier depressive onset, more family history of BD, more atypical features, suicide attempts, treatment resistance, (hypo)manic switches when treated with AD, and higher psychiatric comorbidities.

Obesity

A comparison of patients with or without obesity (body mass index >30) presenting an MDE was conducted in a subanalysis of the BRIDGE-II-Mix study.[39] Obese depressed patients showed higher rates of history of (hypo)manic switches during AD treatment, atypical depressive features, comorbid eating disorders, and anxiety disorders. Psychomotor agitation, distractibility, increased energy, and risky behaviors were the mixed features more frequently presented among obese patients. When hypersomnia was studied with the metabolic aspects in the same sample, the cooccurrence of hypersomnia and overweight/obesity represented a more extreme clinical phenotype of bipolarity complicated by treatment-related adverse effects and mixed features.[40]

Psychiatric Comorbidities

The presence of psychiatric comorbidities, particularly those sharing an important underpinning impulsive component, has been related in a sample of depressed patients with mixed features and bipolarity. The presence of mixed features during an MDE in comorbidity with borderline personality disorder was associated with a more complex course of illness associated with bipolarity, reduced treatment response, and worse outcomes.[41] Similarly, in those patients presenting a comorbid ADHD, mixed features and bipolar clinical course indicators were more represented.[42]

SUMMARY

A proper identification of an MDE with mixed features is of huge importance not only for the diagnostic implications but also for clinical practice due to the worse course and treatment issues associated with this condition.

The DSM-5 made an important step in this sense by introducing the specifier "with mixed features," thus recognizing for the first time that symptoms of opposite polarity may co-occur during an MDE of either BD-I, BD-II, or unipolar MDD and are diagnostically different from pure episodes within these 3 clinical entities. Conversely, the DSM-5 criteria for MFS during an MDE are based on the putative construct of avoiding overdiagnosis due to overlapping symptoms. The definition of MDE with MFS according to DSM-5 is controversial because it includes typical manic symptoms, such as elevated mood and grandiosity, that were found to be rare among patients with mixed depression, whereas it excludes overlapping excitatory symptoms that are frequently reported in mixed depression. Leaving out these 3 symptoms means that only 25% of patients with mixed depression will actually meet DSM-5 criteria. In this sense, the authors agree with Koukopoulos and Sani's position that is to rename the clinical identity of these symptoms as "excitatory" instead of "manic," in order to underline the different nature of this excitatory component from the pure manic symptom presentation in defining mixed features during an MDE.

Indeed, the BRIDGE-II-Mix group claimed at including in the rubric of MFS symptoms, such as psychomotor agitation, mood lability, and aggressiveness, which are not currently considered as mixed features in the DSM-5.

Furthermore, despite the DSM-5 MFS may characterize also a unipolar mixed depression, we argue that the presence of excitatory overlapping symptoms may describe more specifically a subgroup of depressed patients uncovering a bipolar diathesis. This is in line with the findings of the studies mentioned earlier, in which several clinical and course indicators of bipolarity, such as suicidality, AD-induced hypo(mania), treatment resistance or worsening of depression associated with AD, higher rates of depressive recurrences, metabolic issues such as overweight or obesity, and the presence of specific psychiatric comorbidities, ADHD, and borderline personality disorder in particular were found to be associated with the presence of mixed characteristics, mainly overlapping excitatory symptoms, during an MDE.

The aforementioned considerations suggest the need of a deep revision of the MFS in depression for the planned DSM-5 text revision.

DISCLOSURE

Dr I. Pacchiarotti has received CME-related honoraria or consulting fees from ADAMED, Janssen-Cilag, and Lundbeck. Dr A. Murru has received grants, honoraria, or consulting fees from, Janssen, Lundbeck, and Otsuka. Prof. G. Perugi has acted as consultant of Lundbeck, Angelini, FB-Health. He received grant/research support from Lundbeck and Angelini. He is on the speaker/advisory board of Sanofi-Aventis, Lundbeck, FB-Health, and Angelini. Pr E. Vieta has received grants and served as consultant, advisor, or CME speaker for the following entities: AB-Biotics, Abbott, Allergan, Angelini, AstraZeneca, Bristol-Myers Squibb, Dainippon Sumitomo Pharma, Farmindustria, Ferrer, Forest Research Institute, Gedeon Richter, GlaxoSmithKline, Janssen, Lundbeck, Otsuka, Pfizer, Roche, SAGE, sanofi-aventis, Servier, Shire, Sunovion, Takeda, the Brain and Behaviour Foundation, the Spanish Ministry of Science and Innovation (CIBERSAM), the EU Horizon 2020, and the Stanley Medical Research Institute. Dr G.D. Kotzalidis, Dr L. Mazzarini, Dr C. Rapinesi, Dr M. Valentí, Dr G. Anmella, Dr S. Gomes-da-Costa, Dr A. Gimenez, Dr C. Llach, and Dr N. Verdolini has been supported by a BITRECS. BITRECS project has received funding from the European Union's Horizon 2020 research and innovation programme under the Marie Skłodowska-Curie grant agreement No 754550 and from "La Caixa" Foundation.

REFERENCES

1. Grande I, Berk M, Birmaher B, et al. Bipolar disorder. Lancet 2016;387(10027): 1561–72.
2. Solé E, Garriga M, Valentí M, et al. Mixed features in bipolar disorder. CNS Spectr 2017;1–7. https://doi.org/10.1017/S1092852916000869.
3. Vieta E, Berk M, Schulze TG, et al. Bipolar disorders. Nat Rev Dis Prim 2018;4: 18008.
4. Vieta E, Salagre E, Grande I, et al. Early intervention in bipolar disorder. Am J Psychiatry 2018;175(5):411–26.
5. American Psychiatric Association. Diagnostic and statistical manual of mental disorders 3rd edition. Washington, DC; 1980.
6. American Psychiatric Association. Diagnostic and statistical manual of mental disorders. 3rd edition, Rev. Washington, DC: Author.; 1987.
7. American Psychiatric Association. Diagnostic and statistical Manual of mental disorders. 4th edition. Washington, DC: Author.; 1994.
8. American Psychiatric Association. Diagnostic and statistical manual of mental disorders. 4th edition, text revision. Washington, DC: Author.; 2000.

9. World Health Organization. International statistical classification of diseases and related health problems, 10th Revision (ICD-10). Geneva (Switzerland): Author.; 1992.

10. American Psychiatric Association. Diagnostic and statistical manual of mental disorders. 5th edition. Washington, DC: American Psychiatric Association; 2013.

11. Takeshima M, Oka T. DSM-5-defined 'mixed features' and Benazzi's mixed depression: Which is practically useful to discriminate bipolar disorder from unipolar depression in patients with depression? Psychiatry Clin Neurosci 2015; 69(2):109–16.

12. Koukopoulos A, Sani G. DSM-5 criteria for depression with mixed features: a farewell to mixed depression. Acta Psychiatr Scand 2014;129(1):4–16.

13. Angst J, Cui L, Swendsen J, et al. Major depressive disorder with subthreshold bipolarity in the national comorbidity survey replication. Am J Psychiatry 2010; 167(10):1194–201.

14. Smith DJ, Forty L, Russell E, et al. Sub-threshold manic symptoms in recurrent major depressive disorder are a marker for poor outcome. Acta Psychiatr Scand 2009;119(4):325–9.

15. Zimmermann P, Brückl T, Nocon A, et al. Heterogeneity of DSM-IV major depressive disorder as a consequence of subthreshold bipolarity. Arch Gen Psychiatry 2009;66(12):1341.

16. Koukopoulos A, Sani G, Koukopoulos AE, et al. Melancholia agitata and mixed depression. Acta Psychiatr Scand Suppl 2007;115(433):50–7.

17. McIntyre RS, Soczynska JK, Cha D, et al. The prevalence and illness characteristics of DSM-5-defined "mixed feature specifier" in adults with major depressive disorder and bipolar disorder: results from the International Mood Disorders Collaborative Project. J Affect Disord 2015;172:259–64.

18. Perugi G, Angst J, Azorin J-M, et al. Mixed features in patients with a major depressive episode: the BRIDGE-II-MIX study. J Clin Psychiatry 2015;76(3): e351–8.

19. Brancati GE, Vieta E, Azorin J-M, et al. The role of overlapping excitatory symptoms in major depression: are they relevant for the diagnosis of mixed state? J Psychiatr Res 2019;115:151–7.

20. Sato T, Bottlender R, Schröter A, et al. Frequency of manic symptoms during a depressive episode and unipolar "depressive mixed state" as bipolar spectrum. Acta Psychiatr Scand 2003;107(4):268–74. Available at: http://www.ncbi.nlm.nih.gov/pubmed/12662249. Accessed July 11, 2018.

21. Maj M, Pirozzi R, Magliano L, et al. Agitated "unipolar" major depression: prevalence, phenomenology, and outcome. J Clin Psychiatry 2006;67(5):712–9. Available at: http://www.ncbi.nlm.nih.gov/pubmed/16841620. Accessed July 21, 2019.

22. Goldberg JF, Perlis RH, Bowden CL, et al. Manic symptoms during depressive episodes in 1,380 patients with bipolar disorder: findings from the STEP-BD. Am J Psychiatry 2009;166(2):173–81.

23. Malhi GS, Byrow Y, Outhred T, et al. Exclusion of overlapping symptoms in DSM-5 mixed features specifier: heuristic diagnostic and treatment implications. CNS Spectr 2017;22(2):126–33.

24. Perugi G, Quaranta G, Dell'Osso L. The significance of mixed states in depression and mania. Curr Psychiatry Rep 2014;16(10):486.

25. McIntyre RS, Lee Y, Mansur RB. A pragmatic approach to the diagnosis and treatment of mixed features in adults with mood disorders. CNS Spectr 2016; 21(S1):25–33.

26. Vieta E, Valentí M. Mixed states in DSM-5: Implications for clinical care, education, and research. J Affect Disord 2013;148(1):28–36.
27. Stahl SM. Mixed-up about how to diagnose and treat mixed features in major depressive episodes. CNS Spectr 2017;22(02):111–5.
28. Perugi G. ICD-11 mixed episode: nothing new despite the evidence. Bipolar Disord 2019;21(4):376–7.
29. Barbuti M, Mainardi C, Pacchiarotti I, et al. The role of different patterns of psychomotor symptoms in major depressive episode: pooled analysis of the BRIDGE and BRIDGE-II-MIX cohorts. Bipolar Disord 2019. [Epub ahead of print].
30. Mackinnon DF, Pies R. Affective instability as rapid cycling: theoretical and clinical implications for borderline personality and bipolar spectrum disorders. Bipolar Disord 2006;8(1):1–14.
31. Akiskal HS, Maser JD, Zeller PJ, et al. Switching from "unipolar" to bipolar II. An 11-year prospective study of clinical and temperamental predictors in 559 patients. Arch Gen Psychiatry 1995;52(2):114–23.
32. Benazzi F. The relationship of major depressive disorder to bipolar disorder: continuous or discontinuous? Curr Psychiatry Rep 2005;7(6):462–70. Available at: http://www.ncbi.nlm.nih.gov/pubmed/16318825. Accessed July 21, 2019.
33. Verdolini N, Menculini G, Perugi G, et al. Sultans of swing: a reappraisal of the intertwined association between affective lability and mood reactivity in a post hoc analysis of the BRIDGE-II-MIX study. J Clin Psychiatry 2019;80(2). https://doi.org/10.4088/JCP.17m12082.
34. Verdolini N, Perugi G, Samalin L, et al. Aggressiveness in depression: a neglected symptom possibly associated with bipolarity and mixed features. Acta Psychiatr Scand 2017. https://doi.org/10.1111/acps.12777.
35. Popovic D, Vieta E, Azorin J-M, et al. Suicide attempts in major depressive episode: evidence from the BRIDGE-II-Mix study. Bipolar Disord 2015;17(7):795–803.
36. Barbuti M, Pacchiarotti I, Vieta E, et al. Antidepressant-induced hypomania/mania in patients with major depression: evidence from the BRIDGE-II-MIX study. J Affect Disord 2017;219:187–92.
37. Perugi G, Pacchiarotti I, Mainardi C, et al. Patterns of response to antidepressants in major depressive disorder: drug resistance or worsening of depression are associated with a bipolar diathesis. Eur Neuropsychopharmacol 2019;29(7):825–34.
38. Mazzarini L, Kotzalidis GD, Piacentino D, et al. Is recurrence in major depressive disorder related to bipolarity and mixed features? Results from the BRIDGE-II-Mix study. J Affect Disord 2018;229:164–70.
39. Petri E, Bacci O, Barbuti M, et al. Obesity in patients with major depression is related to bipolarity and mixed features: evidence from the BRIDGE-II-Mix study. Bipolar Disord 2017;19(6):458–64.
40. Murru A, Guiso G, Barbuti M, et al. The implications of hypersomnia in the context of major depression: results from a large, international, observational study. Eur Neuropsychopharmacol 2019;29(4):471–81.
41. Perugi G, Angst J, Azorin J-M, et al. Relationships between mixed features and borderline personality disorder in 2811 patients with major depressive episode. Acta Psychiatr Scand 2016;133(2):133–43.
42. Vannucchi G, Medda P, Pallucchini A, et al. The relationship between attention deficit hyperactivity disorder, bipolarity and mixed features in major depressive patients: Evidence from the BRIDGE-II-Mix Study. J Affect Disord 2019;246:346–54.

Clinical Contexts, Complications, and Challenges

The Ring of Fire
Childhood Trauma, Emotional Reactivity, and Mixed States in Mood Disorders

Delfina Janiri, MD[a,b,c], Georgios D. Kotzalidis, MD, PhD[c,d,*],
Lavinia De Chiara, MD[c,d], Alexia Emilia Koukopoulos, MD, PhD[c,e],
Monica Aas, PhD[f], Gabriele Sani, MD[g,h,1]

KEYWORDS

- Mixed states • Childhood trauma • Bipolar disorders • Depression
- Emotional reactivity • Affective lability • Emotional regulation • Mood disorders

KEY POINTS

- Childhood trauma is related to later development of mixed states in bipolar disorder.
- Childhood trauma is related to increased emotional hyperreactivity (EH).
- EH is higher in patients with bipolar disorder and mixed states/symptoms.
- The association between childhood trauma and mixed states is mediated through EH.

INTRODUCTION

Mixed states represent one of the most complex clinical challenges in the course of mood disorders.[1,2] Since Emil Kraepelin and Ewald Hecker,[3] mixed states were described as an affective condition in which depressive and manic symptoms occur simultaneously or alternate within a very narrow time frame. In his original description, Kraepelin[3] observed that in a mixed state, one or more of the main features of

[a] Sapienza School of Medicine and Psychology, Sant'Andrea University Hospital, UOC Psichia-
tria, Via di Grottarossa, 1035-1039, Rome 00189, Italy; [b] ICAHN School of Medicine and Mount
Sinai, New York, NY, USA; [c] Centro Lucio Bini, Via Crescenzio 42, Rome 00193, Italy; [d] School of
Medicine and Psychology, NESMOS Department (Neuroscience, Mental Health and Sensory
Organs) Sapienza University, Sant'Andrea Hospital, Via di Grottarossa 1035-1038, Rome 00189,
Italy; [e] Department of Human Neurosciences, University of Rome "Sapienza", Viale dell'Uni-
versità 30, Roma 00185, Italy; [f] NORMENT K.G Jebsen Centre for Psychosis Research, Division of
Mental Health and Addiction, Institute of Clinical Medicine, University of Oslo, Oslo University
Hospital, Bygg 49, Ullevål Sykehus, PO Box 4956, Nydalen, Oslo 0424, Norway; [g] Institute of
Psychiatry, Università Cattolica del Sacro Cuore, Rome, Italy; [h] Department of Psychiatry, Fon-
dazione Policlinico Universitario "Agostino Gemelli" IRCCS, Rome, Italy
[1] Present address: Institute of Psychiatry, Largo Francesco Vito 1, 00168 Roma
* Corresponding author. NESMOS Department (Neuroscience, Mental Health and Sensory Or-
gans), School of Medicine and Psychology, Sapienza University, Sant'Andrea Hospital, Via di
Grottarossa 1035-1038, Rome 00189, Italy.
E-mail address: giorgio.kotzalidis@uniroma1.it

Psychiatr Clin N Am 43 (2020) 69–82
https://doi.org/10.1016/j.psc.2019.10.007
0193-953X/20/© 2019 Elsevier Inc. All rights reserved.

depression is replaced by one or more of those of mania, and vice versa. Mixed states, recently reconceptualized by the Diagnostic and Statistical Manual of Mental Disorders, Fifth Edition (DSM-5) as depression or mania with mixed features, are frequent in mood disorders, ranging between 20% and 70% depending on setting, samples, diagnostic criteria, and instruments used to assess affective symptoms.[1,4,5] Mixed features are associated with a more severe clinical course, including early age at onset, rapid cycling, long duration of episodes, higher hospitalization rates, and suicidal risk.[5–8]

Among environmental stressors, childhood trauma, conceptualized as abuse or neglect, has emerged as one of the most important course modifiers of mood disorders.[9,10] There is a body of evidence relating the history of childhood maltreatment to severe illness progression.[10,11] A strong association with suicidal behaviors is the most striking clinical outcome of childhood trauma, as related to bipolar disorders (BDs).[9,10,12]

In the early twentieth century, Eugène Minkowski[13] remarked that in affective disorders, "synchronism" with life experiences was excessive and inappropriate. He claimed that patients with affective disorders always retain their contact with the surrounding world and can be overwhelmed by their own sensitivity to these life experiences. Today, recent studies conceptualized this observation as emotional hyperreactivity or reactivity, or also as affective or mood lability, all terms that are used interchangeably. Emotional hyperreactivity refers to the fact that all emotions can be felt with an unusual intensity. Patients feel emotions with a greater intensity as a function of the outer environmental context, rather than inner affective hue, which tends to fluctuate.[14] Affective lability is often used as a synonym of emotional hyperreactivity and has been conceptualized as frequent and intense fluctuations in affect in response to both pleasant and unpleasant events.[15] In a recent study of BD, Aas and colleagues[15] found emotional hyperreactivity/affective lability linked to both mixed states and childhood trauma and hypothesized that this relationship could specifically mediate environmental stress and affective episode polarity.

Aims

Provided that childhood trauma is present at a more than chance rate in mood disorders,[10,11] that emotional hyperreactivity could represent the expression of opposed polarity symptoms and could be related to both mixed states and to early adverse events,[15] we decided to tackle the issue of whether infantile trauma is related to the development of mixed symptoms or states. Therefore, we systematically reviewed the literature with a twofold strategy, that is, a direct approach investigating the association between mixed states and childhood trauma and an indirect approach focusing on emotional hyperreactivity/affective lability as a specific mediator of this association. The latter consisted of 2 arms, one relating hyperreactivity/affective lability to mixed states, the other to childhood trauma.

METHODS

To investigate the role of childhood trauma in the later development of mixed episodes, states, or symptoms, we conducted a series of PubMed searches on the same day (up to and including July 11, 2019) focusing directly or indirectly on this issue. We used the following strategies: ("infantile trauma" OR "childhood trauma" OR "early adverse*" OR "physical abuse" OR "emotional abuse" OR "psychological abuse" OR "sexual abuse" OR neglect OR maltreatment) AND ("mixed state*" OR "mixed symptom*" OR "mixed features" OR "mixed mood" OR "mixed depression" OR "mixed manic" OR "mixed mania" OR "agitated depression" OR "catatonic stupor" OR "dysphoric mania" OR "mixed episode*" OR "mixed specifier*"), that directly investigated the issue (trauma and mixed, direct), and 2 indirect strategies: ("emotional reactivity" OR "emotional hyperreactivity" OR "emotional instability" OR "affective lability") AND ("mixed state*" OR "mixed symptom*" OR "mixed features" OR "mixed mood" OR "mixed depression" OR "mixed manic" OR "mixed mania" OR "agitated depression" OR "catatonic stupor" OR "dysphoric mania" OR "mixed episode*" OR "mixed specifier*") (ie, hyperreactivity and mixed) and ("mood disorder*" OR "affective disorder*" OR "bipolar disorder*" OR "depressive disorder*" OR dysthymi*) AND ("infantile trauma" OR "childhood trauma" OR "early adverse*" OR "physical abuse" OR "emotional abuse" OR "psychological abuse" OR "sexual abuse" OR neglect OR maltreatment) AND ("emotional reactivity" OR "emotional hyperreactivity" OR "emotional instability" OR "affective lability") (ie, hyperreactivity and trauma). The output of each search has been evaluated for inclusion or exclusion through a Delphi procedure by authors DJ, GDK, and GS until complete agreement could be reached. Inclusion criteria were a study being published in a peer-reviewed journal, evaluating patients with mood disorder and including data regarding the presence of mixed episodes, states, or symptoms and the assessment of childhood trauma (direct strategy) or data regarding affective lability and mixed episodes/states/symptoms (first indirect strategy) or regarding affective lability and childhood trauma (second indirect strategy). Excluded were studies pooling data mixed with other diagnostic categories so that effects attributable to mixed states could not be distinguished, studies lacking one of the preceding requirements: opinion papers, editorials, letters to the editor with no data, case reports, congress or conference abstracts, reviews, and meta-analyses. However, the latter 2 were further searched in their reference lists to identify possible further eligible studies. Also excluded were studies reporting on the same sample in different articles.

For our systematic review, we followed the Preferred Reporting Items for Systematic Reviews and Meta-Analyses (PRISMA) Statement.[16] We rated the quality of our review through A Measurement Tool to Assess Systematic Reviews (AMSTAR-2; Shea and colleagues[17]), and completed the Populations/People/Patient/Problem-Intervention(s)-Comparison-Outcome [PICO] form[18] and the Cochrane Risk of Bias Tool.[19]

RESULTS

The direct strategy identified 122 records and the indirect strategies 19, which became 18 after the removal of an overlapping paper, and 12 (11 after duplicate removal), respectively, for a total of 151 records. Through other sources and from reference lists in reviews, we were able to identify 13 further articles to consider for eligibility, for a grand total of 164. Our PRISMA flow chart is shown in **Fig. 1**, which also displays the reasons for exclusion. Briefly, the direct search identified 6 eligible studies, whereas the indirect search identified 4 (hyperreactivity and mixed) and 3 (hyperreactivity and trauma), respectively; finally, the 13 records from other sources added 3 articles those eligible. In all, we included 16 studies. Their results are summarized in **Table 1**.

DISCUSSION

We found in this systematic review that childhood trauma exposure has a higher probability to result in a clinical course characterized by mixed symptomatology than lack of exposure. We also found that this effect was mediated by emotional hyperreactivity to a great extent and quite consistently.

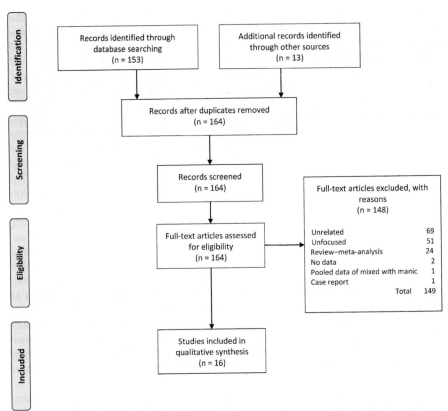

Fig. 1. PRISMA 2009 flow diagram for ("infantile trauma" OR "childhood trauma" OR "early advers*" OR "physical abuse" OR "emotional abuse" OR "psychological abuse" OR "sexual abuse" OR neglect OR maltreatment) AND ("mixed state*" OR "mixed symptom*" OR "mixed features" OR "mixed mood" OR "mixed depression" OR "mixed manic" OR "mixed mania" OR "agitated depression" OR "catatonic stupor" OR "dysphoric mania" OR "mixed episod*" OR "mixed specifier*")/("emotional reactivity" OR "emotional hyperreactivity" OR "emotional instability" OR "affective lability") AND ("mixed state*" OR "mixed symptom*" OR "mixed features" OR "mixed mood" OR "mixed depression" OR "mixed manic" OR "mixed mania" OR "agitated depression" OR "catatonic stupor" OR "dysphoric mania" OR "mixed episod*" OR "mixed specifier*")/("mood disorder*" OR "affective disorder*" OR "bipolar disorder*" OR "depressive disorder*" OR dysthymi*) AND ("infantile trauma" OR "childhood trauma" OR "early advers*" OR "physical abuse" OR "emotional abuse" OR "psychological abuse" OR "sexual abuse" OR neglect OR maltreatment) AND ("emotional reactivity" OR "emotional hyperreactivity" OR "emotional instability" OR "affective lability") on July 11, 2019. (*Adapted from* Moher D, Liberati A, Tetzlaff J, et al. Preferred Reporting Items for Systematic Reviews and Meta Analyses: The PRISMA Statement. PLoS Med 2009;6(7):e1000097; with permission.)

Direct Strategy: Mixed States and Childhood Trauma

We found 6 studies including data regarding mixed states and childhood trauma in patients with mood disorders. One study by Aas and colleagues[15] directly supported this association. The investigators assessed 342 participants with BD for childhood trauma, affective lability, and several clinical variables, including lifetime history of mixed episodes. Using a mediation analysis by *Process*, they found that affective

Table 1
Summary of included studies in chronologic order

Study	Population	Design	Rating	Results	Conclusions/Observations
Goldstein et al,[27] 2005 (D)	405 BD children/adolescents (54% male; 46% female); age range 7–17 y	Retrospective naturalistic, 3-sites	K-SADS, lifetime suicide attempts, history of abuse	Suicide attempters: > physical and/or sexual abuse and > mixed states than nonattempters	Used DSM-IV; mixed state and childhood trauma are independently associated with suicide attempt
Henry et al,[14] 2007 (II)	139 BD (27.3% men; 72.7% women); age range 14–65 y; mean age 40.05, SD ± 11.76	Cross-sectional, 1-site; questionnaire-based cluster analysis	MAThyS	Identified 3 clusters: depressive, manic, and mixed; emotional reactivity highest in the mixed cluster	Used DSM-IV; no reference to trauma or abuse; mixed episodes show more emotional hyperreactivity
Meade et al,[20] 2009 (D)	49 men, 41 women with comorbid BD-I and SUD; age range 18–65 y; mean age 40.6, SD ± 11.7	Longitudinal, 32-wk	SCID, LIFE	Female gender and lifetime abuse significantly more associated with mixed state than depression, mania, and euthymia	Used DSM-IV; mixed states appear to be related to childhood trauma
Henry et al,[32] 2010 (II)	189 BD vs 90 HCs (33% men; 67% women); age range 14–72 y; mean age 39.3, SD ± 13.1	Cross-sectional, 1-site; patients classified as MDE, MDE‡, mixed, manic	MAThyS, DIGS	High emotional reactivity than HCs in MDE‡, mixed, and manic (all similar); lower in MDE than HCs	Used DSM-IV, which restricts mixed states to simultaneous presence of MDE and manic episode; under the DSM-5 specifier, mixed and MDE‡ would have been the same; trauma/abuse not mentioned

(continued on next page)

Table 1
(continued)

Study	Population	Design	Rating	Results	Conclusions/Observations
Erten et al,[31] 2014 (D)	116 BD-I (38.8% male, 61.2% female); mean age 38.34, SD ± 8.46	Cross-sectional, 1-site	CANQ, HDRS, YMRS, SF-36	Childhood trauma related to more depressive symptoms in an episode and low QoL, and rapid cycling/mixed states to low QoL	Used DSM-IV; no apparent relationship between trauma and mixed state
Aas et al,[40] 2014 (I2)	42 BD (BD-I, 37; BD-II, 3; NOS, 2) vs 14 HCs, (45% male, 55% female); mean age 30.87, SD ± 10.6	Cross-sectional, 4-sites	ALS, CTQ, PANSS	Scores on affective lability, which measure the degree of emotional hyperreactivity, correlated with childhood trauma severity	Used DSM-IV; emotional hyperreactivity is related to childhood trauma
Sani et al,[38] 2014 (I1)	435 with MDE (39% male, 61% female); mean age 44.1, SD ± 15.9	Cross-sectional, 40-site network and 1 site; patients classified as MS⁺ (n = 221) or MS⁻ (n = 214) assessed by KCL	SCID; KCL	Emotional hyperreactivity present in 78% of the MS⁺ vs 2% of the MS⁻ sample	Used DSM-IV-TR; people with depression over the mixed symptom threshold had significantly higher emotional hyperreactivity than those with lower symptom scores
Marwaha et al,[41] 2016 (I2)	923 BD-I (75% women, mean age 49.0, SD ± 11.5), 363 BD-II (73.8% women, mean age 46.5, SD ± 12.1), 207 MDD (66.7% women, mean age 50.0 SD ± 10.4)	Cross-sectional, 6-sites recruiting throughout UK	ALS, SCAN, CLEQ, BLEQ	More AL in BD-II > BD-I > MDD; more trauma in BD-II than BD-I and MDD; AL correlated with childhood trauma in BD-I, not in BD-II or MDD	Used DSM-IV; BD-I has more suffered than experienced trauma that in turn could trigger mood swings and instability
Perugi et al,[37] 2016 (I1)	2811 MDE patients from the BRIDGE-II-Mix study; BPD⁺ (75.4% female; mean age 38.0, SD ± 12.1) and BPD⁻ (66.4% female; mean age 44.5 SD ± 13.8)	Cross-sectional, 239-sites; sample subdivided in BPD⁺ (n = 187) and BPD⁻ (n = 2624)	RBDC-MXS	More mixed symptoms among BPD⁺ patients; emotional hyperreactivity higher in MDE patients with mixed features	Used DSM-IV-TR and updated to DSM-5; emotional hyperreactivity is related to DSM-5 mixed features; no mention of trauma, abuse or neglect

	Sample	Design	Measures	Findings	Comments
Etain et al,[23] 2017 (D)	148 euthymic BD (50 male, 89 female; BD-I 112, BD-II 34, BD NOS 2; age not provided)	Retrospective, 3-sites; patients classified as lithium responders (20.3%), partial responders (49.3), and nonresponders (30.4%)	CTQ, Alda scale to rate response retrospectively	People with mixed states and with childhood trauma were more often poor lithium responders	Used DSM-IV mixed state and trauma interact in determining lithium nonresponsiveness, but physical abuse was found to be able alone to determine lithium nonresponsiveness
Etain et al,[42] 2017 (I2)	485 euthymic BD (203 men, 282 women), mean age 40.9, SD ± 12.6.	Cross-sectional and retrospective, 9-sites	SCID, MADRS, YMRS, CTQ, ALS, AIM, BIS, BDHI	AL associated most with emotional abuse, but also with sexual and physical, and impulsiveness	Used DSM-IV; AL used as a proxy for emotional hyperreactivity; AL related to all types of abuse, especially emotional abuse
Aas et al,[15] 2017 (D, I1, I2)	342 BD, (77.2% BD-I; 40% male, 60% female; 300 France, 42 Norway); mean age 41.4, SD ± 13.1	Cross-sectional, 6-sites, bi-national	DIGS, CTQ, ALS	Mixed states in 28.6% of French sample and 20% of the Norwegian sample; the ALS anger subfactor mediated the relationship between emotional hyperreactivity and mixed states	Used DSM-IV; differences between sites: French older, more suicidal, had greater DUI, and had higher levels of emotional reactivity; issue addressed with adding site as a covariate in all analyses; abuse and neglect linked to emotional hyperreactivity; the latter had increased likelihood for occurrence of mixed episodes
Benarous et al,[30] 2017 (D)	158 young inpatients (age range 9–19 y); 81 BD-I (57% female; mean age 15.7 SD ± 1.89), 77 catatonia (55% schizophrenia, 30% MDE, 16% ASD/intellectual disability; 35% female; mean age 15.17 SD ± 2.95)	Cross-sectional, 1-site	DIGS, BFCRS, CGI, YMRS, ACEs, LTEQ	BD-I did not differ from catatonic for symptom severity or treatment response based on prior exposure to adversity; people with mixed episodes had significantly more childhood adversity	Used DSM-IV; although mixed states showed no difference for adversity exposure vs no exposure, they were analyzed pooled with manic episodes

(continued on next page)

Table 1
(continued)

Study	Population	Design	Rating	Results	Conclusions/Observations
Sani et al,[39] 2018 (I1)	350 outpatients with MDE (192 MDD; 158 BD); 50% male; 50% female; mean age, 41.7, SD ± 20.6	Cross-sectional, 3-sites; patients classified as MS+ (n = 169) or MS− (n = 181) assessed by KCL	SCID; KCL; CGI; MADRS, YMRS	Emotional hyperreactivity present in 64% of the MS+ vs 15% of the MS− sample	Used DSM-IV-TR; people with depression and mixed symptoms had significantly higher emotional hyperreactivity than those without
Murru et al,[28] 2019 (I1)	2514 MDE patients from the BRIDGE-II-Mix study; hypersomniacs (mean age 41.08 SD ± 13.03) and insomniacs (mean age 43.96, SD ± 13.80)	Cross-sectional, multisite; patients classified according to sleep disorder hypersomnia (n = 2091, 83.2%) and insomnia (n = 423, 16.8%)	GAS	People with emotional hyperreactivity had hypersomnia more than people without; people with emotional hyperreactivity had more mixed symptoms than people without	Used DSM-IV-TR and updated to DSM-5; there is an indirect link between emotional hyperreactivity and mixed symptoms mediated through sleep disorder
Verdolini et al,[36] 2019 (I1)	2577 MDE patients from the BRIDGE-II-Mix study; men 70.9% in the AL+ sample; men 32.8 and women 67.2% in the AL− sample; mean age not provided	Cross-sectional, 239-sites; patients classified according to AL+ (n = 694, 26.9%) and AL− (n = 1883, 73.1%)	GAS, CGI-BP	Mixed symptoms significantly more present in AL+ sample; the same holds true for the mood reactivity-positive vs mood reactivity-negative samples	Used DSM-IV-TR and updated to DSM-5; affective lability, taken as proxy for emotional hyperreactivity, is related to mixed symptoms; no mention of childhood trauma or abuse

Type of strategy that identified study is shown in brackets (D, direct strategy, ie, mixed-trauma; I1, indirect emotional hyperreactivity-mixed; I2, indirect emotional hyperreactivity-trauma).

Abbreviations: ACEs, adverse childhood experiences scale; AIM, affect intensity measure; AL, affective lability; ALS, affective lability scale; ASD, autistic spectrum disorder; BD, bipolar disorder; BDHI, Buss-Durkee hostility inventory; BFCRS, Bush-Francis catatonia rating scale; BIS, Barratt impulsiveness scale; BLEQ, brief life events questionnaire; BPD, borderline personality disorder; CANQ, childhood abuse and neglect questionnaire; CGI, clinical global impressions scale; CGI-BP, clinical global impressions scale for use in bipolar illness; CLEQ, childhood life events questionnaire; CTQ, childhood trauma questionnaire; DIGS, diagnostic interview for genetic studies; DSM, Diagnostic and Statistical Manual of Mental Disorders; DUI, duration of untreated illness; GAS, global assessment scale; HCs, healthy controls; HDRS, Hamilton depression rating scale; KCL, Koukopoulos' Checklist; K-SADS, schedule for affective disorders and schizophrenia, for school-aged children; LIFE, longitudinal interval follow-up evaluation; LTEQ, list of threatening experiences questionnaire; MADRS, Montgomery-Åsberg depression rating scale; MAThyS, multidimensional assessment of thymic states; MDD, major depressive disorder; MDE, major depressive episode; MDE‡, major depressive episode plus manic symptoms; MS, mixed symptoms; NOS, not otherwise specified; PANSS, positive and negative syndrome scale; QoL, quality of life; RBDC-MXS, research-based diagnostic criteria for depressive mixed states; SCAN, schedules for clinical assessment in neuropsychiatry; SCID, structured clinical interview for DSM-IV; SD, standard deviation; SF-36, 36-item short form health survey; SUD, substance use disorder; UK, United Kingdom; YMRS, young mania rating scale.

lability mediated the relationship between childhood trauma and lifetime history of mixed episodes. Interestingly, the mediation model also showed the same pattern for the relationship between childhood trauma and suicidality. Aas and colleagues[15] suggested that affective lability might represent the psychological dimension specifically moderating the association between childhood traumatic experiences and the risk of more severe and complex clinical expressions of BD. Three additional studies possibly supported the link between childhood trauma and mixed states through an indirect association with other demographic/clinical variables. Meade and colleagues[20] found both mixed states and sexual or physical abuse more frequent in women, compared with men, in a sample of people with co-occurring to be BD-I and substance use disorders. Substance use is likely to switch people with major depressive disorder (MDD) to mixed states or manic excitement,[21] and in turn it is related to childhood trauma,[22] thus establishing a link between the two. This issue has not been thoroughly investigated so far, so it constitutes a target for future research. They hypothesized that adverse events may help explaining the observed gender differences in mood outcomes. Two other studies focused on severe clinical outcome in BD. Etain and colleagues[23] showed that physical abuse and mixed episodes in BD were both associated with poor response to lithium. The association between lithium response and mixed episodes is in line with previous studies showing a direct link between mixed symptoms and worse pharmacologic outcome.[7,8] On the other hand, the impact of childhood trauma on lithium response is an innovative and interesting finding, which may need further considerations. Etain and colleagues[23] hypothesized that an early biological mechanism mediated this important relationship. In the same line, Janiri and colleagues[24,25] recently found a specific effect of childhood trauma on hippocampal volumes in BD. Interestingly, the same group also showed hippocampal volumetric changes in patients with BD with long-term lithium exposure.[26] Therefore, we can hypothesize that the hippocampus may represent a common biological target of both early trauma and lithium activity and may specifically mediate the relationship highlighted by Etain and colleagues.[23] Further studies are needed to confirm this initial speculation.

Goldstein and colleagues[27] investigated factors associated with risk of suicide attempts in pediatric BD. Attempters were more likely to have a history of physical and/or sexual abuse and to present mixed states. These results are in line with a large body of evidence pointing out that suicidal risk is associated with childhood trauma[9,10,12] and mixed symptoms.[6–8,28] Previous studies explained these 2 associations differently. Koukopoulos and Sani[1] linked the high risk of suicide in depression with mixed features to greater energy and impulsivity, which can lead to an attempt to put an end to the unbearable sense of agitation characterizing these states by committing suicide. Because inadequate pharmacologic treatment could worsen agitation and increase the risk of suicide,[8,29] Koukopoulos and Sani[1] suggested approaching this clinical picture with particular caution.[25] Similarly, childhood trauma also has been found to be particularly involved in suicidal risk.[9,12,15] Emotional abuse, with respect to the other types of abuse and neglect, seems to be specifically involved in mood disorders.[9,12,15] A recent study by Janiri and collaborators[12] pointed out that, among several variables, including biological features such as affective temperament, emotional abuse was a direct predictor of suicide attempts in BD. This study speculated that the high risk of suicide attempts found in patients reporting emotional abuse could be related to an inadequate emotional regulation. This is in line with Aas and colleagues,[15] who found affective lability to specifically mediate the relationship between emotional abuse and suicide attempts.

In our search, we found 2 studies disproving a potential association between mixed states and childhood trauma. Benarous and colleagues[30] investigated adverse childhood experiences among inpatient youths with catatonic syndrome or manic and mixed episodes. Looking for clinical correlates they found no differences in number of mixed states in patients with and without early adverse experiences. They also found no differences in treatment response between adversity-exposed and unexposed patients, at odds with what Etain and colleagues[23] found for lithium responsiveness. Erten and colleagues[31] explored how childhood trauma affects the clinical expression of disorder and quality of life in patients with BD-I. Patients with BD were divided into 2 groups according to the presence of childhood trauma. There was no difference between the 2 groups in terms of number of mixed episodes.

Indirect Strategies: Mixed States, Childhood Trauma, and Emotional Reactivity

We found 8 studies including data regarding mixed states and emotional reactivity/affective lability in patients with mood disorders. All studies converged in supporting a strong association between mixed features and emotional dysregulation, conceptualized as emotional hyperreactivity/affective lability. Henry and colleagues[14] assessed patients with BD with a scale evaluating quantitative dimensions of excitatory and inhibition processes and applied a cluster analyses to verify this dimensional approach. They defined 3 clusters, of which the first was characterized by inhibition in all dimensions and corresponded to the depressive cluster; the second showed a general excitation and was observed mainly in manic or hypomanic patients; the third also was characterized by excitation, but included in most cases major depressive episodes (MDEs) with mixed symptoms and mixed states. Emotional reactivity was able to distinguish among diagnostic clusters. In a subsequent study,[32] the same group confirmed these observations in a larger sample, showing that only MDE without manic symptoms had emotional *hypo*reactivity, whereas in contrast, MDE with mixed symptoms, manic and mixed states displayed emotional *hyper*reactivity. They concluded that in patients with manic and mixed states, emotional responses are exacerbated and can lead to emotional hyperreactivity, which emerges as a distinguishing trait of a patient's psychopathology. Interestingly, all these studies corroborated the previous observation of Koukopoulos and colleagues[33] that mixed depression should be considered as a mixed state and that it belongs to the domain of excitation rather than inhibition. Accordingly, excitatory processes could directly link to emotional dysregulation and represent a core dimension of mood disorders, particularly BD.[34,35]

The BRIDGE-II-Mix study provided a reliable estimate of the frequency of mixed states in a large international sample of patients diagnosed with an MDE (n = 2811) according to several sets of criteria. In this context, Verdolini and colleagues[36] found that affective lability was strongly associated with MDE with mixed features and negatively associated with MDE without such features. Specifically, they found that more than half of the patients reporting affective lability were diagnosed with a mixed features specifier. Murru and colleagues[28] further indirectly validated this association in the same sample. For the same BRIDGE-II-Mix study group, Perugi and colleagues[37] specifically focused on comorbidity with borderline personality disorder (BPD). They found that mixed features according to DSM-5 criteria were observed in 27.8% of patients with BPD. Compared with patients without mixed features, the BPD group reported higher levels of emotional lability. Koukopoulos and colleagues[33] originally described a clinical picture of depression characterized, among other symptoms, by emotional reactivity. They postulated the existence of agitated depression with and without psychomotor agitation and proposed criteria for mixed depression without psychomotor agitation, which have been recently validated by Sani and colleagues.[38] These criteria included marked emotional reactivity as one of the 8 symptoms proposed as mixed specifiers for MDE. Sani and colleagues[39] also operationalized them, thus validating the first rating scale specifically aimed at cross-sectional assessment of mixed symptoms, the Koukopoulos Mixed Depression Rating Scale.

We found only 3 eligible studies including data regarding childhood trauma and emotional reactivity/affective lability in patients with mood disorders. Aas and colleagues[40] assessed patients with BD for both childhood trauma and affective lability. Patients with BD-I composed most of the considered sample. Affective lability was significantly and positively correlated with childhood trauma, with the strongest correlation observed for emotional abuse and neglect. In a large sample of patients with BD-I, BD-II, and recurrent MDD, Marwaha and collaborators[41] specified that within the BD-I group, any childhood abuse was significantly associated with higher affective lability scores, but found no association between childhood trauma and affective lability in BD-II and recurrent MDD. Etain and collaborators,[42] using a path analysis, further validated the association between emotional abuse and affective lability. Even if the number of studies supporting this indirect strategy is relatively small so far, neurobiological studies seem to support this approach. A recent study showed alterations in brain activity to an emotional face-processing task in patients with psychosis,[43] diagnosed as either with schizophrenia or BD, who had experienced early trauma. The investigators suggested stronger differentiation in brain responses between negative and positive faces with higher levels of trauma, which could in turn point to emotional hyperreactivity in patients with BD reporting early trauma. Our group recently found that childhood trauma modulated the effect of BD diagnosis on amygdala and hippocampal volumes. Interestingly, limbic structures, and in particular the amygdala and hippocampus, are recognized as key areas in emotion processing/regulation,[44] and could be crucial in explaining the relationship between childhood trauma and emotional hyperreactivity in mood disorders.[45,46] We found no evidence between a link of affective mixed states with prenatal trauma exposure so far, but the latter may induce epigenetic changes that may alter limbic structure that could in turn be detrimental to psychological development and ensue in psychiatric disorders, but the evidence is currently nonspecific.[47,48]

Conclusions, Research Perspective, and Clinical Recommendations

Our results suggested an association between childhood trauma and the development of mixed symptoms or states. Most of the studies, identified by both direct and indirect strategies, supported this association. Further investigations are needed to clarify the grading of the relationship among childhood trauma, emotional hyperreactivity, and mixed states. In particular, we strongly recommend future studies to specifically assess different types of childhood trauma, with particular regard to emotional abuse/neglect. The assessment of emotional hyperreactivity also should be systematically included in the evaluation of early traumatic memories in patients with mood disorders. Furthermore, as all studies we were able to include in this systematic review were cross-sectional and retrospective, there is a need for longitudinal studies adopting a multimodal approach in evaluating the complexity of the previously described association. Future longitudinal studies also could help in exploring the effects of childhood trauma and emotional hyperreactivity on neurobiological patterns and their interplay, so as to understand the mechanisms that render neural networks vulnerable to mixed symptoms/state. This could be used to model the effect of treatments, thereby assisting in the selection of personalized interventions based on their predicted effect.

DISCLOSURE

The authors have nothing to disclose.

REFERENCES

1. Koukopoulos A, Sani G. DSM-5 criteria for depression with mixed features: a fare-well to mixed depression. Acta Psychiatr Scand 2014;129:4–16.
2. Maj M. "Mixed" depression: drawbacks of DSM-5 (and other) polythetic diagnostic criteria. J Clin Psychiatry 2015;76:e381–2.
3. Kraepelin E. Manic depressive insanity and paranoia. Edinburgh (United Kingdom): E. and S. Livingstone; 1921.
4. Akiskal HS, Hantouche EG, Bourgeois ML, et al. Gender, temperament, and the clinical picture in dysphoric mixed mania: findings from a French national study (EPIMAN). J Affect Disord 1998;50:175–86.
5. Goldberg JF, Perlis RH, Bowden CL, et al. Manic symptoms during depressive episodes in 1,380 patients with bipolar disorder: findings from the STEP-BD. Am J Psychiatry 2009;166:173–81.
6. Perugi G, Akiskal HS, Micheli C, et al. Clinical subtypes of bipolar mixed states. J Affect Disord 1997;43:169–80.
7. Perugi G, Angst J, Azorin J, et al. Mixed features in patients with a major depressive episode: the BRIDGE-II-MIX study. J Clin Psychiatry 2015;76. https://doi.org/10.4088/JCP.14m09092.
8. Pacchiarotti I, Mazzarini L, Kotzalidis GD, et al. Mania and depression. Mixed, not stirred. J Affect Disord 2011;133:105–13.
9. Janiri D, Sani G, Danese E, et al. Childhood traumatic experiences of patients with bipolar disorder type I and type II. J Affect Disord 2014;175:92–7.
10. Aas M, Henry C, Andreassen OA, et al. The role of childhood trauma in bipolar disorders. Int J Bipolar Disord 2016;4:2.
11. Paterniti S, Sterner I, Caldwell C, et al. Childhood neglect predicts the course of major depression in a tertiary care sample: a follow-up study. BMC Psychiatry 2017;17. https://doi.org/10.1186/s12888-017-1270-x.
12. Janiri D, De Rossi P, Kotzalidis GD, et al. Psychopathological characteristics and adverse childhood events are differentially associated with suicidal ideation and suicidal acts in mood disorders. Eur Psychiatry 2018;53:31–6.
13. Minkowski E. La schizophrénie: psychopathologie des schizoïdes et des schizophrènes. Paris: Payot; 1927.
14. Henry C, M'Baïlara K, Desage A, et al. Towards a reconceptualization of mixed states, based on an emotional-reactivity dimensional model. J Affect Disord 2007;101:35–41.
15. Aas M, Henry C, Bellivier F, et al. Affective lability mediates the association between childhood trauma and suicide attempts, mixed episodes and co-morbid anxiety disorders in bipolar disorders. Psychol Med 2017;47:902–12.
16. Moher D, Liberati A, Tetzlaff J, et al. Preferred reporting items for systematic reviews and meta-analyses: the PRISMA statement. BMJ 2009;339:2535.
17. Shea BJ, Reeves BC, Wells G, et al. AMSTAR 2: A critical appraisal tool for systematic reviews that include randomised or non-randomised studies of healthcare interventions, or both. BMJ 2017;358. https://doi.org/10.1136/bmj.j4008.
18. Miller SA. PICO worksheet and search strategy. Los Angeles (CA): National Center for Dental Hygiene Research, University of Southern California; 2001.

19. Higgins JPT, Green S. Cochrane handbook for systematic reviews for interventions, version 5.1.0. England, UK: Wiley-Blackwell; 2008. p. 1–639. Available at: handbook-5-1.cochrane.org/.

20. Meade CS, McDonald LJ, Graff FS, et al. A prospective study examining the effects of gender and sexual/physical abuse on mood outcomes in patients with co-occurring bipolar I and substance use disorders. Bipolar Disord 2009;11: 425–33.

21. Ostacher MJ, Perlis RH, Nierenberg AA, et al, STEP-BD Investigators. Impact of substance use disorders on recovery from episodes of depression in bipolar disorder patients: prospective data from the Systematic Treatment Enhancement Program for Bipolar Disorder (STEP-BD). Am J Psychiatry 2010;167(3):289–97.

22. Daruy-Filho L, Brietzke E, Lafer B, et al. Childhood maltreatment and clinical outcomes of bipolar disorder. Acta Psychiatr Scand 2011;124(6):427–34.

23. Etain B, Lajnef M, Brichant-Petitjean C, et al. Childhood trauma sbipolar disorders. Acta Psychiatr Scand 2017;135:319–27.

24. Janiri D, Sani G, De Rossi P, et al. Amygdala and hippocampus volumes are differently affected by childhood trauma in patients with bipolar disorders and healthy controls. Bipolar Disord 2017;19:353–62.

25. Janiri D, Sani G, De Rossi P, et al. Hippocampal subfield volumes and childhood trauma in bipolar disorders. J Affect Disord 2019;253:35–43.

26. Sani G, Simonetti A, Janiri D, et al. Association between duration of lithium exposure and hippocampus/amygdala volumes in type I bipolar disorder. J Affect Disord 2018;232:341–8.

27. Goldstein TR, Birmaher B, Axelson D, et al. History of suicide attempts in pediatric bipolar disorder: factors associated with increased risk. Bipolar Disord 2005;7: 525–35.

28. Murru A, Guiso G, Barbuti M, et al. The implications of hypersomnia in the context of major depression: results from a large, international, observational study. Eur Neuropsychopharmacol 2019;29:471–81.

29. Rapinesi C, Kotzalidis GD, Scatena P, et al. Alcohol and suicidality: could deep transcranial magnetic stimulation (DTMS) be a possible treatment? Psychiatr Danub 2014;26:281–4.

30. Benarous X, Raffin M, Bodeau N, et al. Adverse childhood experiences among inpatient youths with severe and early-onset psychiatric disorders: prevalence and clinical correlates. Child Psychiatry Hum Dev 2017;48:248–59.

31. Erten E, Funda Uney A, Saatçioğlu Ö, et al. Effects of childhood trauma and clinical features on determining quality of life in patients with bipolar i disorder. J Affect Disord 2014;162:107–13.

32. Henry C, M'Bailara K, Lépine JP, et al. Defining bipolar mood states with quantitative measurement of inhibition/activation and emotional reactivity. J Affect Disord 2010;127:300–4.

33. Koukopoulos A, Sani G, Koukopoulos AE, et al. Melancholia agitata and mixed depression. Acta Psychiatr Scand 2007;115(Suppl. 433):50–7.

34. Kotzalidis GD, Rapinesi C, Savoja V, et al. Neurobiological evidence for the primacy of mania hypothesis. Curr Neuropharmacol 2017;339–52. https://doi.org/10.2174/1570159X14666160708231.

35. Janiri D, Di Nicola M, Martinotti G, et al. Who's the leader, mania or depression? Predominant polarity and alcohol/polysubstance use in bipolar disorders. Curr Neuropharmacol 2016. https://doi.org/10.2174/1570159X14666160607101400.

36. Verdolini N, Menculini G, Perugi G, et al. Sultans of swing: a reappraisal of the intertwined association between affective lability and mood reactivity in a post

hoc analysis of the BRIDGE-II-MIX study. J Clin Psychiatry 2019;80. https://doi.org/10.4088/JCP.17m12082.

37. Perugi G, Angst J, Azorin JM, et al. Relationships between mixed features and borderline personality disorder in 2811 patients with major depressive episode. Acta Psychiatr Scand 2016;133:133–43.

38. Sani G, Vöhringer PA, Napoletano F, et al. Koukopoulos' diagnostic criteria for mixed depression: a validation study. J Affect Disord 2014;164:14–8.

39. Sani G, Vöhringer PA, Barroilhet SA, et al. The Koukopoulos mixed depression rating scale (KMDRS): an international mood network (IMN) validation study of a new mixed mood rating scale. J Affect Disord 2018;232:9–16.

40. Aas M, Aminoff SR, Vik Lagerberg T, et al. Affective lability in patients with bipolar disorders is associated with high levels of childhood trauma. Psychiatry Res 2014;218:252–5.

41. Marwaha S, Gordon-Smith K, Broome M, et al. Affective instability, childhood trauma and major affective disorders. J Affect Disord 2016;190:764–71.

42. Etain B, Lajnef M, Henry C, et al. Childhood trauma, dimensions of psychopathology and the clinical expression of bipolar disorders: a pathway analysis. J Psychiatr Res 2017;95:37–45.

43. Aas M, Kauppi K, Brandt CL, et al. Childhood trauma is associated with increased brain responses to emotionally negative as compared with positive faces in patients with psychotic disorders. Psychol Med 2017;47:669–79.

44. Del Casale A, Kotzalidis GD, Rapinesi C, et al. Neural functional correlates of empathic face processing. Neurosci Lett 2017;655:68–75.

45. Janiri D, Ambrosi E, Danese E, et al. Bipolar disorders. In: Spalletta G, Piras F, Gili T, editors. Brain morphometry. New York: Springer; 2018. p. 339–83.

46. Janiri D, Sani G, Piras F, et al. Understanding trauma-induced hippocampal subfield volume changes in the context of age and health. Response to Malhi et al. J Affect Disord 2019;260:24–5.

47. Vinkers CH, Kalafateli AL, Rutten BP, et al. Traumatic stress and human DNA methylation: a critical review. Epigenomics 2015;7(4):593–608.

48. Provenzi L, Giorda R, Beri S, et al. SLC6A4 methylation as an epigenetic marker of life adversity exposures in humans: a systematic review of literature. Neurosci Biobehav Rev 2016;71:7–20.

Suicidal Behavior Associated with Mixed Features in Major Mood Disorders

Leonardo Tondo, MD[a,b,c,d,*],
Gustavo H. Vazquez, MD, PhD, FRCPC[a,b,e],
Ross J. Baldessarini, MD[a,b,c]

KEYWORDS

- Attempt • Depression • Ideation • Lethality • Mixed features • Risk rates • Suicide
- Treatment

KEY POINTS

- Mixed features of the opposite nominal mood-polarity are increasingly recognized in both depressive and [hypo]manic phases of major affective disorders. They are associated with major increases of risk of suicidal behaviors.
- Mixed states of agitated depression and dysphoric [hypo]mania are associated with much higher rates of suicidal behavior than when such factors are not present. Antidepressants can occasionally induce or worsen agitation, with potential risk of increasing suicidal risk. Their replacement with antipsychotic or mood-stabilizing medicines can reduce agitation and may reduce suicidal risk.
- Mixed features can arise spontaneously in major affective episodes or be induced or worsened by antidepressant treatment. Use of antipsychotic or mood-stabilizing treatments can benefit mood episodes with mixed features and so may reduce associated suicidal risk.

INTRODUCTION: SUICIDAL RISK FACTORS

Psychiatric disorders vary greatly in suicidal risks, although major mood, psychotic, and substance abuse disorders are associated with particularly high suicide rates.[1–3] Bipolar disorders (BDs) generally, as well as major depressive disorder (MDD) severe enough to require hospitalization, bear among the highest reported rates of suicides and attempts of all psychiatric disorders.[2,4–7] Suicide risk as standardized mortality ratio for BD and severe MDD can reach 20 times the suicide rates in the general

[a] International Consortium for Research on Mood & Psychotic Disorders, McLean Hospital, Belmont, MA, USA; [b] Mailman Research Center 3, McLean Hospital, 115 Mill Street, Belmont, MA 02478-9106, USA; [c] Department of Psychiatry, Harvard Medical School, Boston, MA, USA; [d] Lucio Bini Mood Disorders Center, Cagliari, Italy; [e] Department of Psychiatry, Queen's University, Kingston, Ontario, Canada
* Corresponding author. Mailman Research Center 3, McLean Hospital, 115 Mill Street, Belmont, MA 02478-9106.
E-mail address: ltondo@aol.com

Psychiatr Clin N Am 43 (2020) 83–93
https://doi.org/10.1016/j.psc.2019.10.008
0193-953X/20/© 2019 Elsevier Inc. All rights reserved.

population, which average 10 to 15 per 100,000 per year internationally.[2,8,9] Importantly, a high proportion of patients with BD, perhaps one-third, attempt suicide at least once, often when they are undertreated, in part possibly due to nondiagnosis or misdiagnosis, and they have ominously high risk early in the illness course, often years before diagnosis and treatment are established.[7,10]

Suicide as a cause of death is more prevalent among men than women in most cultures, commonly in association with a diagnosable mood disorder, substance abuse, or previous suicide attempts.[2,7,8,11–16] Family history of suicidal behavior, as well as childhood trauma, emotional abuse, and neglect also are important predictors of later suicidal behavior.[8,17–26] Suicide attempts and suicides probably are more prevalent among patients diagnosed with BD than with unipolar MDD, particularly moderately severely ill, never-hospitalized patients with MDD.[27–29] Of note, among patients with BD, rates of suicidal acts are similar in types I and II[1,7,16] and higher in women with either BD-I or BD-II.[7] Age can also affect suicidal risks: rates of suicide are higher at older ages, whereas attempts are especially prevalent in young adult years.[4,8,30–32]

Current morbid states also represent risk factors for suicides and attempts, most often current depression, depressive or dysphoric states following depression as an initial episode, more time spent in depression, treatment-resistant depressive episodes in both BD and MDD, and with mixed features.[11,20,33–40]

MIXED FEATURES IN MOOD DISORDERS

Mixed features have been recognized by the *Diagnostic and Statistical Manual of Mental Disorders, Fifth Edition* (DSM-5) as specifiers for hypomanic or manic ("[hypo]manic") syndromes, as well as for depression, essentially representing dysphoric manic and agitated depressive states. Suicidal risk in BD is far more strongly associated with depressive than [hypo]manic states, but mixed states of dysphoric mania as well as of depression can present elevated risk of suicidal behaviors.[41–43] However, hypomanic features that can occur in depression in either BD or MDD have been more extensively studied. They include the following:

a. Elevated or expansive mood
b. Inflated self-esteem or grandiosity
c. Talkativeness or pressure to talk
d. Flight-of-ideas or experience of racing thoughts
e. Increase in energy or goal-directed activity
f. Increased or excessive involvement in activities with high potential for painful consequences, including excessive spending, sexual promiscuity or risky business decisions
g. Decreased need for sleep

Four other symptoms are not usually included among mixed features, as they can arise in either [hypo]manic or depressive syndromes: distractibility, irritability, insomnia, and indecisiveness [DSM-5]. Nevertheless, Koukopoulos and colleagues[44–49] proposed that such "overlapping" symptoms, possibly associated with suicide risk, can arise in either depression or [hypo]mania and should be considered mixed features when identified in depressive episodes, in which they add to indications of the presence of agitated or mixed depression. This proposal is also supported by more recent studies.[50,51] Koukopoulos recognized 7 symptoms as indicative of mixed or agitated depression,[52] ranking by frequency as follows:

a. Psychic agitation or inner tension
b. Absence of retardation

c. Experience of suffering or spells of weeping
d. Talkativeness
e. Racing or crowded thoughts
f. Irritability
g. Mood lability

The most recent report of his views did not include 3 symptoms (distractibility, insomnia, and indecisiveness) included previously,[46] because they were less reliably associated with agitated depression.[52]

MIXED FEATURES AS A SUICIDAL RISK FACTOR

Interest in identifying mixed symptoms is justified by their strong association with suicidal risk. Early associations of mixed symptoms in depression with suicidal ideation or behavior date to the early 1990s,[53] and suggested that active treatment of patients with major depression for co-occurring clinical anxiety could modify suicide risk. Koukopoulos and his colleagues[54] [1992] examined and treated 361 mood disorder patients for 6 months. Of these, 178 were depressed at intake and 34 women (28.6%) and 11 men (15.9%) presented with mixed features, including irritability, internal tension, psychomotor agitation, emotional lability, racing thoughts, sleep disturbance, severe suffering, and talkativeness. These symptoms were associated with suicidal thoughts or attempting suicide, often impulsively. Moreover, these investigators proposed that the syndrome of *agitated depression* be considered a relatively distinct mood disorder, with prognostic and therapeutic implications. The same conclusion was reached later by a study requiring a new category when the combination of depressive and [hypo]manic symptoms did not meet the relatively narrow criteria for a "mixed state" according to the DSM-IV-TR, which required meeting diagnostic criteria for both a major depressive and [hypo]manic episode simultaneously.[55] A newer study suggested that the definition of "mixed states" in mood disorders include prognostic severity, risk of suicide, lower therapeutic response, co-occurrence of other psychiatric disorders, and particular temperamental traits.[56]

Indeed, temperament has emerged as an important characteristic accompanying mixed features and associated with suicidal behavior. Affective temperamental traits (cyclothymic, dysthymic, irritable, hyperthymic, and anxious) can readily be assessed with the TEMPS-A questionnaire.[57] With this tool, we found significant associations of suicidal behavior with cyclothymic, dysthymic, and irritable temperamental traits, whereas the presence of hyperthymic traits had an apparent protective effect against suicide risk.[19,58,59] Irritable temperament was especially strongly associated with suicidal acts,[58] and along with cyclothymic traits, also associated with mixed features.[58] These findings suggest that irritable traits be considered as risk factors for suicidal ideation and acts, and even more so when mixed features are present.

In [hypo]mania, risk of suicidal behavior has been greater among patients with mixed symptoms than without.[41–43,60–67] However, in [hypo]manias with or without depressive symptoms, treatment typically is based on use of antipsychotics and mood stabilizers, which are likely to be safe by avoiding use of antidepressants.

Several studies have noted increased suicidal risk in depressed patients when mixed symptoms are present.[12,32,39,50,68–80] However, a recent study of 290 patients with BD reported that suicidal risk was associated with depressive symptoms but not significantly increased by the presence of mixed features defined as the simultaneous presence of depressive and manic symptoms.[81]

Among 3099 patients with MDD or BD, in association with mixed features, suicidal acts were 3.37 times more prevalent (30.3% vs 8.98%) and average age at a first-lifetime suicidal act 4.40 years younger (33.1 vs 37.5 years).[39] We further evaluated suicidal risks in 3284 subjects with a DSM-5 major mood of 14.0 years' average duration.[19] The rate of suicidal acts (suicide and attempts) was 20.6% among patients with BD and 5.26% with MDD, and was 1.70 times greater (29.5% vs 17.4%), overall, among depressed subjects with mixed features. In that study, mixed features in depressive episodes were identified by multivariable regression modeling as an independent risk factor associated with suicidal acts. Finally, in a recent analysis of 6050 psychiatric patients, among the highest rates of suicidal behavior were found with BD-I disorder, and especially if mixed or psychotic features were present.[1]

SUICIDAL RISKS AND MIXED FEATURES ASSOCIATED WITH ANTIDEPRESSANT TREATMENT

The clinical relevance of ascertaining the boundaries of mixed features and their presence in depressive episodes includes the concern that antidepressants may worsen the clinical condition by increasing agitation, with potentially increased risk of suicidal behavior.[45,82–85] Moreover, it has been suggested that antidepressants may exacerbate suicidal tendencies more broadly, at least in young patents. Based on post hoc reanalysis of findings from hundreds of placebo-controlled trials of antidepressants in which suicidal ideation or behavior was sometimes noted among "adverse effects," the Food and Drug Administration proposed that such outcomes, although uncommon, were most likely to arise among depressed juveniles and young adults, although with decreased risk in older adults.[86,87] This finding of age-related variance in suicidal risks during antidepressant treatment was supported by an analysis of clinical observations in large numbers of depressed patients treated with modern antidepressants.[88] These associations have been reviewed critically.[89,90]

At least 8 possible clinical mechanisms have been proposed to explain worsening of suicidal risk during treatment with an antidepressant:

a. Energizing depressed patients to act on suicidal ideation
b. Paradoxically worsening depression
c. Inducing akathisia with associated self-destructive or aggressive impulses
d. Inducing panic attacks
e. Switching patients into agitated or mixed states
f. Producing severe insomnia or interfering with sleep architecture
g. Inducing an obsessional state
h. Producing cerebrotoxic psychopathological states, including electroencephalographic or other neurologic disturbances[85]

TREATMENTS TO LIMIT SUICIDAL RISK WITH MIXED AFFECTIVE FEATURES

Some findings support the proposal that several alternative treatments may limit potential worsening of mixed features and of suicidal risk during treatment with an antidepressant. In early observations, Koukopoulos and colleagues[54] reported that, whereas antidepressants can increase agitation and suicidal risk in depression with mixed features, antipsychotics, anticonvulsants, lithium, and electroconvulsive therapy (ECT) were relatively safe and effective in such circumstances. Their findings are supported by several later studies.[91–101] They have been extended to include minimizing risk of antidepressant-associated increases in suicidal ideation or behavior even without mixed features in depressive episodes by use of treatments lacking in arousal-enhancing properties, often to replace antidepressants. These include use of *second generation antipsychotics*,[102–110] *anticonvulsants*,[43,104,108,110–113]

ECT,[114–116] and *psychotherapies*.[115] Rare among psychiatric treatments, long-term use of lithium has been strongly associated with reduction of suicidal risk[117–120] and it is also found to be effective in the treatment of both depressive and [hypo]manic mixed states of BD.[106,109,121,122] Therefore, lithium should be considered a first-line treatment when suicidal behavior and major affective episodes with mixed features are present.

SUMMARY

Rates of suicidal behavior are especially high in mood disorders, and extensive research has found consistently that risk of suicide is greater when mixed features are present, especially in depressive episodes. Identification of mixed features in mood disorders is becoming increasingly relevant to efforts to improve treatment and to prevent suicidal behavior. Antidepressant treatments are generally useful for both treatment and prevention of recurrences in MDD, but continue to have a controversial place in the treatment of depression in bipolar disorder. In all patients with mood disorder, antidepressants can occasionally induce activation and agitation which can represent mixed features and may lead in some cases to suicidal ideation and behavior. Other treatments, including antipsychotics, anticonvulsants, ECT, and psychotherapies may be helpful in spontaneous or antidepressant-associated affective episodes with mixed features, and long-term treatment with lithium may have a particularly beneficial role owing to substantial evidence of its antisuicidal effects in patients with BD and perhaps in patients with MDD, as well as its useful effects in episodes with mixed features.

ACKNOWLEDGMENTS

Supported by a grant from the Aretaeus Foundation of Rome (to L. Tondo), and a grant from the Bruce J Anderson Foundation and by the McLean Private Donors Psychiatric Research Fund (to R.J. Baldessarini).

DECLARATION OF INTEREST

No author or immediate family member has financial relationships with commercial entities that might appear to represent potential conflicts of interest with the information presented.

REFERENCES

1. Baldessarini RJ, Tondo L. Suicidal risk in psychiatric disorders. Am J Psychiatry, in press.
2. Harris EC, Barraclough B. Suicide as an outcome for mental disorders: a meta-analysis. Br J Psychiatry 1997;170:205–28.
3. Rihmer Z, Kiss K. Bipolar disorders and suicidal behavior. Bipolar Disord 2002; 4:21–5.
4. Goodwin FK, Jamison KR. Manic-depressive illness: bipolar disorders and recurrent depression. 2nd edition. New York: Oxford University Press; 2007.
5. Schaffer A, Isometsä ET, Tondo L, et al. International Society for Bipolar Disorders Task Force on Suicide: meta-analyses and meta-regression of correlates of suicide attempts and suicide deaths in bipolar disorder. Bipolar Disord 2015;17:1–16.

6. Tondo L, Baldessarini RJ. Suicide in bipolar disorder. In: Yildiz A, Nemeroff C, Ruiz P, editors. Chapt 37 in the Bipolar book: history, neurobiology, and treatment. New York: Oxford University Press; 2015. p. 509–28.
7. Tondo L, Pompili M, Forte A, et al. Suicide attempts in bipolar disorders: comprehensive review of 101 reports. Acta Psychiatr Scand 2016;133:174–86.
8. Simon GE, Hunkeler E, Fireman B, et al. Risk of suicide attempt and suicide death in patients treated for bipolar disorder. Bipolar Disord 2007;9:526–30.
9. Tondo L, Lepri B, Baldessarini RJ. Risks of suicidal ideation, attempts and suicides among 2826 men and women with types I and II bipolar, and recurrent major depressive disorders. Acta Psychiatr Scand 2007;116:419–28.
10. Valtonen HM, Suominen K, Mantere O, et al. Suicidal behavior during different phases of bipolar disorder. J Affect Disord 2007;97:101–7.
11. Hawton K, Comabella CC, Haw C, et al. Risk factors for suicide in individuals with depression: systematic review. J Affect Disord 2013;147:17–28.
12. Isometsä E. Suicidal behavior in mood disorders–who, when, and why? Can J Psychiatry 2014;59:120–30.
13. Mccullumsmith CB, Williamson DJ, May RS, et al. Simple measures of hopelessness and impulsivity are associated with acute suicidal ideation and attempts in patients in psychiatric crisis. Innov Clin Neurosci 2014;11:47–53.
14. McElroy SL, Kotwal R, Kaneria R, et al. Antidepressants and suicidal behavior in bipolar disorder. Bipolar Disord 2006;8:596–617.
15. McIntyre RS, Cucchiaro J, Pikalov A, et al. Lurasidone in the treatment of bipolar depression with mixed (subsyndromal hypomanic) features: post hoc analysis of a randomized placebo-controlled trial. J Clin Psychiatry 2015;76:398–405.
16. Novick DM, Swartz HA, Frank E. Suicide attempts in bipolar I and bipolar II disorder: review and meta-analysis of the evidence. Bipolar Disord 2010;12:1–9.
17. Altamura AC, Dell'Osso B, Berlin HA, et al. Duration of untreated illness and suicide in bipolar disorder: a naturalistic study. Eur Arch Psychiatry Clin Neurosci 2010;260:385–91.
18. Antypa N, Serretti A, Rujescu D. Serotonergic genes and suicide: systematic review. Eur Neuropsychopharmacol 2013;23:1125–42.
19. Baldessarini RJ, Tondo L, Pinna M, et al. Suicidal risk factors in major affective disorders. Br J Psychiatry 2019;1–6.
20. Bellivier F, Yon L, Luquiens A, et al. Suicidal attempts in bipolar disorder: results from an observational study (EMBLEM). Bipolar Disord 2011;13:377–86.
21. Dalton EJ, Cate-Carter TD, Mundo E, et al. Suicide risk in bipolar patients: the role of co-morbid substance use disorders. Bipolar Disord 2003;5:58–61.
22. de Abreu LN, Nery FG, Harkavy-Friedman JM, et al. Suicide attempts are associated with worse quality of life in patients with bipolar disorder type I. Compr Psychiatry 2012;53:125–9.
23. de Mattos-Souza LD, Molina ML, da Silva RA, et al. History of childhood trauma as risk factors to suicide risk in major depression. Psychiatry Res 2016;246: 612–6.
24. Gonda X, Pompili M, Serafini G, et al. Suicidal behavior in bipolar disorder: epidemiology, characteristics and major risk factors. J Affect Disord 2012;143: 16–26.
25. Leverich GS, Altshuler LL, Frye MA, et al. Factors associated with suicide attempts in 648 patients with bipolar disorder in the Stanley Foundation Bipolar Network. J Clin Psychiatry 2003;64:506–15.
26. Neves FS, Malloy-Diniz LF, Correa H. Suicidal behavior in bipolar disorder: what is the influence of psychiatric comorbidities? J Clin Psychiatry 2009;70:13–8.

27. Lester D. Suicidal behavior in bipolar and unipolar affective disorders: a meta-analysis. J Affect Disord 1993;27:117–21.
28. Pawlak J, Dmitrzak-Węglarz M, Skibińska M, et al. Suicide attempts and clinical risk factors in patients with bipolar and unipolar affective disorders. Gen Hosp Psychiatry 2013;35:427–32.
29. Zalsman G, Braun M, Arendt M, et al. Comparison of the medical lethality of suicide attempts in bipolar and major depressive disorders. Bipolar Disord 2006;8:558–65.
30. Conwell Y, Duberstein PR, Caine ED. Risk factors for suicide in later life. Biol Psychiatry 2002;52:193–204.
31. Goldring N, Fieve RR. Attempted suicide in manic-depressive disorder. Am J Psychother 1984;38:373–83.
32. Hawton K, Sutton L, Haw C, et al. Suicide and attempted suicide in bipolar disorder: systematic review of risk factors. J Clin Psychiatry 2005;66:693–704.
33. Chaudhury SR, Grunebaum MF, Galfalvy HC, et al. Does first episode polarity predict risk for suicide attempt in bipolar disorder? J Affect Disord 2007;104:245–50.
34. Galfalvy H, Oquendo MA, Carballo JJ, et al. Clinical predictors of suicidal acts after major depression in bipolar disorder: prospective study. Bipolar Disord 2006;8:586–95.
35. Ghaemi SN, Vohringer PA. Athanasios Koukopoulos' Psychiatry: primacy of mania and the limits of antidepressants. Curr Neuropharmacol 2017;15:402–8.
36. Holma KM, Haukka J, Suominen K, et al. Differences in incidence of suicide attempts between bipolar I and II disorders and major depressive disorder. Bipolar Disord 2014;16:652–61.
37. Oquendo MA, Currier D, Mann JJ. Prospective studies of suicidal behavior in major depressive and bipolar disorders: what is the evidence for predictive risk factors? Acta Psychiatr Scand 2006;114:151–8.
38. Ryu V, Jon D-I, Cho HS, et al. Initial depressive episodes affect the risk of suicide attempts in Korean patients with bipolar disorder. Yonsei Med J 2010;51:641–7.
39. Tondo L, Vázquez GH, Pinna M, et al. Characteristics of depressive and bipolar patients with mixed features. Acta Psychiatr Scand 2018;138:243–52.
40. Undurraga J, Baldessarini RJ, Valenti M, et al. Suicidal risk factors in bipolar I and II disorder patients. J Clin Psychiatry 2012;73:778–82.
41. Eberhard J, Weiller E. Suicidality and symptoms of anxiety, irritability, and agitation in patients experiencing manic episodes with depressive symptoms: naturalistic study. Neuropsychiatr Dis Treat 2016;12:2265–71.
42. Lage RR, Santana CMT, Nardi AE, et al. Mixed states and suicidal behavior: systematic review. Trends Psychiatry Psychother 2019;41:191–200.
43. Reinares M, Bonnín-Cdel M, Hidalgo-Mazzei D, et al. Making sense of DSM-5 mania with depressive features. Aust N Z J Psychiatry 2015;49:540–9.
44. Faedda GL, Marangoni C, Reginaldi D. Depressive mixed states: reappraisal of Koukopoulos' criteria. J Affect Disord 2015;176:18–23.
45. Koukopoulos A, Albert MJ, Sani G, et al. Mixed depressive states: nosologic and therapeutic issues. Int Rev Psychiatry 2005;17:21–37.
46. Koukopoulos A, Koukopoulos A. Agitated depression as a mixed state and the problem of melancholia. Psychiatr Clin North Am 1999;22:547–64.
47. Koukopoulos A, Sani G, Koukopoulos AE, et al. Melancholia agitata and mixed depression. Acta Psychiatr Scand Suppl 2007;433:50–7.

48. Koukopoulos A, Sani G. DSM-5 criteria for depression with mixed features: a farewell to mixed depression. Acta Psychiatr Scand 2014;129:4–16.

49. Koukopoulos A, Sani G, Ghaemi SN. Mixed features of depression: why DSM-5 is wrong (and so was DSM-IV). Br J Psychiatry 2013;203:3–5.

50. Brancati GE, Vieta E, Azorin JM, et al. Role of overlapping excitatory symptoms in major depression: are they relevant for the diagnosis of mixed state? J Psychiatr Res 2019;115:151–7.

51. Solé E, Garriga M, Valentí M, et al. Mixed features in bipolar disorder. CNS Spectr 2017;22:134–40.

52. Sani G, Vöhringer PA, Napoletano F, et al. Koukopoulos' diagnostic criteria for mixed depression: a validation study. J Affect Disord 2014;164:14–8.

53. Fawcett J. Targeting treatment in patients with mixed symptoms of anxiety and depression. J Clin Psychiatry 1990;51(Suppl):40–3.

54. Koukopoulos A, Faedda G, Proietti R, et al. Mixed depressive syndrome. Encephale 1992;18(Special issue 1):19–21.

55. M'Bailara K, Van den Bulke D, Demazeau N, et al. Depressive mixed state: evidence for a new form of depressive state in type I and II bipolar patients. Neuropsychiatr Dis Treat 2007;3:899–902.

56. Pringuey D, Cherikh F, Giordana B, et al. Mixed states: evolution of classifications. Encephale 2013;39(Suppl 3):S134–8.

57. Vázquez GH, Kahn C, Schiavo CE, et al. Bipolar disorders and affective temperaments: a national family study testing the "endophenotype" and "subaffective" theses using the TEMPS-A Buenos Aires. J Affect Disord 2008;108:25–32.

58. Tondo L, Vázquez GH, Sani G, et al. Association of suicidal risk with ratings of affective temperaments. J Affect Disord 2018;229:322–7.

59. Vázquez GH, Gonda X, Lolich M, et al. Suicidal risk and affective temperaments evaluated with the TEMPS-A scale: systematic review. Harv Rev Psychiatry 2018;26:8–18.

60. Azorin JM, Aubrun E, Bertsch J, et al. Mixed states vs. pure mania in the French sample of the EMBLEM study: results at baseline and 24 months: European mania in bipolar longitudinal evaluation of medication. BMC Psychiatry 2009; 9:33.

61. Johnson SL, McMurrich SL, Yates M. Suicidality in bipolar I disorder. Suicide Life Threat Behav 2005;35:681–9.

62. Perugi G, Akiskal HS, Micheli C, et al. Clinical subtypes of bipolar mixed states: validating a broader European definition in 143 cases. J Affect Disord 1997;43: 169–80.

63. Sato T, Bottlender R, Tanabe A, et al. Cincinnati criteria for mixed mania and suicidality in patients with acute mania. Compr Psychiatry 2004;45:62–9.

64. Schwartzmann AM, Amaral JA, Issler C, et al. A clinical study comparing manic and mixed episodes in patients with bipolar disorder. Braz J Psychiatry 2007;29: 130–3.

65. Shim IH, Woo YS, Jun TY, et al. Reevaluation of the possibility and characteristics in bipolar mania with mixed features: a retrospective chart review. Psychiatry Res 2014;215:335–40.

66. Strakowski SM, McElroy SL, Keck PE Jr, et al. Suicidality among patients with mixed and manic bipolar disorder. Am J Psychiatry 1996;153:674–6.

67. Kim KR, Cho HS, Kim SJ, et al. Reevaluation of patients with bipolar disorder on manic episode: improving the diagnosing of mixed episode. J Nerv Ment Dis 2013;201:686–90.

68. Fawcett J. Diagnosis, traits, states, and comorbidity in suicide. In: Dwivedi Y, editor. The neurobiological basis of suicide. Boca Raton (FL): CRC Press/Taylor & Francis; 2012 [Chapter 1].

69. Goldberg JF, Perlis RH, Bowden CL, et al. Manic symptoms during depressive episodes in 1380 patients with bipolar disorder: findings from the STEP-BD. Am J Psychiatry 2009;166:173–81.

70. Maj M, Pirozzi R, Magliano L, et al. Agitated "unipolar" major depression: prevalence, phenomenology, and outcome. J Clin Psychiatry 2006;67:712–9.

71. Maron M, Vaiva G. Predominant polarity, mixed states and suicide. Encephale 2012;38(Suppl 4):S155–9.

72. Oquendo MA, Waternaux C, Brodsky B, et al. Suicidal behavior in bipolar mood disorder: clinical characteristics of attempters and nonattempters. J Affect Disord 2000;59:107–17.

73. Pallaskorpi S, Suominen K, Ketokivi M, et al. Incidence and predictors of suicide attempts in bipolar I and II disorders: a 5-year follow-up study. Bipolar Disord 2017;19:13–22.

74. Persons JE, Coryell WH, Solomon DA, et al. Mixed state and suicide: Is the effect of mixed state on suicidal behavior more than the sum of its parts? Bipolar Disord 2018;20:35–41.

75. Rihmer A, Gonda X, Balazs J, et al. The importance of depressive mixed states in suicidal behavior. Neuropsychopharmacol Hung 2008;10:45–9.

76. Serra F, Gordon-Smith K, Perry A, et al. Agitated depression in bipolar disorder. Bipolar Disord 2019;21(6):547–55.

77. Shim IH, Woo YS, Bahk WM. Prevalence rates and clinical implications of bipolar disorder "with mixed features" as defined by DSM-5. J Affect Disord 2015;173:120–5.

78. Shim IH, Woo YS, Kim MD, et al. Antidepressants and mood-stabilizers: novel research avenues and clinical insights for bipolar depression. Int J Mol Sci 2017;18:E2406.

79. Song JY, Yu HY, Kim SH, et al. Assessment of risk factors related to suicide attempts in patients with bipolar disorder. J Nerv Ment Dis 2012;200:978–84.

80. Swann AC, Lafer B, Perugi G, et al. Bipolar mixed states: an International Society for Bipolar Disorders task force report of symptom structure, course of illness, and diagnosis. Am J Psychiatry 2013;170:31–42.

81. Fiedorowicz JG, Persons JE, Assari S, et al. Depressive symptoms carry an increased risk for suicidal ideation and behavior in bipolar disorder without any additional contribution of mixed symptoms. J Affect Disord 2019;246:775–82.

82. Akiskal HS, Akiskal KK, Haykal RF, et al. Progress towards validation of a self-rated clinical version of the Temperament Evaluation of the Memphis, Pisa, Paris, and San Diego Auto-questionnaire. J Affect Disord 2005;85:3–16.

83. Akiskal HS, Benazzi F, Perugi G, et al. Agitated "unipolar" depression reconceptualized as a depressive mixed state: implications for the antidepressant-suicide controversy. J Affect Disord 2005;85:245–58.

84. Rihmer Z, Gonda X. Suicide behavior of patients treated with antidepressants. Neuropsychopharmacol Hung 2006;8:13–6.

85. Teicher MH, Glod CA, Cole JO. Antidepressant drugs and the emergence of suicidal tendencies. Drug Saf 1993;8:186–212.

86. Hamad T. Relationship between psychotropic drugs and pediatric suicidality: review and evaluation of clinical data. Silver Spring (MD): Food and Drug

Administration; 2004. Available at: http://www.fda.gov/ohrms/dockets/ac/04/briefing/2004-4065b1-10-TAB08-Hammads-Review.pdf.

87. Laughren TP. Proceedings of a meeting of the Psychopharmacology Drug Advisory Committee (PDAC) concerning suicidal risk in trials of antidepressant drugs in juvenile and adult patients. 2006. Available at: http://www.fda.gov/ohrms/dockets/ac/06/briefing//2006-4272b1-01-fda.pdf. Accessed December 22, 2018.

88. Barbui C, Esposito E, Cipriani A. Selective serotonin reuptake inhibitors and risk of suicide: systematic review of observational studies. CMAJ 2009;180:291-7.

89. Baldessarini RJ, Tondo L, Strombom IM, et al. Ecological studies of antidepressant treatment and suicidal risks. Harv Rev Psychiatry 2007;15:133-45.

90. Friedman RA. Antidepressants' black-box warning–10 years later. N Engl J Med 2014;371:1666-8.

91. Berk M, Dodd S. Are treatment emergent suicidality and decreased response to antidepressants in younger patients due to bipolar disorder being misdiagnosed as unipolar depression? Med Hypotheses 2005;65:39-43.

92. Faedda GL, Marangoni C. What is the role of conventional antidepressants in the treatment of major depressive episodes with the mixed features specifier? CNS Spectr 2017;22:120-5.

93. McIntyre RS, Lee Y, Mansur RB. Pragmatic approach to the diagnosis and treatment of mixed features in adults with mood disorders. CNS Spectr 2016;21:25-33.

94. Perugi G, Pacchiarotti I, Mainardi C, et al. Patterns of response to antidepressants in major depressive disorder: drug resistance or worsening of depression are associated with a bipolar diathesis. Eur Neuropsychopharmacol 2019;29:825-34.

95. Popovic D, Vieta E, Azorin JM, et al. Suicide attempts in major depressive episode: evidence from the BRIDGE-II-Mix study. Bipolar Disord 2015;17:795-803.

96. Raja M, Azzoni A, Koukopoulos AE. Psychopharmacological treatment before suicide attempt among patients admitted to a psychiatric intensive care unit. J Affect Disord 2009;113:37-44.

97. Stahl SM. Mixed-up about how to diagnose and treat mixed features in major depressive episodes. CNS Spectr 2017;22:111-5.

98. Stahl SM, Morrissette DA, Faedda G, et al. Guidelines for the recognition and management of mixed depression. CNS Spectr 2017;22:203-19.

99. Takeshima M, Oka T. Association between the so-called "activation syndrome" and bipolar II disorder, a related disorder, and bipolar suggestive features in outpatients with depression. J Affect Disord 2013;151:196-202.

100. Valentí M, Pacchiarotti I, Rosa AR, et al. Bipolar mixed episodes and antidepressants: a cohort study of bipolar I disorder patients. Bipolar Disord 2011;13:145-54.

101. Sani G, Napoletano F, Vöhringer PA, et al. Mixed depression: clinical features and predictors of its onset associated with antidepressant use. Psychother Psychosom 2014;83:213-21.

102. Berk M, Tiller JW, Zhao J, et al. Effects of asenapine in bipolar I patients meeting proxy criteria for moderate-to-severe mixed major depressive episodes: post hoc analysis. J Clin Psychiatry 2015;76:728-34.

103. Houston JP, Ahl J, Meyers AL, et al. Reduced suicidal ideation in bipolar I disorder mixed-episode patients in a placebo-controlled trial of olanzapine combined with lithium or divalproex. J Clin Psychiatry 2006;67:1246-52.

104. Köhler S, Stöver LA, Sterzer P. Mixed episodes in bipolar disorders: changes in DSM-5 and treatment recommendations. Fortschr Neurol Psychiatr 2015;83: 606–15.
105. Nishiyama A, Matsumoto H. Quetiapine reduces irritability and risk of suicide in patients with agitated depression. Tokai J Exp Clin Med 2013;38:93–6.
106. Rosenblat JD, McIntyre RS. Treatment of mixed features in bipolar disorder. CNS Spectr 2017;22:141–6.
107. Suppes T, Silva R, Cucchiaro J, et al. Lurasidone for the treatment of major depressive disorder with mixed features: randomized, double-blind, placebo-controlled study. Am J Psychiatry 2016;173:400–7.
108. Takeshima M. Treating mixed mania/hypomania: review and synthesis of the evidence. CNS Spectr 2017;22:177–85.
109. Grunze H, Vieta E, Goodwin GM, et al. The World Federation of Societies of Biological Psychiatry (WFSBP) Guidelines for the Biological Treatment of Bipolar Disorders: Acute and long-term treatment of mixed states in bipolar disorder. World J Biol Psychiatry 2018;19:2–58.
110. Dassa D, Dubois M, Maurel M, et al. [Antimanic treatments in bipolar mixed states]. Encephale 2013;39(Suppl 3):S172–8.
111. Kiloh LG. The trials of ECT. Psychiatr Dev 1985;3:205–18.
112. Liu CC. Adjuvant valproate therapy for patients with suspected mixed-depressive features. Ther Adv Psychopharmacol 2014;4:143–8.
113. Thuile J, Even C, Guelfi JD. Mixed states in bipolar disorders: a review of current therapeutic strategies. Encephale 2005;31:617–23.
114. Ciapparelli A, Dell'Osso L, Tundo A, et al. Electroconvulsive therapy in medication-nonresponsive patients with mixed mania and bipolar depression. J Clin Psychiatry 2001;62:552–5.
115. Dubois M, Dassa D, Belzeaux R, et al. Treatment of depressive mixed states. Encephale 2013;39(Suppl 3):S179–84.
116. Liang CS, Chung CH, Ho PS, et al. Superior anti-suicidal effects of electroconvulsive therapy in unipolar disorder and bipolar depression. Bipolar Disord 2018;20:539–46.
117. Guzzetta F, Tondo L, Centorrino F, et al. Lithium treatment reduces suicide risk in recurrent major depressive disorder. J Clin Psychiatry 2007;68(3):380–3.
118. Müller-Oerlinghausen B, Grof P, Schou M. Lithium and suicide prevention. Br J Psychiatry 1999;175:90–1.
119. Müller-Oerlinghausen B, Lewitzka U. Lithium reduces pathological aggression and suicidality: a mini-review. Neuropsychobiology 2010;62:43–9.
120. Tondo L, Baldessarini RJ. Antisuicidal Effects in Mood Disorders: Are They Unique to Lithium Pharmacopsychiatry 2018;51:177–88.
121. Fagiolini a, Coluccia A, Maina G, et al. Diagnosis, epidemiology and management of mixed states in bipolar disorder. CNS Drugs 2015;29:725–40.
122. McKnight RF, de La Motte de Broöns de Vauvert SJGN, Chesney E, et al. Lithium for acute mania. Cochrane Database Syst Rev 2019;(6):CD004048.

Mixed States in Early-Onset Bipolar Disorder

Kirti Saxena, MD[a,b],*, Sherin Kurian, MD[a,b], Johanna Saxena, BS, BA[a,b], Adam Goldberg, MD[c], Eugenia Chen, BS[a], Alessio Simonetti, MD[a,d,e,f]

KEYWORDS

- Mixed states • Bipolar disorder • Children • Adolescents • Diagnosis • Comorbidity
- Treatment

KEY POINTS

- Youth with mixed features of pediatric bipolar disorder (PBD) have a younger age of onset of bipolar disorder (BD), more severe symptoms, and a more severe course of illness.
- Criteria used to diagnose BD using the Diagnostic and Statistical Manual of Mental Disorders (DSM), Fifth Edition are the same in children, adolescents, and adults. In DSM-IV–Text Revision (TR), mixed episodes are one of the mood states in BD type I, whereas DSM-5 provides a mixed-features specifier to its definition of BD I, BD II, and major depressive disorders. Clinical presentations of PBD differ developmentally between children and adolescents.
- Clinical trials to date have focused on manic or mixed states in PBD using the DSM-IV or DSM-IV-TR criteria. Psychotropics for PBD during the mixed or manic phase have been approved by the US Food and Drug Administration. However, clinical trials using DSM-5 criteria for mixed states need to be conducted.

INTRODUCTION

Pediatric bipolar disorder (PBD) is a chronic affective disorder affecting psychosocial and academic functioning, and increasing the risk for psychotic episodes, substance abuse, and legal problems.[1] Youth diagnosed with PBD represent a unique population at increased risk of recurrence, treatment resistance, and suicidality. The co-occurrence of depressive and manic/hypomanic symptoms is related to more severe symptoms, younger age of onset of bipolar disorder (BD), and a more severe course of illness.[2,3]

[a] Menninger Department of Psychiatry and Behavioral Sciences, Baylor College of Medicine, 1 Baylor Plaza, Houston, TX 77030, USA; [b] Department of Psychiatry, Texas Children's Hospital, Houston, TX, USA; [c] Department of Psychiatry & Behavioral Sciences, McGovern Medical School at the University of Texas Health Science Center, 1941 East Road, Houston, TX 77054, USA; [d] Department of Neurology and Psychiatry, Sapienza University of Rome, Rome, Italy; [e] Centro Lucio Bini, Rome, Italy; [f] Department of Psychiatry, Baylor College of Medicine, 1977 Butler Boulevard Suite E4.400, Houston, TX 77030, USA
* Corresponding author. One Baylor Plaza, Mail Stop: BCM350, Houston, TX 77030.
E-mail address: Kirti.Saxena@bcm.edu

Psychiatr Clin N Am 43 (2020) 95–111
https://doi.org/10.1016/j.psc.2019.10.009
0193-953X/20/© 2019 Elsevier Inc. All rights reserved.

Therefore, the recognition of mixed symptoms and specific treatments needs to be undertaken to impede illness progression and reduce future illness burden. This article provides an update on the epidemiology, clinical profile, and treatment of youth with PBD with mixed states.

EPIDEMIOLOGY

As defined by the Diagnostic and Statistical Manual of Mental Disorders, Fifth Edition (DSM-5), bipolar spectrum disorder (ie, BD type I, BD II, cyclothymic disorder, BD not otherwise specified, and unspecified BD and other-specified BD and related disorder) is a prevalent condition in adults, children, and adolescents.[4]

Global community surveys suggest lifetime prevalence of bipolar spectrum disorders to be approximately 2%.[5] Specifically, even though there are no current data on the prevalence of mixed states in PBD, studies report that a significant percentage of youth with PBD present with this mood phase. Indeed, 98% of 279 youth (6–15 years old) diagnosed with DSM-IV had mixed features[6]; 62% of 237 youth (10–17 years old) diagnosed with DSM-IV–Text Revision (TR) had mixed features[7]; mixed features were present in more than 50% of 115 youth with mania (aged 7–16 years)[8]; in 3 randomized treatment trials that each enrolled more than 200 youth with DSM-IV–diagnosed mania, mixed features were present at baseline in 42% to 98% of the youth.[6,7,9] Furthermore, mixed states were the most common presentation for outpatient youth with PBD in a major depressive episode,[10] and, among youth with BD II, mixed hypomania was a common presentation.[11]

CLINICAL PROFILE OF PEDIATRIC BIPOLAR DISORDER

Mixed features of PBD are present in children[12,13] and adolescents. However, clinicians should consider the developmental age of children/adolescents and place the symptoms they are presenting with in a developmental context. For example, manic symptoms in children take the shape of running out into the street, jumping from high places, and trying to jump out of a moving vehicle. Adolescents may have access to cars, credit cards, drugs, and alcohol and use these means to engage in high-risk behaviors. With regard to the grandiose criterion, children may state, "I teach better than the teacher," but, in reality they are failing the class. Or they describe themselves as being very good piano players, but in reality they are not. Or they may to try to jump off a roof like Superman and not recognize this as being a very dangerous behavior.[14] In contrast, depressive symptoms in children may manifest in different forms. For instance, children younger than 7 years of age may not be able to describe their internal mood states and may express their distress through vague somatic symptoms or pain. In adolescence, irritable mood may be the cause of angry, hostile behavior. Impaired attention, poor concentration, and anxiety may resemble attention-deficit/hyperactivity disorder, and substance abuse may be a means of self-medication for this subgroup of patients.[15] As a consequence, mixed features might also present in atypical forms, and this clinical picture is probably underestimated in this population. Therefore, an accurate and specific diagnosis is vital in children and adolescents presenting with mood symptoms. However, criteria used to diagnose BD using the DSM-5[3] are the same in children, adolescents, and adults,[16] thus biasing the impact of mixed states in the developmental age.

Compared with studies of adults with BD, youth with BD spend more time symptomatic and with mixed/rapid cycling, subsyndromal symptoms, and with more mood changes.[17] Adults and older adolescents are more likely to have classic manic and depressive symptoms and distinct episodes, whereas children with PBD tend to have more mood variations within an episode.[18] For example, a child experiencing an episode with mixed features may be irritable, grandiose, depressed, euthymic, or sometimes happy, and the distinct onset and offset of the episode may be difficult to determine. This clinical presentation may make it difficult to tease out the episodicity and symptoms of PBD with mixed features.

To clinicians, parents and caregivers state things such as, "My child is always irritable and aggressive and never sleeps; it is a roller-coaster of mood changes all the time." Moreover, children may not be able to vocalize symptoms clearly and it can be difficult to tease out normal behavior from manic and depressive mood states.[18] To this extent, it is for the clinician to tease out the specific duration of the mood episode, noticeable changes in symptoms and everyday functioning, over days to weeks, to ascertain true episodic mood changes.

Distinct episodes with manic and depressive symptoms can be elicited and endorsed by adolescents and their caregivers, allowing a clearer clinical presentation of mixed features in adolescents.[18]

Of significance, both children and adolescents with PBD are at significantly greater risk of suicide than other youth, and studies have reported higher rates of mixed episodes in suicidal than nonsuicidal children/adolescents.[19,20] In 407 adolescents (aged 12–18 years), of whom 38 had depression with mixed features (MXD), 79 had consensus bipolar, and 145 had depression only, patients in the MXD group were more likely to be suicidal at admission and showed overall greater impairment than the other 2 groups.[21] Also, female patients with PBD experiencing mixed states had nearly 4 times the risk of having made a suicide attempt compared with those without mixed states. Furthermore, they have 4 times higher risk of having a recent suicide attempt.[22]

It has been suggested that oscillating moods characterizing unipolar MXD could be a childhood precursor to bipolar spectrum disorders,[23] or mixed states may be a prodrome to PBD, possibly indicating features leading to a future manic episode.[21,24] Illness course of those experiencing mixed symptoms seems to be more severe, and chronic: in a 4-year longitudinal study of 413 youth (aged 7–17 years) with DSM-IV–diagnosed PBD, youth spent nearly 25% of follow-up time in syndromal or subsyndromal mixed episodes.[17,25]

Clinically, it is important to assess the specific features of mood states in children and adolescents. This assessment allows both the clinician and family to be aware of the course of the illness and prepare for the necessary levels of care possibly needed (ie, intensive outpatient and inpatient services).

COMORBIDITY

Comorbidity is defined as the occurrence of 2 syndromes in an individual, and implies that they are distinct categorical entities. Conditions comorbid with PBD include attention-deficit/hyperactivity disorder, anxiety disorder, oppositional defiant disorder, conduct disorder, and substance abuse.[26] In youth experiencing mood episode with mixed features, significantly higher levels of anger, anger expression, and posttraumatic stress disorder have been reported.[21]

In clinical practice, comorbidity is more the rule than the exception in youth with mixed states. Comorbid conditions add to the illness burden for both family and children, and require targeted intervention.

DIAGNOSING MIXED STATES IN PEDIATRIC BIPOLAR DISORDER

As noted earlier, DSM-5 criteria used to diagnose BD are the same in children, adolescents, and adults. However, while making a diagnosis of PBD in youth, developmental differences need to be taken into consideration. In the transition from DSM-IV-TR to DSM-5, the mixed states criteria for BD were revised.

Transition from Diagnostic and Statistical Manual of Mental Disorders, Fourth Edition, Text Revision, to Diagnostic and Statistical Manual of Mental Disorders, Fifth Edition

In DSM-IV-TR, mixed episodes are one of the mood states in BD I.[27] The DSM-IV-TR definition of a mixed state or episode requires meeting criteria both for a manic episode and for a major depressive episode almost every day for 1 week, thus limiting mixed states to only those patients who had depressive symptoms when manic (DSM-IV-TR). Using these criteria, individuals may be missed as having mixed states of BD, and may be diagnosed as BD, not otherwise specified. Further, the definition stated that the individual experiences rapidly altering moods, thus, capturing individuals experiencing mood lability or rapid cycling.[28]

In contrast, DSM-5 provides a mixed-features specifier to its definition of bipolar I, bipolar II and major depression.

During an episode of mania/hypomania, to be diagnosed as being in a mixed state using the DSM-5 specifier requires the presence of at least 3 symptoms of depression together with the episode of mania/hypomania. Depressive symptoms may include:

1. Prominent dysphoria or depressed mood
2. Anhedonia
3. Psychomotor retardation
4. Fatigue or low energy
5. Feelings of worthlessness or excessive guilt
6. Recurrent thoughts of death

During the most recent week of a manic episode or during the most recent 4 days of a hypomanic episode, at least 3 of these depressive symptoms must be present nearly every day.

Similarly, during an episode of major depression, to be diagnosed as having MXD using the DSM-5 specifier requires the presence of at least 3 manic/hypomanic symptoms that do not overlap with symptoms of major depression. Manic/hypomanic symptoms can include:

1. Elevated mood
2. Inflated self-esteem
3. More talkative
4. Flight of ideas
5. An increase in energy or goal-directed activity
6. Increased or excessive involvement in activities that have a high potential for painful consequences
7. Decreased need for sleep

In addition, during the most recent 2 weeks of the major depressive episode, at least 3 of these symptoms must be present nearly every day.[16]

The transition from mixed episodes to mixed features in the DSM-5 allows for individuals previously not diagnosed with mixed states using the DSM-IV-TR criteria to now be recognized as having mixed states. In addition, this specifier for mixed states in the DSM-5 may allow the identification of patients with unipolar depressive states more likely to progress to BD.[16]

The International Statistical Classification of Diseases and Related Health Problems (ICD-10) defines mixed states in bipolar affective disorder when an individual has had at least 1 hypomanic, manic, depressive, or mixed affective episode in the past, and the current episode by either a mixture or a rapid alternation (ie, within a few hours) of hypomanic, manic, and depressive symptoms. During a period of at least 2 weeks, both manic and depressive symptoms must be prominent most of the time. There is no specification for the severity of the episode.[29]

PHARMACOTHERAPY FOR MIXED OR MANIC STATES IN PEDIATRIC BIPOLAR DISORDER

There are no specific clinical trials only on mixed states in PBD. The clinical trials conducted to date have focused on manic/mixed states in PBD. Data on subgroup analyses of mixed states have not been described. With regard to medications approved by the US Food and Drug Administration (FDA) for the treatment of PBD, mixed or manic states, lithium and some atypical antipsychotics have FDA approval:[30]

For patients 10 to 17 years old
- Risperidone: 0.25 to 4 mg/d
- Aripiprazole: 2 to 30 mg/d
- Quetiapine: 50 to 600 mg/d
For patients 12 to 17 years old
- Lithium: 300 to 2400 mg/d
For patients 13 to 17 years old
- Olanzapine: 2.5 to 20 mg/d

In 2018, asenapine (sublingual) was also FDA approved for PBD, mixed or manic phase for patients 10 to 17 years old at a dose of 5 to 20 mg/d[31]

Clinical trials have documented the efficacy of lithium, anticonvulsants, and atypical antipsychotics in the treatment of manic and mixed symptoms in youth (10–17 years old).[30] Adverse effects (AEs) and toxicity of these drugs are important factors to consider while conducting clinical trials within the pediatric population. Among studies, the most common AEs for those participants who received lithium were headache, vomiting, gastrointestinal discomfort, enuresis, initial insomnia, upper respiratory tract infection, decreased appetite, and nasopharyngitis.[32–34] Less common potential side effects included leukocytosis, hypothyroidism, and renal tubular dysfunction. With lithium, it is important to monitor lithium blood levels, kidney and thyroid function, and electrocardiograms. With anticonvulsants, the most common AEs noted were headaches, nausea, and vomiting. Weight gain was associated more specifically with divalproex sodium (DVPX) and carbamazepine. More serious AEs included hyperammonemia (DVPX), thrombocytopenia (DVPX, carbamazepine), hepatotoxicity (carbamazepine, lamotrigine), and serious dermatologic reactions (Stevens-Johnson syndrome or toxic epidermal necrolysis with lamotrigine). However, trials have not reported any hyperammonemia. Overall, the AE profiles of antipsychotics differ from those of lithium and anticonvulsants. Abnormal involuntary movements such as tardive dyskinesia and extrapyramidal symptoms (EPSs) are a common concern with atypical antipsychotics. Trials that included treatment with quetiapine, lurasidone, risperidone, asenapine, and higher doses of aripiprazole associated them with a greater risk of EPSs. Risperidone, quetiapine, and olanzapine may increase prolactin levels, contribute to weight gain, and cause metabolic abnormalities (metabolic syndrome). Ziprasidone may also increase prolactin levels. Therefore, clinicians should monitor carefully for these adverse metabolic effects from these drugs.[30]

To date, clinical trials have been conducted using the DSM-IV or DSM-IV-TR criteria for diagnosing PBD, manic or mixed states (**Table 1**).

CLINICAL TRIALS WITH LITHIUM IN PEDIATRIC BIPOLAR DISORDER, MIXED OR MANIC STATES

Findling and colleagues[32] (2013) designed a clinical trial of the effectiveness of lithium over a period of 16 weeks. Youth (N = 41; 7–17 years old) who partially responded to 8 weeks of treatment with lithium (phase I) continued to be treated with lithium for another 16 weeks (phase II). During the continuation phase, mood remained stabilized in those youth who had initially responded to lithium as assessed by the Young Mania Rating Scale (YMRS) and Clinical Global Impressions–Improvement (CGI-I) scale. Notably, even with adjunctive medications, the youth who partially responded to lithium did not show more improvement during phase II.[32] In another 8-week randomized controlled trial (N = 81; 7–17 years old), compared with placebo, lithium significantly decreased manic symptoms and improved global functioning in youth with mixed or manic states.[33] To study whether lithium is effective in the maintenance treatment of youth with PBD, Findling and colleagues[34] (2019) designed a multicenter, double-blind, placebo-controlled discontinuation study. Youth in a manic or mixed state were treated for 24 weeks with lithium in one of 2 phases, the Collaborative Lithium Trials (CoLT phase 1 and CoLT phase 2). After being prerandomized to lithium for 24 weeks, which included completing 8 weeks of open-label lithium treatment followed by 16 weeks of open-label lithium treatment, 21 youth entered the study from CoLT phase 1. Also, 10 youth entered the study from CoLT phase 2, in which, before randomization, they received treatment with (1) 8 weeks of double-blind lithium, followed by 16 weeks of open-label lithium; or (2) 8 weeks of double-blind placebo followed by 24 weeks of open-label lithium. Youth who responded to lithium as determined by remaining euthymic for a period of 6 weeks based on YMRS and Children's Depression Rating Scale–Revised (CDRS-R) scores were randomized to continue lithium or be cross-titrated to placebo for up to 28 weeks. Any reason to discontinue the study was the primary outcome measure. In the 28-week discontinuation trial there were 31 youth, of whom 17 were randomized to lithium and 14 were randomized to placebo. Eleven lithium-treated youth completed the 28-week discontinuation trial.

Most youth discontinued the trial because of the emergence of mood symptoms. Overall, the safety and tolerability of the use of lithium as a maintenance treatment of youth with PBD is supported by this study.[34]

Clinical Trials with Anticonvulsants in Pediatric Bipolar Disorder, Mixed or Manic States

Anticonvulsants, namely DVPX, lamotrigine, and carbamazepine, do not have FDA approval for the treatment of children and adolescents with PBD, mixed or manic states. However, clinical trials have shown efficacy of these medications in the management of PBD, mixed or manic states.

Youth (N = 20 PBD type I and N = 22 PBD type II; 8–18 years old) received 6 weeks of open treatment with lithium, DVPX, or carbamazepine, and all 3 mood stabilizers showed a large effect size in treatment of these youth.[35]

In another study, youth (N = 40; 7–19 years old) participating in a 2-week to 8-week open-label study of DVPX followed by an 8-week double-blind, placebo-controlled study reported significant reduction in mood symptoms from baseline as assessed by the Mania Rating Scale, Manic Syndrome Scale, Behavior and Ideation Scale, Brief

Table 1
Randomized control trials

Title	Age (y)	N	DSM Diagnosis	Methods	Clinical Outcomes
Kowatch et al,[35] 2000: Effect Size of Lithium, Divalproex Sodium, and Carbamazepine in Children and Adolescents with Bipolar Disorder	8–18	42 youth (20 PBDI and 22 PBDII), mixed or manic	DSM-IV	6-wk open treatment with lithium, divalproex sodium, or carbamazepine	All 3 mood stabilizers showed a large effect size in treatment of these youth
Wagner et al,[36] 2002: An Open-Label Trial of Divalproex in Children and Adolescents with Bipolar Disorder	7–19	40 youth with PBD, manic, hypomanic, or mixed	DSM-IV	Open-label study (2–8 wk) of divalproex sodium followed by an 8-wk double-blind, placebo-controlled study	Significant reduction in mood symptoms from baseline as assessed by the MRS, Manic Syndrome Scale, Behavior and Ideation Scale, BPRS, CGI-S, and HAM-D
Findling et al,[37] 2003: Combination Lithium and Divalproex Sodium in Pediatric Bipolarity	5–17	96 youth with PBDI or PBDII, mixed, manic, hypomanic, depressed, euthymic	DSM-IV	20-wk open-label combination study of lithium and divalproex	Significant reduction in mood symptoms and improvement in functioning as assessed by the YMRS, CDRS-R and CGAS
Findling et al,[38] 2005: Double-Blind 18-Month Trial of Lithium vs Divalproex Maintenance Treatment in Pediatric Bipolar Disorder	5–17	60 youth with PBDI and PBDII, mania, hypomania, mixed	DSM-IV	Youth randomized to receive monotherapy with lithium (n = 30) or divalproex (n = 30) in an 18-mo randomized, double-blind comparison study	Divalproex was not found to be superior to lithium in youths that stabilized on combination therapy with lithium and divalproex
Pavuluri et al,[39] 2005: Divalproex Sodium for Pediatric Mixed Mania: A 6-month Prospective Trial	Mean, 12.3	34 youth with PBDI, mixed	DSM-IV	6-mo, open-label study	Significant reductions in YMRS and CDRS-R scores over the 6 mo

(continued on next page)

Table 1
(continued)

Title	Age (y)	N	DSM Diagnosis	Methods	Clinical Outcomes
DelBello et al,[40] 2006: A double-blind Randomized Pilot Study Comparing Quetiapine and Divalproex for Adolescent Mania	12–18	50 youth with PBDI, manic or mixed	DSM-IV-TR	28-d, double-blind, randomized study of quetiapine vs divalproex	Manic symptoms may decrease faster with quetiapine than divalproex sodium
Tohen et al,[45] 2007: Olanzapine Versus Placebo in the Treatment of Adolescents with Bipolar Mania	13–17	161 youth with PBD, manic or mixed	DSM-IV-TR	3-wk multicenter, parallel, double-blind, randomized, placebo-controlled trial. Youth randomized to olanzapine (2.5–20 mg/d [N = 107]) or placebo (N = 54)	Significant reduction in YMRS scores from baseline to end point in youth taking olanzapine compared with youth on placebo
Findling et al,[9] 2009: Acute Treatment of Pediatric Bipolar I Disorder, Manic or Mixed Episode, with Aripiprazole: A Randomized, Double-blind, Placebo-controlled Study	10–17	296 youth with PBDI, manic or mixed, with or without psychotic features	DSM-IV	Randomized, double-blind 4-wk study of aripiprazole 10 mg/d and 30 mg/d, and placebo	Aripiprazole found to be effective in reducing mania in doses of 10 mg/d or 30 mg/d compared with placebo
Haas et al,[47] 2009: Risperidone for the Treatment of Acute Mania in Children and Adolescents with Bipolar Disorder: A Randomized, Double-blind, Placebo-controlled Study	10–17	169 youth with PBDI, manic or mixed	DSM-IV	Randomized, placebo-controlled, double-blind study with placebo, risperidone (0.5–2.5 mg/d) or risperidone 3–6 mg/d for 3 wk	YMRS scores significantly reduced in youth treated with risperidone vs youth on placebo

Wagner et al,[41] 2009: A Double-blind, Randomized, Placebo-controlled Trial of Divalproex Extended-release in the Treatment of Bipolar Disorder in Children and Adolescents	10–17	150 youth with PBDI, manic or mixed	DSM-IV-TR	28-d double-blind study. Youth randomized to once-daily placebo or divalproex ER	From baseline to the end point, no statistically significant difference between divalproex ER and placebo
Biederman et al,[42] 2010: A Prospective Open-Label Trial of Lamotrigine Monotherapy in Children and Adolescents with Bipolar Disorder	6–17	39 youth with PBDI, PBDII, or PBD-NOS, manic, hypomanic, or mixed	DSM-IV	12-wk, open-label, prospective trial of lamotrigine monotherapy	Significant reduction in manic symptoms as assessed by mean YMRS scores and significant reduction in depressive, attention-deficit/hyperactivity disorder, and psychotic symptoms
Geller et al,[6] 2012: A Randomized Controlled Trial of Risperidone, Lithium, or Divalproex Sodium for Initial Treatment of Bipolar I Disorder, Manic or Mixed Phase, in Children and Adolescents	6–15	279 youth with PBDI, manic or mixed	DSM-IV	Controlled, randomized 8-wk parallel comparison of risperidone, lithium carbonate, and divalproex sodium in manic medication-naive youth	Risperidone found to be significantly more efficacious than lithium or divalproex sodium
Findling et al,[46] 2013: Aripiprazole for the Treatment of Pediatric Bipolar I Disorder: a 30-wk, Randomized, Placebo-controlled Study	10–17	296 PBDI, manic or mixed with or without psychotic features	DSM-IV	Randomized, double-blind, 30-wk, placebo-controlled study of aripiprazole (10 or 30 mg/d)	Both doses of aripiprazole (10 mg/d and 30 mg/d) at week 30 significantly improved mania and functioning compared with placebo

(continued on next page)

Table 1
(continued)

Title	Age (y)	N	DSM Diagnosis	Methods	Clinical Outcomes
Findling et al,[7] 2013: Efficacy, Long-Term Safety, and Tolerability of Ziprasidone in Children and Adolescents with Bipolar Disorder	10–17	237 youth with PBDI manic or mixed episodes	DSM-IV-TR	4-wk, randomized, double-blind, placebo-controlled multicenter study followed by a 26-wk open-label extension study	Ziprasidone resulted in a significant improvement in YMRS compared with placebo. In a subgroup of youth with symptoms of elation/euphoria and with a parental history of BD, posthoc analyses found ziprasidone to be efficacious
Findling et al,[32] 2013: Post-acute Effectiveness of Lithium in Pediatric Bipolar I Disorder	7–17	41 youth with PBDI, manic or mixed	DSM-IV	Youth who partially responded to 8 wk of treatment with lithium (phase I) were eligible to get lithium for an additional 16 wk	Youth who initially responded to lithium as assessed by YMRS and CGI-I maintained mood stabilization during continuation treatment. Youth who partially responded to lithium did not show more improvement during phase II, even with adjunctive medications
Findling et al,[33] 2015: Lithium in the Acute Treatment of Bipolar I Disorder: A Double-Blind, Placebo-Controlled Study	7–17	81 youth with PBDI/manic or mixed episodes	DSM-IV	8-wk randomized, double-blind, placebo-controlled study compared lithium vs placebo	Significant reduction in YMRS in lithium-treated youth compared with youth on placebo

Study	Age	Sample	Diagnostic criteria	Study design	Findings
Findling et al,[48] 2015: Asenapine for the Acute Treatment of Pediatric Manic or Mixed Episodes of Bipolar I Disorder	10–17	403 youth with PBDI in manic or mixed episodes	DSM-IV-TR	Double-blind, placebo-controlled. Youth randomized to placebo, asenapine 2.5, 5, or 10 mg twice daily	Significant reduction in YMRS with all asenapine doses vs placebo
Findling et al,[43] 2015: Adjunctive Maintenance Lamotrigine for Pediatric Bipolar I Disorder: A Placebo-Controlled, Randomized Withdrawal Study	10–17	298 youth with PBDI, depressed, manic/hypomanic, mixed mood states	DSM-IV-TR	A parallel-group, placebo-controlled, double-blind, randomized withdrawal study, open-label (up to 18 wk), and randomized (up to 36 wk)	Time to occurrence of mood episodes was delayed with the addition of lamotrigine with treatment effect favoring the use of lamotrigine in youth aged 13–17 y
Findling et al,[34] 2019: Lithium for the Maintenance Treatment of Bipolar I Disorder: A Double-Blind, Placebo-Controlled Discontinuation Study	7–17	31 youth with PBDI mixed or manic episodes	DSM-IV	Youth received 24 wk of lithium in either CoLT 1 or CoLT 2 in a double-blind, placebo-controlled discontinuation study. Responders randomized to continue lithium or be cross-titrated to placebo for up to 28 wk	Overall, the safety and tolerability and the use of lithium as a maintenance treatment of youth with PBD is supported by this study

Abbreviations: BPRS, Brief Psychiatric Rating Scale; CDRS-R, Children's Depression Rating Scale–Revised; CGAS, Children's Global Assessment Scale; CGI-S, Clinical Global Impression–Severity; CoLT, Collaborative Lithium Trial; ER, extended release; HAM-D, Hamilton Depression Rating Scale; MRS, Mania Rating Scale; PBDI, pediatric bipolar disorder I; PBDII, pediatric bipolar disorder II; PBD-NOS, pediatric bipolar disorder not otherwise specified; YMRS, Young Mania Rating Scale.

Psychiatric Rating Scale, Clinical Global Impressions Scale, and the Hamilton Depression Rating Scale.[36] Also, youth (N = 96; 5–17 years old) in mixed, manic, hypomanic, depressed, or euthymic states were enrolled into a 20-week open-label combination study of lithium and DVPX. Results revealed significant reductions in mood symptoms and improvement in functioning as assessed by the YMRS, CDRS-R, and Children's Global Assessment Scale.[37]

In 60 youth (5–17 years) who were randomized to receive monotherapy with lithium (n = 30) or DVPX (n = 30) in an 18-month randomized, double-blind comparison study, DVPX was not found to be superior to lithium in youths that stabilized on a combination therapy of lithium and DVPX.[38]

In a 6-month, open-label study using DVPX monotherapy in youth (N = 34; mean age 12.3 years), DVPX showed significant reductions in manic and depressive symptoms as assessed by the YMRS and the CDRS-R scores over 6 months.[39] Also, a 28-day, double-blind, randomized study of quetiapine versus divalproex in 50 youth (aged 12–18 years) with DSM-IV-TR–diagnosed PBD type I, manic or mixed episodes, revealed faster decrease in manic symptoms with quetiapine than with DVPX.[40]

In a 28-day double-blind study, youth (N = 150; 10–17 years old) were randomized to once-daily placebo or divalproex extended release (ER). From baseline to the end point, results reported no statistically significant difference between divalproex ER and placebo.[41]

A 12-week, open-label study with lamotrigine monotherapy reported significant reductions in manic, depressive, attention-deficit/hyperactivity disorder, and psychotic symptoms in youth (N = 39; 6–17 years old) with PBD.[42]

The Treatment of Early Age Mania (TEAM) study randomized medication-naive youth (N = 279; 10–15 years old) to risperidone, lithium, or DVPX for 8 weeks. At the end of week 8, 68.5% of youth randomized to risperidone were much or very much improved on the Clinical Global Impression for Bipolar Illness Improvement–Mania scale (CGI-BP), compared with 35.6% of those on lithium and 24.4% of those on DVPX.[6]

Findling and colleagues[43] (2015) conducted a multicenter study of the efficacy of adjunctive lamotrigine in youth in moderate manic/hypomanic, depressed, or mixed mood episodes. In an 18-week open-label phase, youth (N = 298; 10–17 years old) received lamotrigine. Those who remained on a stable dose of lamotrigine for 2 weeks with 6 consecutive weeks of having a score of 3 (mildly ill) on the CGI-BP were randomized for 36 weeks to double-blind lamotrigine or placebo. Because lamotrigine or placebo were adjunctive treatments, youth remained on a stable dose of their concomitant medications for treatment of BD. Time to occurrence of mood episodes was delayed with the addition of lamotrigine, with treatment effect favoring the use of lamotrigine in youth aged 13 to 17 years.

Clinical Trials with Atypical Antipsychotics in Pediatric Bipolar Disorder, Mixed or Manic States

As of 2009, risperidone, aripiprazole, and quetiapine have received FDA approval as monotherapy for the treatment of acute manic and mixed episodes in youth aged 10 to 17 years. Olanzapine has been approved for a similar indication in adolescents aged 13 to 17 years.[44]

In a 3-week multicenter, parallel, double-blind, randomized, placebo-controlled trial, youth (N = 161; 13–17 years old) were randomized to olanzapine (2.5–20 mg/d; N = 107) or placebo (N = 54). In youth taking olanzapine, there was a significant reduction in YMRS scores from baseline to end point compared with youth on placebo.[45]

Aripiprazole effectively decreased manic symptoms compared with placebo in youth (N = 296; 10–17 years old) enrolled in a randomized, double-blind, 4-week study of aripiprazole.[9] In a randomized, double-blind, 30-week, placebo-controlled study of aripiprazole (10 mg/d or 30 mg/d), both doses of aripiprazole at week 30 significantly improved mania and functioning in youth (N = 296; 10–17 years old) with PBD, compared with placebo.[46]

Risperidone effectively decreased manic symptoms compared with placebo in a 3-week randomized, double-blind, placebo-controlled study in youth (10–17 years) with DSM-IV diagnosis of BD I, manic or mixed episode.[47]

Ziprasidone was studied in a 4-week, randomized, double-blind, placebo-controlled, multicenter study followed by a 26-week open-label extension (OLE) study in youth (N = 237; 10–17 years old) with PBD. Compared with placebo, ziprasidone significantly decreased manic symptoms as assessed by the YMRS. The OLE phase showed that this improvement in manic symptoms remained over 6 months. In addition, in a subgroup of youth with symptoms of elation/euphoria and with a parental history of BD, posthoc analyses found ziprasidone to be efficacious.[7]

Asenapine was effective in reducing manic and mixed symptoms compared with placebo in a double-blind, placebo-controlled, parallel-group study conducted in 403 youth (10–17 years old) with PBD.[48]

Studies have not specifically investigated the effect of psychotropics on the mixed states of PBD. More studies need to be conducted specifically of the effectiveness and tolerability of psychotropics for youth in mixed states of PBD, with a focus on the long-term benefits and risks of these medications in youth.

Also, clinical trials conducted to date have used the DSM-IV or DSM-IV-TR criteria to diagnose PBD with mixed states. Using the DSM-5 criteria in future studies will allow a more distinct phenotype of mixed features. The diagnostic clarity of the mixed-features episode will allow targeted interventions. Then, clinical trials can further specifically recognize clinical responses to psychotropics in youth with mixed features.

RANDOMIZED CONTROLLED TRIAL
Guidelines for the Treatment of Mixed Features in Pediatric Bipolar Disorder

In randomized trials that established the efficacy of second-generation antipsychotics (SGAs) for PBD, a significant number of youth at baseline had mixed features.[40] SGAs have been noted to improve depressive symptoms in PBD with mixed features.[49] Thus, second-generation antipsychotics are suggested as first-line therapy for PBD, mixed features.[50] In youth with mania, a randomized trial comparing quetiapine with placebo showed improvement in depressive symptoms[6]; risperidone was superior to lithium or divalproex[6] in the TEAM study, in which 98% of the youth presented with mixed features; ziprasidone was superior to placebo in DSM-IV-TR–diagnosed mania,[7] of which mixed features were present in 62% of the youth; 42% of youth had DSM-IV–diagnosed mixed features in a study comparing aripiprazole with placebo, in which aripiprazole (10 mg or 30 mg daily) was effective and well tolerated for the acute treatment of PBD I, mania/mixed episodes.[9]

Differences in treatment response based on episode subtype (mania vs depression) in youth with mixed features have not been reported to date. Possibly, differences were not examined or insufficient power did not permit these analyses.

Electroconvulsive therapy (ECT) is used infrequently for adolescents and rarely for younger children,[51] and is used before a trial of clozapine for mania with mixed features. It may be beneficial for severe, persistent, and significantly disabling mania with mixed features that is refractory to multiple (at least 5) pharmacotherapy trials. Evidence supporting the use of ECT includes retrospective studies in youth as well as randomized trials in adults with mania.

FUTURE DIRECTIONS

Mixed features in children/adolescents are related to higher rates of chronicity, comorbidity, and suicide, as are mixed features in adults with BD. However, the continuing evolving development of the definition, course, diagnosis, and treatment of both PBD and mixed states substantially impedes a clear definition of specific diagnostic criteria and treatment strategies for such conditions. The use of the DSM-5 criteria will allow a more defined phenotype of mixed features in PBD and a more defined approach toward specific interventions. In addition, further research using biological markers such as neuroimaging, neurophysiology, neurocognition, and genetics can pave the way to study the underlying pathophysiology of mixed states in PBD.

DISCLOSURE

The authors have nothing to disclose.

REFERENCES

1. Danner S, Fristad MA, Arnold LE, et al. Early-onset bipolar spectrum disorders: diagnostic issues. Clin Child Fam Psychol Rev 2009;12(3):271–93.
2. Mazza M, Mandelli L, Zaninotto L, et al. Bipolar disorder: "pure" versus mixed depression over a 1-year follow-up. Int J Psychiatry Clin Pract 2012;16(2):113–20.
3. Sole E, Garriga M, Valenti M, et al. Mixed features in bipolar disorder. CNS Spectr 2017;22(2):134–40.
4. Goldstein BI, Birmaher B, Carlson GA, et al. The International Society for Bipolar Disorders Task Force report on pediatric bipolar disorder: Knowledge to date and directions for future research. Bipolar Disord 2017;19(7):524–43.
5. Birmaher B. Pediatric bipolar disorder: epidemiology and pathogenesis 2019. Available at: https://www.uptodate.com/contents/pediatric-bipolar-disorder-epidemiology-and-pathogenesis. Accessed April 25, 2019.
6. Geller B, Luby JL, Joshi P, et al. A randomized controlled trial of risperidone, lithium, or divalproex sodium for initial treatment of bipolar I disorder, manic or mixed phase, in children and adolescents. Arch Gen Psychiatry 2012;69(5): 515–28.
7. Findling RL, Cavus I, Pappadopulos E, et al. Efficacy, long-term safety, and tolerability of ziprasidone in children and adolescents with bipolar disorder. J Child Adolesc Psychopharmacol 2013;23(8):545–57.
8. Geller B, Tillman R, Bolhofner K, et al. Pharmacological and non-drug treatment of child bipolar I disorder during prospective eight-year follow-up. Bipolar Disord 2010;12(2):164–71.
9. Findling RL, Nyilas M, Forbes RA, et al. Acute treatment of pediatric bipolar I disorder, manic or mixed episode, with aripiprazole: a randomized, double-blind, placebo-controlled study. J Clin Psychiatry 2009;70(10):1441–51.
10. Dilsaver SC, Benazzi F, Akiskal HS. Mixed states: the most common outpatient presentation of bipolar depressed adolescents? Psychopathology 2005;38(5): 268–72.

11. Dilsaver SC, Akiskal HS. "Mixed hypomania" in children and adolescents: is it a pediatric bipolar phenotype with extreme diurnal variation between depression and hypomania? J Affect Disord 2009;116(1–2):12–7.

12. Renk K, White R, Lauer BA, et al. Bipolar disorder in children. Psychiatry J 2014; 2014:928685.

13. Carlson GA, Kotov R, Chang SW, et al. Early determinants of four-year clinical outcomes in bipolar disorder with psychosis. Bipolar Disord 2012;14(1):19–30.

14. Geller B, Zimerman B, Williams M, et al. Phenomenology of prepubertal and early adolescent bipolar disorder: examples of elated mood, grandiose behaviors, decreased need for sleep, racing thoughts and hypersexuality. J Child Adolesc Psychopharmacol 2002;12(1):3–9.

15. Bhatia SK, Bhatia SC. Childhood and adolescent depression. Am Fam Physician 2007;75(1):73–80.

16. American Psychiatric Association. Diagnostic and statistical manual of mental disorders, fifth edition. 5th edition. Washington, DC: American Psychiatric Association; 2013.

17. Birmaher B, Axelson D, Goldstein G, et al. Four-year longitudinal course of children and adolescents with bipolar spectrum disorders: the Course and Outcome of Bipolar Youth (COBY) study. Am J Psychiatry 2009;166(7):795–804.

18. Birmaher B. Bipolar disorder in children and adolescents. Child Adolesc Ment Health 2013;18(3):1–15.

19. Algorta GP, Youngstrom EA, Frazier TW, et al. Suicidality in pediatric bipolar disorder: predictor or outcome of family processes and mixed mood presentation? Bipolar Disord 2011;13(1):76–86.

20. Hauser M, Correll CU. The significance of at-risk or prodromal symptoms for bipolar I disorder in children and adolescents. Can J Psychiatry 2013;58(1):22–31.

21. Frazier EA, Swenson LP, Mullare T, et al. Depression with mixed features in adolescent psychiatric patients. Child Psychiatry Hum Dev 2017;48(3):393–9.

22. Dilsaver SC, Benazzi F, Rihmer Z, et al. Gender, suicidality and bipolar mixed states in adolescents. J Affect Disord 2005;87(1):11–6.

23. Singh MK, Chang KD, Kelley RG, et al. Early signs of anomalous neural functional connectivity in healthy offspring of parents with bipolar disorder. Bipolar Disord 2014;16(7):678–89.

24. Hunt J, Schwarz CM, Nye P, et al. Is there a bipolar prodrome among children and adolescents? Curr Psychiatry Rep 2016;18(4):35.

25. Birmaher B, Axelson D, Strober M, et al. Clinical course of children and adolescents with bipolar spectrum disorders. Arch Gen Psychiatry 2006;63(2):175–83.

26. Birmaher B. Pediatric bipolar disorder: comorbidity 2018. Available at: https://www.uptodate.com/contents/pediatric-bipolar-disorder-comorbidity/print. Accessed April 13, 2019.

27. Subramaniam M, Abdin E, Vaingankar JA, et al. Prevalence, correlates, comorbidity and severity of bipolar disorder: results from the Singapore Mental Health Study. J Affect Disord 2013;146(2):189–96.

28. American Psychiatric Association. In: Diagnostic and statistical manual of mental disorders, Fourth Edition, text revision. 4th edition. Washington, DC: American Psychiatric Association; 2000.

29. Grunze H, Vieta E, Goodwin GM, et al. The World Federation of Societies of Biological Psychiatry (WFSBP) guidelines for the biological treatment of bipolar disorders: acute and long-term treatment of mixed states in bipolar disorder. World J Biol Psychiatry 2018;19(1):2–58.

30. Sun AY, Woods S, Findling RL, et al. Safety considerations in the psychopharmacology of pediatric bipolar disorder. Expert Opin Drug Saf 2019;1–18.
31. Stepanova E, Grant B, Findling RL. Asenapine treatment in pediatric patients with bipolar I disorder or schizophrenia: a review. Paediatr Drugs 2018;20(2):121–34.
32. Findling RL, Kafantaris V, Pavuluri M, et al. Post-acute effectiveness of lithium in pediatric bipolar I disorder. J Child Adolesc Psychopharmacol 2013;23(2):80–90.
33. Findling RL, Robb A, McNamara NK, et al. Lithium in the acute treatment of bipolar I disorder: a double-blind, placebo-controlled study. Pediatrics 2015;136(5): 885–94.
34. Findling RL, McNamara NK, Pavuluri M, et al. Lithium for the maintenance treatment of bipolar I disorder: a double-blind, placebo-controlled discontinuation study. J Am Acad Child Adolesc Psychiatry 2019;58(2):287–296 e4.
35. Kowatch RA, Suppes T, Carmody TJ, et al. Effect size of lithium, divalproex sodium, and carbamazepine in children and adolescents with bipolar disorder. J Am Acad Child Adolesc Psychiatry 2000;39(6):713–20.
36. Wagner KD, Weller EB, Carlson GA, et al. An open-label trial of divalproex in children and adolescents with bipolar disorder. J Am Acad Child Adolesc Psychiatry 2002;41(10):1224–30.
37. Findling RL, McNamara NK, Gracious BL, et al. Combination lithium and divalproex sodium in pediatric bipolarity. J Am Acad Child Adolesc Psychiatry 2003;42(8):895–901.
38. Findling RL, McNamara NK, Youngstrom EA, et al. Double-blind 18-month trial of lithium versus divalproex maintenance treatment in pediatric bipolar disorder. J Am Acad Child Adolesc Psychiatry 2005;44(5):409–17.
39. Pavuluri MN, Henry DB, Carbray JA, et al. Divalproex sodium for pediatric mixed mania: a 6-month prospective trial. Bipolar Disord 2005;7(3):266–73.
40. DelBello MP, Kowatch RA, Adler CM, et al. A double-blind randomized pilot study comparing quetiapine and divalproex for adolescent mania. J Am Acad Child Adolesc Psychiatry 2006;45(3):305–13.
41. Wagner KD, Redden L, Kowatch RA, et al. A double-blind, randomized, placebo-controlled trial of divalproex extended-release in the treatment of bipolar disorder in children and adolescents. J Am Acad Child Adolesc Psychiatry 2009;48(5): 519–32.
42. Biederman J, Joshi G, Mick E, et al. A prospective open-label trial of lamotrigine monotherapy in children and adolescents with bipolar disorder. CNS Neurosci Ther 2010;16(2):91–102.
43. Findling RL, Chang K, Robb A, et al. Adjunctive maintenance lamotrigine for pediatric bipolar I disorder: a placebo-controlled, randomized withdrawal study. J Am Acad Child Adolesc Psychiatry 2015;54(12):1020–31.e3.
44. Physicians' desk reference. 63rd edition. Montvale (NJ): Thomson PDR, Inc; 2009.
45. Tohen M, Kryzhanovskaya L, Carlson G, et al. Olanzapine versus placebo in the treatment of adolescents with bipolar mania. Am J Psychiatry 2007;164(10): 1547–56.
46. Findling RL, Correll CU, Nyilas M, et al. Aripiprazole for the treatment of pediatric bipolar I disorder: a 30-week, randomized, placebo-controlled study. Bipolar Disord 2013;15(2):138–49.
47. Haas M, Delbello MP, Pandina G, et al. Risperidone for the treatment of acute mania in children and adolescents with bipolar disorder: a randomized, double-blind, placebo-controlled study. Bipolar Disord 2009;11(7):687–700.

48. Findling RL, Landbloom RL, Szegedi A, et al. Asenapine for the acute treatment of pediatric manic or mixed episode of bipolar I disorder. J Am Acad Child Adolesc Psychiatry 2015;54(12):1032–41.
49. Liu HY, Potter MP, Woodworth KY, et al. Pharmacologic treatments for pediatric bipolar disorder: a review and meta-analysis. J Am Acad Child Adolesc Psychiatry 2011;50(8):749–762 e39.
50. Axelson D. Pediatric bipolar disorder: overview of choosing treatment 2019. Available at: https://www.uptodate.com/contents/pediatric-bipolar-disorder-overview-of-choosing-treatment#H299888. Accessed April 24, 2019.
51. Connor DF. Electroconvulsive therapy, transcranial magnetic stimulation, and deep brain stimulation. In: Dulcan MK, editor. Dulcan's textbook of child and adolescent psychiatry. Washington, DC: American Psychiatric Publishing, Inc.; 2010. p. 795.

Perinatal Mixed Affective State: Wherefore Art Thou?

Alexia Emilia Koukopoulos, MD, PhD[a,b,c,]*,
Gloria Angeletti, MD[b,c,d], Gabriele Sani, MD[e,f,1],
Delfina Janiri, MD[b,c,d], Giovanni Manfredi, MD, PhD[b,c,d],
Georgios D. Kotzalidis, MD, PhD[b,c,d], Lavinia De Chiara, MD[b,c,d]

KEYWORDS

- Perinatal period • Postpartum • Peripartum • Pregnancy • Mixed affective state
- Mixed depression • Bipolar disorder • Women

KEY POINTS

- The mixed affective state during the perinatal period is the least studied affective mood state.
- The perinatal period is most vulnerable for the emergence of mood episodes in women.
- Depression with symptoms of an excitatory nature is common in clinical practice.
- Women present higher rates then men of mixed episodes during their life span; the perinatal period could be a time of particularly high risk for mixed episodes.

It is known to every clinician that at about the fifth or sixth day of the lying in period many women get nervous, irritable, depressed and demanding. This mood is somewhat similar to premenstrual tension.

—S. Haas, 1952[1]

…the phrase thinking too much ("kufungisisa") was also identified as both a cause and a symptom of depression by new mothers of the Shona people in Zimbabwe
—Thandi Davies et al., 2016[2]

INTRODUCTION

The perinatal period is the time frame in childbearing women's lives that includes the whole duration of pregnancy and the first 4 weeks (*Diagnostic and Statistical Manual of*

---

[a] SPDC, Azienda Ospedaliera Universitaria Policlinico Umberto I, Sapienza School of Medicine and Dentistry, Rome, Italy; [b] Centro Lucio Bini, Rome, Italy; [c] Azienda Ospedaliera Sant'Andrea, UOC di Psichiatria, Via di Grottarossa 1035, CAP 00189, Rome 00185, Italy; [d] NESMOS Department, Sapienza School of Medicine and Psychology, Sant'Andrea University Hospital, Rome, Italy; [e] Institute of Psychiatry, Università Cattolica del Sacro Cuore, Roma, Italy; [f] Department of Psychiatry, Fondazione Policlinico Universitario "Agostino Gemelli" IRCCS, Roma, Italy
[1] Present address: Institute of Psychiatry, Largo Francesco Vito 1, 00168 Roma
* Corresponding author. Viale dell'Università 30, Rome 00185, Italy.
E-mail address: alexiakoukopoulos@gmail.com

Psychiatr Clin N Am 43 (2020) 113–126
https://doi.org/10.1016/j.psc.2019.10.004
0193-953X/20/© 2019 Elsevier Inc. All rights reserved.

Mental Disorders, 5th edition [DSM-5] criteria) or up to the first year (commonly used in research and clinical practice) postpartum. This loosely defined window is universally considered the most vulnerable time for emergence of psychiatric disturbances in women.

The literature regarding perinatal psychiatric disorders has focused primarily on typical postpartum depression and on postpartum psychosis. The excitatory symptoms that often accompany depressive states has received less attention. The least studied affective mood state during the perinatal period is certainly the mixed affective state. However, major depression with symptoms of an excitatory nature is common in clinical practice.[3–5] The most striking difference is found between depressive syndromes characterized by inhibitory symptoms and those marked by disinhibition, which are of an opposite polarity. Symptoms like irritable mood, mood lability, inner tension, distractibility, psychomotor agitation, impulsivity, aggressiveness, racing or crowded thoughts, talkativeness, early insomnia, dramatic description of suffering, or weeping spells are frequently observed among patients diagnosed with a major depressive episode[6,7]; they are, in our view, symptoms of nervous excitability and constitute the essence of a mixed affective episode. In contrast, hypomanic symptoms of euphoria, grandiosity, and hypersexuality have been found less frequently.[8–12]

Compared with nonmixed depression, mixed depression (MxD) is considered to be more severe and worse in its clinical presentation, is more common in bipolar disorders (BD) and is more frequently associated with a family history of BD, younger age at onset, longer duration, higher prevalence of suicide attempts, and comorbidities, worse outcome, poorer response to treatments,[5,6,8,10] and higher switch rates with antidepressant treatment.[9,11–14]

Unlike unipolar disorder, where depression is twice as common in women, gender distribution in BD is more balanced; however, women have an increased risk of BD type II (BDII)/hypomania, rapid cycling, and mixed episodes.[15] Compared with men, women have higher rates of depressive mixed episodes,[16] mixed hypomania,[17] mixed episodes,[18–20] rapid cycling,[21] and atypical depressive features,[22] despite differences in applied criteria. Between 5% and 7% of men and 6.7% and 18.2% women show such symptoms.[20] Among patients with MxD, female gender has been associated with BDII diagnosis and hyperthymic temperament.[7]

Women with mood episodes during reproductive-related events (ie, premenstrual, perinatal, and menopausal transition) may be particularly sensitive to intense hormonal fluctuations,[23] which could influence neurochemical pathways linked to depression.[24,25] Early recognition and clinical diagnosis of perinatal excitatory symptoms is an important prerequisite to offer adequate treatment and to prevent the possible negative impact on child development.[26] Given the high rates of mixed affective states in women[7,22] and the high rates of mood recurrences during the perinatal period,[27,28] we hypothesized that the perinatal period would be a critical time for the onset of mixed affective states.

METHODS

We conducted a PubMed search (1974–2019) on July 3, 2019, using the following Boolean search strategy: (depressive[ti] OR depression[ti] OR "bipolar disorder"[ti] OR "mood disorder*"[ti] OR "affective disorder*"[ti] OR Psychosis[ti] OR Psychotic [ti]) AND (puerperal[ti] OR pregnan*[ti] OR postpartum[ti] OR perinatal[ti] OR child-birth[ti] OR postnatal[ti] OR peripartum[ti] OR delivery[ti]) AND (hyperactivity OR rest-lessness OR "mood lability" OR Irritability OR "racing thoughts" OR "inner tension" OR suicid* OR Impulsiv* OR dysphori* OR anger OR "increased libido" OR "mixed feature*" OR "mixed state*" OR "mixed symptom*" OR "mixed episode*" OR Insomnia OR hypomani* OR euphori* OR highs OR agitat*).

All authors viewed the search output and examined eligibility independently. Eligibility was determined through Delphi rounds, until complete consensus was reached. Eligible were studies focusing on depressive episodes in the perinatal period including pregnancy up to 1 year postpartum and/or detailing affective symptomatology in which the simultaneous presence of excitatory and inhibitory mood symptoms was reported. Excluded were studies reporting on perinatal nonmixed mood episodes without describing symptoms, and any unfocused or unrelated study. We excluded single case reports, reviews/meta-analyses, opinion papers without data such as letters and editorials, nonclinical studies, and animal studies. However, we used reviews for possibly identifying additional relevant studies from their reference lists.

We did not use the DSM-5 MxD mixed symptoms definition, but rather the psychopathology-oriented diagnostic definition (**Box 1**).[4,6,7,29–31] According to the DSM-5, at least 3 hypomanic or manic symptoms that do not overlap with major depression symptoms are needed to apply the "with mixed features" specifier to an major depressive episode case. In case of mania or hypomania, the presence of at least 3 depressive symptoms is required during the hypomanic or manic episodes to apply the specifier. In our clinical practice, we have seen the third and fourth criteria (namely, more talkative than usual or pressure to keep talking, and flight of ideas or subjective experience that thoughts are racing) frequently in MxD, but the other 5 criteria are extremely rare, if ever present. Furthermore, these criteria are closer to the research-based diagnostic criteria, which proved to be more reliable than the DSM-5 in a large sample.[32]

RESULTS

Mixed Affective States in the Perinatal Period

In contrast with the lack of data examining a relationship with the menstrual cycle or the menopause,[15] there is consistent evidence of a strong temporal relationship

---

Box 1
Koukopoulos' diagnostic criteria for mixed depression

Major depressive episode plus at least 3 of the following 8 items:
   Psychic agitation or inner tension
   Racing or crowded thoughts
   Irritability or unprovoked rage
   Absence of retardation
   Talkativeness
   Dramatic description of suffering or frequent spells of weeping
   Mood lability or marked reactivity
   Early insomnia

Adapted from Sani G, Vöhringer PA, Napoletano F, et al. Koukopoulos' diagnostic criteria for mixed depression: a validation study. J Affect Disord 2014;164:15; with permission.

between depressive,[33] manic, or mixed episodes of BD[34–39] and childbirth,[28,40–42] particularly in the first postpartum month.[43] Women with BD are at particular risk for developing mood symptoms postpartum.[44]

A mood episode during the perinatal period has been suggested as an indicator for BD.[45–47] Unlike depression, which can occur anytime postpartum, manic or mixed episodes are more likely to occur soon after delivery.[36,46,48]

The postpartum period also seems to be a time of high risk for a conversion from major depressive disorder to BD, which is more than 6%,[3,36] considerably higher than the about 1% per year in the general population, which fades away during longer follow-ups.[49] Furthermore, women at their first delivery are at a higher risk for BD diagnosis than women at their second or higher parity.[36]

Retrospective as well as prospective studies indicate that approximately 60% to 70% of women with BD experienced a mood episode during pregnancy and the postpartum period.[28,33,50] Rates as high as 67% were found for postpartum depression,[50] and between 25% and 50% for postpartum mania and psychosis.[39,41] Women in nonclinical populations who show hypo/manic symptoms immediately after delivery range from 9.6% to 20.4% across studies.[51–56]

Mixed episodes may occur during the perinatal period either in women with previously diagnosed BD or in those without a previous history of mood disorder, the 4-week criteria allowed by the DSM-5 seems to be insufficient.[57] Furthermore, depressive or dysphoric-mixed episodes seem to be more prevalent in pregnant than nonpregnant bipolar women.[58]

A hallmark study by Viguera and colleagues[28] estimated the risk of recurrence of mood episodes in BD women who continued or discontinued treatment with mood stabilizers during pregnancy in a prospective observational clinical cohort study. Most recurrences were depressive or dysphoric/mixed (74%), especially early in pregnancy, and exceeded by far manic-hypomanic episodes. The depressive-dysphoric versus manic-hypomanic prevalence became even more prominent after discontinuation of mood stabilizer treatment, compared with continued treatment. Predictors of recurrence included BDII disorder diagnosis, earlier onset, more recurrences/y, recent illness, use of antidepressants, and use of anticonvulsants rather than lithium.[28] The authors confirmed Marcé's 1858 original observations that pregnancy predisposed vulnerable patients to depressive-dysphoric recurrences.[59]

Within the international BRIDGE study,[60] higher BD rates in first episode postpartum depression were shown compared with first episode nonpostpartum depression. Women with first episode postpartum depression showed significantly more psychotic symptoms, atypical features, and MxD. They had younger age at onset, more prior episodes, episodes of short duration, first-degree relatives with BD, switches while on antidepressants, and seasonality of mood episodes.[60] Furthermore, first episode postpartum depression women scored significantly higher on the active/elated subscore of the 32-item self-rated Hypomania Checklist (HCL-32).[60]

Data from 276 BD women untreated during pregnancy showed 75.0% of them developing psychiatric episodes after delivery, with depressive episodes being the most frequent (79.7%), followed by DSM-IV-TR manic (13.5%), mixed (3.9%), and hypomanic episodes (2.9%). A history of psychotic symptoms during postpartum was associated with depression in 22.4% of patients, with mania in 67.8%, and with mixed episodes in 87.5%.[43] Younger age at onset, type I disorder, MDI cycle, and psychotic symptoms were associated with (hypo)manic or mixed postpartum episodes.[43,61]

In a recent study focusing on the prevalence of MxD during the postpartum period, Çelik and colleagues[62] included 63 postpartum women. The participants were administered the Beck Depression Inventory, the Edinburgh Postnatal Depression Scale (EPDS), the Mood Disorders Questionnaire, and the Modified HCL-32. The Mood Disorder Questionnaire scores of women "depressive" according to the EPDS cut-off scores, were significantly higher than those of women with EPDS scores lower than the cut-off. The modified hypomania scores were significantly higher in the women with higher depression scores compared with those scoring under the EPDS cut-off. According to the Modified HCL-32 results, 79.4% of women had at least 1 symptom, 71.4% of women had at least 3 symptoms, and 68.3% of women had at least 5 symptoms of MxD.[62] In other words, hypomanic symptoms were more prevalent in severe depression, which suggests that MxD is a more severe type of depression, in line with Koukopoulos, Sani, Ghaemi, and their colleagues.[29,30]

Clinical Characteristics

There is no consensus in the literature on what the typical clinical presentation of perinatal depressive episodes is. Some authors support that perinatal depression is indistinguishable from depressive episodes occurring at other times in a woman's life span,[63,64] whereas others point to particular symptom clusters in perinatal depressive episodes.[65] We sought studies describing perinatal episode symptomatology to highlight the importance and frequency of symptoms that would pertain to mixed affective episodes according to these broader criteria (see **Box 1**).[7] Overlapping manic symptoms as psychomotor agitation, irritability and mood lability were reported to be the most prevalent symptoms in MxD in nonperinatal populations, despite being all excluded from the DSM-5 specifier.[7,29,30]

Unfortunately, the great majority of studies in the perinatal research area uses the EPDS as the sole instrument both as screening and as diagnostic tool. Although the EPDS is valid and useful for the detection of depressive symptomatology, it is not designed to capture mixed or atypical symptomatology. At this time, there is no specific validated screening method to confirm the presence of postpartum mania or postpartum mixed episodes; hence, we review here studies that used instruments able to detect a broader spectrum of symptoms that included symptoms typically present in mixed affective states. The most common symptoms reported were dysphoria, irritability, anger, agitation, mood lability, early insomnia, racing thoughts, and impulsivity; we discuss these symptoms in detail.

Mood lability

Several studies reported that excitatory symptoms are common in women in the early postpartum period,[52,54,55,66–69] with an 8-fold increase in hypomanic symptoms soon after delivery, compared with pregnancy.[56] The emergence of these symptoms should not be confused with the physiologic happiness usually surrounding the arrival of a baby; a strong correlation has in fact been frequently observed between hypomanic symptoms in the early postpartum and depressive symptoms.[33,51,52,66,70–72] The prevalence rates of postpartum hypomanic symptoms ranged from 9.6% to 29% across studies 2 to 4 days after delivery.[33,51,73] In a South African sample, 17.5% of women met both cut-off scores for depression and hypomania on postpartum day 3. This subgroup had significantly higher depression scores at week 6 postpartum than the rest of the sample. The lability of mood, typically observed in women after birth, has been described as follows: they were "giggly," "excited," "oversensitive," "cried at nothing," "laughed at nothing," or were "up and down."[68]

Although detecting mood lability in the early postpartum period may require expert observation and interviewing, it has important implications for clinical management and longitudinal diagnosis.[74] In fact, a striking 83% of women with combined postpartum depression and postpartum hypomania on the Highs Scale had an BD diagnosis based on the Structured Clinical Interview for DSM-IV in 1 study.[75]

Irritability and anger

Irritability is the single mixed symptom most commonly reported in perinatal depressive episodes by these reviewed reports.[71,76] A depressive episode characterized by irritability or anger or aggressiveness could be defined as dysphoric depression.[77] Feelings of anger are reported in 75% of women meeting the criteria for postpartum depression.[78] High anger scores were reported both in the antenatal and in the postnatal periods, and anger was directed both inward (manifesting itself as self-denigration or suicidality) or outward (manifesting as anger attacks).[79] In the perinatal population, irritability that is manifested outwards has especially important consequences because it is mainly directed on children and/or partner, thus creating a negative familial environment.[80] A study of the effects of prenatal depression of the mother on the neonate noted many more correlations between prenatal anger than prenatal depression and neonatal outcomes.[81,82] Irritability, which may be considered as a proxy to anger, could be a hallmark of perinatal depressive episodes,[83,84] although, being excluded from DSM-5 criteria for depression and not being considered in the EPDS, it is not assessed routinely.

Agitation

The few studies we found that assessed agitation during perinatal episodes found higher rates of agitation in these episodes as compared with nonperinatal depressive episodes,[65] especially in patients with BD.[85] Lack of psychomotor retardation is also reported in depressive postpartum episodes, which should be considered a clue for mixicity.[86,87] Agitation is frequently correlated with suicidal ideation and thoughts of self-harm and should therefore always be taken into serious consideration.[88,89]

Early insomnia

Sleep disturbances are characteristic of the perinatal period for most women in the general population. Sleep is usually impaired during the last part of pregnancy owing to physical discomfort and even more so after delivery owing to neonate care, which is usually performed by the new mother, whether breastfeeding or not. Postpartum sleep, especially in patients with BD, may protect from perinatal episodes and its derangement may constitute a trigger for such episodes.[90] Insomnia is defined as difficulty falling asleep or returning to sleep in the absence of physical discomfort or environmental disturbances (eg, noise or demands from the infant). Insomnia is present in more than 50% of women seeking psychiatric help in the perinatal period and severe insomnia is present in 12%.[91] Early insomnia or difficulty falling asleep is in particular highly correlated with postpartum depressive symptoms,[92] which is a distinctive trait of atypical depressive episodes and may herald psychosis in women with BD.[90]

Suicidality

Suicide is the second leading cause of death in postpartum women, accounting for approximately 20% of postpartum mortality.[93,94] A prospective study found that 16.97% of women with major depressive disorder or BDII had thoughts of self-harm and 6.16% reported suicidal ideation during the first year postpartum.[95] Interestingly, women with thoughts of self-harm or suicidal ideation also reported higher levels of depression and hypomanic symptoms. High suicidality in depressed mothers has been associated with more sleep and eating problems, more anxiety, and more emotional lability compared with depressed mothers with low suicidality; the former also scored significantly higher on psychoticism scales.[96] Importantly, those who made actual attempts to take their lives used more violent and lethal methods (eg, jumping from a building, self-incineration, or intentional traffic accidents), indicating high intent.[97–99]

Racing or crowded thoughts

Even though racing or crowded thoughts are frequently observed in clinical practice among women during the perinatal period, it is a symptom that is scarcely reported in the literature. Interesting descriptions are given in a study by Davies and colleagues,[2] who examined experiences and explanations of depression among Xhosa-speaking pregnant women, mothers, and health workers in an urban township in Cape Town, South Africa. Interestingly, many of the expressions used by the women are descriptive of what we would label MxD. Here follow some of their descriptions:

- "It's when your brain is, is cramped … It's not focused on who I'm talking to, the brain is busy, it's under suffocation, and everything can just blow up right now."
- They are angry, and when they talk about their problems they cry.
- Thinking too much, and when she is thinking, it's like she is going to go mad, and lose control. For example, when she thinks, she can even scream thinking about committing suicide.
- Interestingly, the phrase thinking too much ("kufungisisa") was also identified as both a cause and a symptom of depression by the Shona people in Zimbabwe.
- One mother said that she knew she was depressed because she thinks until her "brain is tired."[2]

This example makes clear that racing thoughts are present across cultures and are perceived as part of a not better specified "depression."

Screening

Screening for the presence of mixed episodes in the perinatal period is currently performed with classical clinical interviews when there are suspicions for their presence. Routine mood assessments during the perinatal period focuses on depression and the sole instrument used is the EPDS,[100] yet many an investigator calls for careful screening for BD in women with their first onset of depression in the postpartum period, in cases of recurrence of depression immediately after delivery,[39] in treatment-resistant postpartum depression,[33] in depression with psychotic features, or in cases of a positive family history for BD.[27,75] To avoid missing the diagnosis of postpartum MxD, appropriate diagnostic tools should be used.

For the time being, several instruments validated in nonperinatal populations have been used and proved useful. The HCL-32 can be helpful in detecting hypomania and proved to be reliable and easy to administer, with measurement properties largely invariant across cultures.[101] The Highs Scale[51] addresses cognitive and affective symptoms of hypomania assessing feeling elated, being more active and/or more talkative than usual, racing thoughts, feeling like an especially important person, decreased sleep requirement, and difficult concentration. The Mood Disorder Questionnaire is a 15-item self-report inventory that assesses the lifetime prevalence of hypomanic or manic symptoms based on DSM-IV criteria.[102] The Koukopoulos Mixed Depression Rating Scale is the first rating scale specifically designed to assess MxD. It was developed to enable clinicians and research investigators to collect data assessing the presence and severity of symptoms of excitatory or mixed nature in people with a DSM-IV major depressive episode. It consists of 14 clinician-rated items and recently received validation.[103]

The conjoint application of these assessment tools may be useful in completing our knowledge of patients who all too often suffer undiagnosed BD and whose mixed states are missed, with deleterious consequences on their optimal treatment.

Limitations

Because this is not a systematic review, caveats of nonsystematic reviews such as the lack of exhaustive review of the literature and formal data extraction apply.

SUMMARY AND FUTURE PERSPECTIVES

Mixed symptoms seem to be common in the perinatal period, even though they are scarcely noted in the literature. The neglect of modern psychiatry on mixed affective states is probably rooted in our current nosologic approach and this holds true, especially in the perinatal area where the term postpartum depression has encompassed all types depressive episodes and the term postpartum psychosis all types of manic episodes with a clear cut distinction between the two.

It is not easy to resolve the puzzle why the perinatal period is a vulnerable one, beginning with the third trimester of pregnancy, for the expression of MxD, but it could be related to excitability changes in the stress system and in particular, in GABAergic activity, which is influenced by neurosteroids. This has been shown in the mouse[104,105] and may occur also in the human; recent data point to the efficacy of the allopregnanolone analog, brexanolone, in treating postpartum depression.[1] Future studies should address whether GABAergic instability in late pregnancy and puerperium is related with a higher rate of mixed symptoms.

In our view, the diagnostic evaluation, even for women who present for depression should include questions on manic, hypomanic, and mixed symptoms to differentiate MxD from the classic melancholic states. We propose to carefully evaluate any case of perinatal depression that raises clinical suspicions for bipolarity and to consider the Koukopoulos' scale, or other similar criteria, for identifying mixed states. This should impact the treatment of women with MxD, because commonly prescribed antidepressants, which are associated with cycle acceleration and switch to opposite polarity, would not be the optimal treatment for this condition.

REFERENCES

1. Haas S. Psychiatric complications in gynecology and obstetrics. In: Bellack L, editor. Psychology of physical illness: psychiatry applied to medicine, surgery and the specialties. New York: Grune & Stratton; 1952.
2. Davies T, Schneider M, Nyatsanza M, et al. The sun has set even though it is morning": experiences and explanations of perinatal depression in an urban township, Cape Town. Transcult Psychiatry 2016;53(3):286–312.
3. Sharma V, Xie B, Campbell MK, et al. A prospective study of diagnostic conversion of major depressive disorder to bipolar disorder in pregnancy and postpartum. Bipolar Disord 2014;16(1):16–21.
4. Koukopoulos A, Sani G, Koukopoulos AE, et al. Melancholia agitata and mixed depression. Acta Psychiatr Scand 2007;115(Suppl. 433):50–7.
5. Maj M, Pirozzi R, Magliano L, et al. Agitated depression in bipolar I disorder: prevalence, phenomenology, and outcome. Am J Psychiatry 2003;160:2134–40.
6. Koukopoulos A, Albert MJ, Sani G, et al. Mixed depressive states: nosologic and therapeutic issues. Int Rev Psychiatry 2005;17:21–37.
7. Sani G, Vöhringer PA, Napoletano F, et al. Koukopoulos diagnostic criteria for mixed depression: a validation study. J Affect Disord 2014;164:14–8.

8. Akiskal HS, Benazzi F. Family history validation of the bipolar nature of depressive mixed states. J Affect Disord 2003;73:113–22.
9. Sato T, Bottlender R, Schröter A, et al. Frequency of manic symptoms during a depressive episode and unipolar 'depressive mixed state' as bipolar spectrum. Acta Psychiatr Scand 2003;107(4):268–74.
10. Maj M, Pirozzi R, Magliano L, et al. Agitated "unipolar" major depression: prevalence, phenomenology, and outcome. J Clin Psychiatry 2006;67(5):712–9.
11. Goldberg JF, Perlis RH, Bowden CL, et al. Manic symptoms during depressive episodes in 1,380 patients with bipolar disorder: findings from the STEP-BD. Am J Psychiatry 2009;166(2):173–81.
12. Perugi G, Angst J, Azorin JM, et al, BRIDGE-II-Mix Study Group. Mixed features in patients with a major depressive episode: the BRIDGE-II-MIX study. J Clin Psychiatry 2015;76(3):e351–8.
13. Bottlender R, Sato T, Kleindienst N, et al. Mixed depressive features predict maniform switch during treatment of depression in bipolar I disorder. J Affect Disord 2004;78(2):149–52.
14. Vieta E, Grunze H, Azorin JM, et al. Phenomenology of manic episodes according to the presence or absence of depressive features as defined in DSM-5: results from the IMPACT self-reported online survey. J Affect Disord 2014;156:206–13.
15. Diflorio A, Jones I. Is sex important? Gender differences in bipolar disorder. Int Rev Psychiatry 2010;22(5):437–52.
16. Cassidy F, Carroll BJ. The clinical epidemiology of pure and mixed manic episodes. Bipolar Disord 2001;3:35–40.
17. Suppes T, Mintz J, McElroy SL, et al. Mixed hypomania in 908 patients with bipolar disorder evaluated prospectively in the Stanley Foundation Bipolar Treatment Network: a sex-specific phenomenon. Arch Gen Psychiatry 2005;62:1089–96.
18. Grant BF, Stinson FS, Hasin DS, et al. Prevalence, correlates, and comorbidity of bipolar I disorder and axis I and II disorders: results from the National Epidemiologic Survey on alcohol and related conditions. J Clin Psychiatry 2005;66:1205–15.
19. Kessing LV. Gender differences in the phenomenology of bipolar disorder. Bipolar Disord 2004;6:421–5.
20. Kessing LV. The prevalence of mixed episodes during the course of illness in bipolar disorder. Acta Psychiatr Scand 2008;117:216–24.
21. Robb JC, Young LT, Cooke RG, et al. Gender differences in patients with bipolar disorder influence outcome in the medical outcomes survey (SF-20) subscale scores. J Affect Disord 1998;49:189–93.
22. Benazzi F. The role of gender in depressive mixed state. Psychopathology 2003;36:213–7.
23. Soares CN, Zitek B. Reproductive hormone sensitivity and risk for depression across the female life cycle: a continuum of vulnerability? J Psychiatry Neurosci 2008;33:331–43.
24. Schmidt PJ, Nieman LK, Danaceau MA, et al. Differential behavioral effects of gonadal steroids in women with and in those without premenstrual syndrome. N Engl J Med 1998;338:209–16.
25. Bloch M, Schmidt PJ, Danaceau M, et al. Effects of gonadal steroids in women with a history of postpartum depression. Am J Psychiatry 2000;157:924–30.
26. Rusner M, Berg M, Begley C. Bipolar disorder in pregnancy and childbirth: a systematic review of outcomes. BMC Pregnancy Childbirth 2016;16(1):331.

27. Sharma V, Khan M, Corpse C, et al. Missed bipolarity and psychiatric comorbidity in women with postpartum depression. Bipolar Disord 2008;10:742–7.

28. Viguera AC, Whitfield T, Baldessarini RJ, et al. Risk of recurrence in women with bipolar disorder during pregnancy: prospective study of mood stabilizer discontinuation. Am J Psychiatry 2007;164:1817–24.

29. Koukopoulos A, Sani G, Ghaemi SN. Mixed features of depression: why DSM-5 is wrong (and so was DSM-IV). Br J Psychiatry 2013;203(1):3–5.

30. Koukopoulos A, Sani G. DSM-5 criteria for depression with mixed features: a farewell to mixed depression. Acta Psychiatr Scand 2014;129(1):4–16.

31. Sani G, Tondo L, Koukopoulos A, et al. Suicide in a large population of former psychiatric inpatients. Psychiatry Clin Neurosci 2011;65(3):286–95.

32. Mazzarini L, Kotzalidis GD, Piacentino D, et al, BRIDGE-II-Mix Study Group. Is recurrence in major depressive disorder related to bipolarity and mixed features? Results from the BRIDGE-II-Mix study. J Affect Disord 2018;229:164–70.

33. Sharma V, Khan M. Identification of bipolar disorder in women with postpartum depression. Bipolar Disord 2010;12:335–40.

34. Kendell RE, Chalmers JC, Platz C. Epidemiology of puerperal psychosis. Br J Psychiatry 1987;150:662–73.

35. Kadrmas A, Winokur G, Crowe R. Postpartum mania. Br J Psychiatry 1979;135: 551–4.

36. Munk-Olsen T, Jones I, Laursen TM. Birth order and postpartum psychiatric disorders. Bipolar Disord 2014;16(3):300–7.

37. Hunt N, Silverstone T. Does puerperal illness distinguish a subgroup of bipolar patients? J Affect Disord 1995;34:101–7.

38. Valdimarsdottir U, Hultman CM, Harlow B, et al. Psychotic illness in first-time mothers with no previous psychiatric hospitalizations: a population-based study. PLoS Med 2009;6:e13.

39. Brockington I, Margison F, Schofield E, et al. The clinical picture of the depressed form of puerperal psychosis. J Affect Disord 1998;15:29–37.

40. Heron J, Robertson Blackmore E, McGuinness M, et al. No 'latent period' in the onset of bipolar affective puerperal psychosis. Arch Womens Ment Health 2007; 10(2):79–81.

41. Jones I, Craddock N. Bipolar disorder and childbirth: the importance of recognising risk. Br J Psychiatry 2005;186:453–4.

42. Viguera AC, Nonacs R, Cohen LS, et al. Risk of recurrence of bipolar disorder in pregnant and nonpregnant women after discontinuing lithium maintenance. Am J Psychiatry 2000;157:179–84.

43. Maina G, Rosso G, Aguglia A, et al. Recurrence rates of bipolar disorder during the postpartum period: a study on 276 medication-free Italian women. Arch Womens Ment Health 2014;17(5):367–72.

44. Viguera AC, Tondo L, Koukopoulos AE, et al. Episodes of mood disorders in 2,252 pregnancies and postpartum periods. Am J Psychiatry 2011;168(11): 1179–85.

45. Howard LM, Molyneaux E, Dennis C-L, et al. Non-psychotic mental disorders in the perinatal period. Lancet 2014;384:1775–88.

46. Jones I, Chandra PS, Dazzan P, et al. Bipolar disorder, affective psychosis, and schizophrenia in pregnancy and the postpartum period. Lancet 2014;384: 1789–99.

47. Khan M, Sharma V. Post-partum depressive episodes and bipolar disorder. Lancet 2015;385:771–2.

48. Wesseloo R, Kamperman AM, Munk-Olsen T, et al. Risk of postpartum relapse in bipolar disorder and postpartum psychosis: a systematic review and meta-analysis. Am J Psychiatry 2016;173(2):117–27.
49. Musliner KL, Østergaard SD. Patterns and predictors of conversion to bipolar disorder in 91 587 individuals diagnosed with unipolar depression. Acta Psychiatr Scand 2018;137(5):422–32.
50. Freeman MP, Smith KW, Freeman SA, et al. The impact of reproductive events on the course of bipolar disorder in women. J Clin Psychiatry 2002;63(4):284–7.
51. Glover V, Liddle P, Taylor A, et al. Mild hypomania (the highs) can be a feature of the first postpartum week: association with later depression. Br J Psychiatry 1994;164:517–21.
52. Lane A, Keville R, Morris M, et al. Postnatal depression and elation among mothers and their partners: prevalence and predictors. Br J Psychiatry 1997; 171:550–5.
53. Hasegawa M. Mild hypomania phenomenon in Japanese puerperal women. Nurs Health Sci 2000;2:231–5.
54. Webster J, Pritchard MA, Creedy D, et al. A simplified predictive index for the detection of women at risk for postnatal depression. Birth 2003;30:101–8.
55. Farias ME, Wenk E, Cordero M. Adaptacion de la escala highs para la deteccion de sintomatologia hipomaniaca en el puerperio. Trastornos Del Animo 2007;3: 27–36.
56. Heron J, Haque S, Oyebode F, et al. A longitudinal study of hypomania and depression symptoms in pregnancy and the postpartum period. Bipolar Disord 2009;11:410–7.
57. Sharma V, Mazmanian D. The DSM-5 peripartum specifier: prospects and pitfalls. Arch Womens Ment Health 2014;17(2):171–3.
58. Viguera AC, Baldessarini RJ, Tondo L. Response to lithium maintenance treatment in bipolar disorders: comparison of women and men. Bipolar Disord 2001;3(5):245–52.
59. Marcé LV. Traité de la Folie des Femmes Enceintes: Des Nouvelles Accouchés et des Nourrices. Paris: Baillière et Fils; 1858.
60. Azorin JM, Angst J, Gamma A, et al. Identifying features of bipolarity in patients with first-episode postpartum depression: findings from the international BRIDGE study. J Affect Disord 2012;136(3):710–5.
61. Rybakowski JK, Suwalska A, Lojko D, et al. Types of depression more frequent in bipolar than in unipolar affective illness: results of the Polish DEP-BI study. Psychopathology 2007;40(3):153–8.
62. Çelik SB, Bucaktepe GE, Uludağ A, et al. Screening mixed depression and bipolarity in the postpartum period at a primary health care center. Compr Psychiatry 2016;71:57–62.
63. Colom F, Cruz N, Pacchiarotti I, et al. Postpartum bipolar episodes are not distinct from spontaneous episodes: implications for DSM-V. J Affect Disord 2010;126(1–2):61–4.
64. Whiffen VE, Gotlib IH. Comparison of postpartum and nonpostpartum depression: clinical presentation, psychiatric history, and psychosocial functioning. J Consult Clin Psychol 1993;61(3):485–94.
65. Bernstein IH, Rush AJ, Yonkers K, et al. Symptom features of postpartum depression: are they distinct? Depress Anxiety 2008;25(1):20–6.
66. Sharma V, Burt VK, Ritchie HL. Bipolar II postpartum depression: detection, diagnosis, and treatment. Am J Psychiatry 2009;166(11):1217–21.

67. Smith S, Heron J, Haque S, et al. Measuring hypomania in the postpartum: a comparison of the Highs Scale and the Altman Mania Rating Scale. Arch Womens Ment Health 2009;12(5):323–7.

68. Pingo J, van den Heuvel LL, Vythylingum B, et al. Probable postpartum hypomania and depression in a South African cohort. Arch Womens Ment Health 2017; 20(3):427–37.

69. Leight KL, Fitelson EM, Weston CA, et al. Childbirth and mental disorders. Int Rev Psychiatry 2010;22:453–71.

70. O'Hara MW. Postpartum depression: what we know. J Clin Psychol 2009;65: 1258–69.

71. Pitt B. Atypical depression following childbirth. Br J Psychiatry 1968;114: 1325–35.

72. McCoy SJG, Beal JM, Payton ME, et al. Correlations of visual analog scales with Edinburgh Postnatal Depression Scale. J Affect Disord 2005;86(2–3):295–7.

73. Ballinger CB, Kay DS, Naylor GJ, et al. Some biochemical findings during pregnancy and after delivery in relation to mood change. Psychol Med 1982;12: 549–56.

74. Robin AA. The psychological changes of normal parturition. Psychiatr Q 1962; 36:129–50.

75. Sharma V. Management of bipolar II disorder during pregnancy and the postpartum period–Motherisk Update 2008. Can J Clin Pharmacol 2009;16(1): e33–41.

76. Andrews-Fike C. A review of postpartum depression. Prim Care Companion J Clin Psychiatry 1999;1(1):9–14.

77. Maloni JA, Park S, Anthony MK, et al. Measurement of antepartum depressive symptoms during high-risk pregnancy. Res Nurs Health 2005;28(1):16–26.

78. Shlomi Polachek I, Huller Harari L, Baum M, et al. Postpartum anxiety in a cohort of women from the general population: risk factors and association with depression during last week of pregnancy, postpartum depression and postpartum PTSD. Isr J Psychiatry Relat Sci 2014;51(2):128–34.

79. Field T, Diego M, Hernandez-Reif M, et al. Pregnancy anxiety and comorbid depression and anger: effects on the fetus and neonate. Depress Anxiety 2003;17(3):140–51.

80. Ou CH, Hall WA. Anger in the context of postnatal depression: an integrative review. Birth 2018;45(4):336–46.

81. Field T, Diego M, Hernandez-Reif M, et al. Prenatal anger effects on the fetus and neonate. J Obstet Gynaecol 2002;22(3):260–6.

82. Slomian J, Honvo G, Emonts P, et al. Consequences of maternal postpartum depression: a systematic review of maternal and infant outcomes. Womens Health (Lond) 2019;15. 1745506519844044. [Erratum appears in Womens Health (Lond) 2019;15:1745506519854864].

83. Williamson JA, O'Hara MW, Stuart S, et al. Assessment of postpartum depressive symptoms: the importance of somatic symptoms and irritability. Assessment 2015;22(3):309–18.

84. Kettunen P, Koistinen E, Hintikka J. Is postpartum depression a homogenous disorder: time of onset, severity, symptoms and hopelessness in relation to the course of depression. BMC Pregnancy Childbirth 2014;14:402.

85. Fisher SD, Wisner KL, Clark CT, et al. Factors associated with onset timing, symptoms, and severity of depression identified in the postpartum period. J Affect Disord 2016;203:111–20.

86. Fox M, Sandman CA, Davis EP, et al. A longitudinal study of women's depression symptom profiles during and after the postpartum phase. Depress Anxiety 2018;35(4):292–304.

87. Hoertel N, López S, Peyre H, et al. Are symptom features of depression during pregnancy, the postpartum period and outside the peripartum period distinct? Results from a nationally representative sample using item response theory (IRT). Depress Anxiety 2015;32(2):129–40.

88. Serra F, Gordon-Smith K, Perry A, et al. Agitated depression in bipolar disorder. Bipolar Disord 2019. https://doi.org/10.1111/bdi.12778.

89. Kamperman AM, Veldman-Hoek MJ, Wesseloo R, et al. Phenotypical characteristics of postpartum psychosis: a clinical cohort study. Bipolar Disord 2017; 19(6):450–7.

90. Sharma V, Mazmanian D. Sleep loss and postpartum psychosis. Bipolar Disord 2003;5(2):98–105.

91. Swanson LM, Pickett SM, Flynn H, et al. Relationships among depression, anxiety, and insomnia symptoms in perinatal women seeking mental health treatment. J Womens Health (Larchmt) 2011;20(4):553–8.

92. Goyal D, Gay C, Lee K. Fragmented maternal sleep is more strongly correlated with depressive symptoms than infant temperament at three months postpartum. Arch Womens Ment Health 2009;12(4):229–37.

93. Lindahl V, Pearson JL, Colpe L. Prevalence of suicidality during pregnancy and the postpartum. Arch Womens Ment Health 2005;8(2):77–87.

94. Cantwell R, Clutton-Brock T, Cooper G, et al. Saving Mothers' Lives: reviewing maternal deaths to make motherhood safer: 2006-2008. The Eighth Report of the Confidential Enquiries into Maternal Deaths in the United Kingdom. BJOG 2011;118(Suppl 1):1–203 [Erratum appears in BJOG. 2015;122(5):e1].

95. Dudek D, Jaeschke R, Siwek M, et al. Postpartum depression: identifying associations with bipolarity and personality traits. Preliminary results from a cross-sectional study in Poland. Psychiatry Res 2014;215(1):69–74.

96. Paris R, Bolton RE, Weinberg MK. Postpartum depression, suicidality, and mother-infant interactions. Arch Womens Ment Health 2009;12(5):309–21.

97. Henshaw C. Maternal suicide. In: Cockburn J, Pawson M, editors. Psychological challenges in obstetrics and gynecology: the clinical Management. New York: Springer; 2007. p. 157–64.

98. Högberg U, Innala E, Sandström A. Maternal mortality in Sweden, 1980–1988. Obstet Gynecol 1994;84:240–4.

99. Appleby L. Suicide after pregnancy and the first postnatal year. Br Med J 1991; 302:137–40.

100. Cox JL, Holden JM, Sagovsky R. Detection of postnatal depression. Development of the 10-item Edinburgh Postnatal Depression Scale. Br J Psychiatry 1987;150:782–6.

101. Angst J, Meyer TD, Adolfsson R, et al. Hypomania: a transcultural perspective. World Psychiatry 2010;9(1):41–9.

102. Hirschfeld RM, Williams JB, Spitzer RL, et al. Development and validation of a screening instrument for bipolar spectrum disorder: the Mood Disorder Questionnaire. Am J Psychiatry 2000;157(11):1873–5.

103. Sani G, Vöhringer PA, Barroilhet SA, et al. The Koukopoulos Mixed Depression Rating Scale (KMDRS): an International Mood Network (IMN) validation study of a new mixed mood rating scale. J Affect Disord 2018;232:9–16.

104. Maguire J, Ferando I, Simonsen C, et al. Excitability changes related to GABAA receptor plasticity during pregnancy. J Neurosci 2009;29(30): 9592–601.
105. Zheng W, Cai DB, Zheng W, et al. Brexanolone for postpartum depression: a meta-analysis of randomized controlled studies. Psychiatry Res 2019; 279:83–9.

Mixed States in Patients with Substance and Behavioral Addictions

Marco Di Nicola, MD, PhD[a],*, Maria Pepe, MD[a],
Marco Modica, MD[a], Pierluigi Lanzotti, MD[a],
Isabella Panaccione, MD, PhD[b,c], Lorenzo Moccia, MD[a],
Luigi Janiri, MD[a],*

KEYWORDS

- Mixed features • Bipolar disorders • Addictive behaviors • Personalized medicine

KEY POINTS

- Mixed states, affecting approximately 40% of patients with mood disorders, frequently co-occur with addictive disorders (AD). Substance misuse modifies the clinical presentation, promoting the onset of mixed features.
- Mixed symptoms and AD are associated with poor outcome, treatment resistance, more frequent recurrences and hospitalizations, susceptibility to rapid cycling, higher health care costs, and increased risk of suicide.
- AD and mood disorders share some neurobehavioral underpinnings, such as monoamine dysregulation, circadian rhythm alterations, predisposing genetic factors, abnormalities in the hypothalamic-pituitary-adrenal axis, specific impaired Response Inhibition and Salience Attribution (iRISA) networks.
- Increased impulsivity and affective instability seem to be common psychopathological features of bipolar disorder and AD, being involved in the onset of both diseases and correlating with detrimental outcome.
- Treating mixed states, especially with comorbid AD, can be particularly challenging because of increased clinical vulnerability and less favorable response to currently available pharmacotherapeutic agents.

INTRODUCTION

The occurrence of mixed affective states throughout the whole spectrum of mood disorders represents a challenge for clinicians at diagnostic, nosographic, and

[a] Fondazione Policlinico Universitario "A. Gemelli" IRCCS, Università Cattolica del Sacro Cuore, L.go Agostino Gemelli 8, Rome 00168, Italy; [b] Mental Health Department, ASL Roma1, Piazza di Santa Maria della Pietà 5, Rome 00135, Italy; [c] Centro Lucio Bini, via Crescenzio 42, Rome 00193, Italy
* Corresponding authors.
E-mail addresses: marcodinicola.md@gmail.com (M.D.N.); luigi.janiri@unicatt.it (L.J.)

Psychiatr Clin N Am 43 (2020) 127–137
https://doi.org/10.1016/j.psc.2019.10.012
0193-953X/20/© 2019 Elsevier Inc. All rights reserved.

therapeutic levels.[1] Mixed episodes were first described by Kraepelin and Weygandt and repeatedly reconceptualized over the years.[2] In the Diagnostic and Statistical Manual of Mental Disorders, Fifth Edition (DSM-5), the term "mixed episode" was eventually replaced by the "with mixed features" specifier, which can be applied to episodes of major depression, hypomania, or mania.[3] This change allows clinicians to diagnose mixed features even in subjects without an established bipolar disorder (BD), reflecting the increasing relevance that researchers are attributing to these peculiar presentations. In fact, mixed states are common (affecting approximately 40% of patients with mood disorders),[4,5] predict a poor symptomatic and functional outcome, and are associated with treatment resistance, more frequent recurrences and hospitalizations, susceptibility to rapid cycling, higher health care costs, and increased risk of suicide.[6,7] In addition, subjects developing mixed episodes during the course of illness are more likely to have experienced early-life stressors and to suffer from psychiatric comorbidities, including addictive disorders (AD).[6,7] Winokur and colleagues[8] described back in 1969 that the percentage of patients with BD increasing alcohol consumption was higher during mixed states than during depression. A few years later, Himmelhoch and colleagues[9] found that mixed forms of BD were correlated with higher rates of alcohol and drug abuse, especially sedatives. Subsequent reports on mixed bipolar affective disorders further confirmed these observations.[10] Goldberg and colleagues[11] also found that clinical remission during hospitalization was less likely for patients with BD with mixed features and past substance abuse. However, other investigators obtained different results.[12] Several studies described that the comorbid misuse of alcohol, sedatives, or stimulants might modify the clinical presentation of both (hypo)manic and depressive episodes, leading to the onset of mixed states.[13-16] However, although the relation between AD, especially substance use disorders (SUD), and mixed episodes has been investigated, the determinants underlying the increased proneness to both substance and non-substance addictive behaviors in these individuals have not been fully elucidated yet.

MIXED STATES AND ADDICTIVE DISORDERS: COMMON PATHOGENETIC PATHWAYS
Neurobiological Underpinnings

An increased understanding of the detrimental neurobiological effects of chronic substance abuse on the central nervous system (CNS) explains how SUD might adversely affect long-term mood stability in subjects with BD, leading to a heightened vulnerability toward mixed affective states. Monoamine dysregulation is among the most influential hypothesis in BD pathophysiology.[17] Evidence suggests that depressive symptoms may involve functional deficiency of brain monoaminergic neurotransmitters, such as norepinephrine, serotonin, and/or dopamine, whereas a functional excess of monoamines at critical synapses may trigger mania. Some investigators hypothesized that mixed states might arise from more complex alterations, that is, an imbalance between catecholaminergic and cholinergic neurotransmission.[6] Acute stimulant consumption, likewise elation symptoms, is linked with an increased catecholaminergic function, and there is evidence that patients with BD are more sensitive than healthy controls to the behavioral effects of amphetamines. In addition, it is well-established that dopamine and norepinephrine have a prominent role in the rewarding and behavioral effects of addictive behaviors, as well as in the sensitization process that may contribute to maintain AD. Consistently with this conceptual framework, chronic substance exposure may negatively affect the function of the previously mentioned neurotransmitters, contributing to trigger an abnormal switch into different affective states (eg, mania and/or depression). Growing evidence suggests that distinct abnormalities in the glutamatergic system also play an important role in the pathophysiology of certain bipolar mixed features, including impulsivity, affective instability, and dysphoria.[18] Previous studies found that homocysteine, which has been involved in synaptic dysfunction and neurodegeneration, is increased during mixed states in patients with BD with comorbid SUD.[19] Homocysteine may act as an excitatory amino acid and interfere with glutamatergic neurotransmission, leading to instability of the affective symptomatology. Interestingly, previous studies on major depressive disorder detected higher levels of homocysteine in the serum of depressed patients with increased anger and hostility traits.[20]

Circadian rhythm dysregulation is involved in the pathogenesis of various affective disorders, including BD, with relevance to mixed affective states induction and perpetuation.[6] Sleep alterations with concomitant increases in catecholamine release have been observed at the time of the switch to mania in euthymic unmedicated patients with BD, and are also thought to underlie the onset of mixed states.[6] Intriguingly, altered sleep patterns have been shown to be linked to the development of AD through dysfunctions in the mesolimbic dopaminergic system.[21] Studies suggest a critical role of circadian rhythms and specific chronotypes in the regulation of cortico-striatal reward-related dopaminergic pathways and indicate that substances of abuse directly affect the suprachiasmatic nucleus, which represents the central circadian pacemaker. Conversely, individuals with AD display disrupted circadian rhythms or pathologic chronotypes that may increase the risk for substance abuse and consequent relapses.[21,22] Polymorphisms in several CLOCK (Circadian Locomotor Output Cycles Kaput) genes, involved in chronobiological regulation, have been repeatedly found in patients with BD with and without comorbid AD. These mechanisms continuously interplay, so chronic substance abuse can induce a disruption in sleep architecture that, in turn, might have an impairing effect on long-term mood stability.

The concept of allostasis may provide further insights in the understanding of certain pathogenetic mechanisms underlying BD-AD comorbidity.[23] From the addiction perspective, allostasis is defined as the process of maintaining apparent reward function stability through changes in brain reward mechanisms.[24] AD are characterized by the occurrence of an allostatic state in the brain reward system, reflected in a chronic deviation of reward thresholds. The allostatic state is fueled not only by dysregulation of reward circuits per se, but also by brain dynorphin/kappa opioid receptor (KOR) system activation and hypothalamic-pituitary-adrenal (HPA) axis stress responses.[25] Mixed episodes frequently occur in the context of prolonged affective instability and increased stressors, and there is evidence that mixed states combine the HPA activation found in depression with increased catecholamine function.[6] Glucocorticoids play an important role in this process, whereby the allostasis mediators interact with neurotransmitter systems and brain peptides resulting in neuroplastic alterations in brain areas involved in emotional processing, such as hippocampus, amygdala, and prefrontal cortex.[26,27] Stress is recognized as a main trigger for both AD and BD recurrences, as well as for mood switches, thus exposing patients to increased transition episodes that are frequently characterized by mixed features.[28] Evidence suggests that the endogenous opioid neuropeptide dynorphin is involved in neurobiological processes underlying mood modulation and increasing the rewarding effects of drugs of abuse. The activation of the dynorphin/KOR system is also likely to play a major role in the pro-addictive effects of stress.[29] Interestingly, several studies reported that different substance and non–substance-related addictive behaviors, including alcohol, cocaine, gambling, and food addiction, impair the activity of dynorphin, which seems to induce dysphoric symptoms by affecting dopaminergic and noradrenergic neurotransmission.[30,31] It is possible to hypothesize that abnormal emotional processing and/or affective instability may trigger drug intake, leading to an intense activity of the dopaminergic system, followed by both a compensatory decrease in dopaminergic activity and an increase in HPA axis and dynorphin/KOR system response, to reestablish the allostatic set point.[32] This same process might sustain the onset and maintenance of mixed features.

Functional neuroimaging studies identified specific networks in the brain, that is, Default Mode Network, also named self-directed network (DMN), ventral Fronto-Parietal Network (FPN), and Salience/Reward Network (SN), involved in self-focus processing and metacognitive functions.[33] These networks show abnormalities both in BD and AD, representing a possible common trademark in the physiopathology of these disorders.[34] DMN also correlates with self-reported needs and pathologic urges, like craving in substance and behavioral addiction.[35] The dysfunctional balance between the previously mentioned systems seems to contribute to a pathophysiological paradigm known in the literature as iRISA, "impaired Response Inhibition and Salience Attribution".[36,37] This model suggests that impairments of certain neuropsychological functions (ie, response inhibition and salience attribution) may contribute to the main phenomenology underlying substances and behavioral addiction, as well as several psychiatric disorders.[38,39] Functional neuroimaging studies, involving patients with mixed states with BD, highlighted abnormalities in prefrontal–subcortical networks and an altered DMN-SN communication, suggesting a connection between failure in response inhibition (ie, behavioral impulsivity) and deficit in counterbalancing subcortical aberrant salience attribution.[36,40] Indeed, an incentive and aberrant salience plays a role in promoting a suboptimal choice behavior, like in gambling and other addictions. Both FPN and SN attribute cognitive and emotional salience to any stimulus, either environmental or internal, reaching the CNS.[41–43] Communication between these networks is involved in reinforcement learning and in the elaboration of a goal-directed behavioral scheme in response to a stimulus that alters the internal homeostasis.[44]

Behavioral[45] and substance[46] addictions, as well as BD,[47] seem to share alterations in the functional connectivity from and to the anterior insula, which belongs to FPN and mediates DMN-SN dynamic activity and the transition from environmental stimuli to DMN-centered functions.[48] Taken together, these alterations translate into failure in basic neurocognitive and metacognitive functions of self-awareness and self-agency and therefore may represent a common pathophysiological substrate of both behavioral addictions and mood episodes, especially with mixed features.

Clinical and Psychopathological Features

According to the self-medication hypothesis, both substance misuse and addictive behaviors could be conceptualized as an attempt to cope with distressing affective states. Mixed bipolar symptomatology may be therefore associated with divergent psychological factors that may represent distinct pathways to substance abuse and maladaptive behaviors.[49] Patients with BD might misuse stimulants, such as amphetamines and cocaine, to enhance, lengthen, or restore symptoms of elation, rather than to self-medicate depressive states. Instead, subjects experiencing dysphoria during hypomanic or manic phases show increased preference for opiates or other CNS depressants, including alcohol. Likewise, alcohol and sedative compounds may be abused to alleviate insomnia, anxiety, and agitation symptoms during mixed episodes.[50] Some investigators postulated that, in subjects undergoing mixed states, the misuse of sedative compounds is an attempt to counter the "psychologically disorganizing effects of overwhelming rage".[51] Other investigators questioned the self-medication theory and suggested instead that the increased substance misuse in these patients might simply be another manifestation of the current affective episode.[52]

The preceding considerations could be extended to behavioral addictions. In fact, increasing evidence suggests that vulnerable individuals may engage in potentially addictive activities (eg, gambling, gaming) to mitigate a variety of negative affective states,[31] and patients with BD show high rates of comorbid behavioral addictions.[53–55] However, studies specifically investigating the implications of behavioral addictions across the different phases of BD are still lacking.

Mixed episodes are also reported to occur with higher frequency during switches into other affective states. Therefore, it is possible to hypothesize that subjects with BD may increase substance consumption or addictive behaviors during switching phases to maintain "desired" elation symptoms or to counterbalance the unpleasant effects arising from symptoms cycling across opposite affective polarity.[56] This might contribute to explain, at least in part, the high co-occurrence of substance use during mixed states, although the direction of this association remains unclear. In fact, substance misuse is known to modify the course and clinical expression of BD. Mixed symptoms could arise as a direct pharmacologic effect of both substance intoxication and withdrawal within a "pure" affective state. Also, drug consumption might facilitate switching between opposite polarities and increase the number of recurrences, exposing patients more frequently to mixed episodes.[57]

The association between addictive disorders and mixed episodes also supports the hypothesis of shared underlying psychopathological mechanisms that may affect BD clinical presentation. Affect dysregulation, usually defined as "rapid oscillations of intense affect, with a difficulty in regulating these oscillations or their behavioral consequences", is a common psychopathological feature of both BD and AD.[58] Mixed states frequently occur in the context of prolonged affective instability, including ultradian mood cycling. Likewise, affect dysregulation has been proposed as a critical component in the development and maintenance of mood disorders by triggering a recursive and dynamic loop that reinforces affective instability. In subjects with BD, increased interepisodic affective instability has been correlated with the presence of a lifetime SUD.[59] Moreover, affective dysregulation is considered a susceptibility factor for problematic substance use independently from psychiatric diagnoses. Impulsivity, broadly defined as the tendency to act rapidly, without premeditation or conscious judgment, may represent a further potential biological and behavioral overlap.[60] Impulsivity is prominent in both BD and SUD and evidence suggests that depressed patients with mixed symptoms have a long-term susceptibility to impulsivity, not limited to the current affective episode. Interepisode impulsivity is heightened in patients with BD with a past history of substance abuse.[61] Impulsivity and increased psychomotricity are often considered hallmark features of certain bipolar mixed presentation, such as agitated depression. Furthermore, the combination of depression and impulsivity is associated with behavioral risk in BD, reflecting the tendency to make rapid, unplanned responses, like in subjects with a history of suicide attempts.[53] Suicide risk is known to be elevated in both AD and mixed mood episodes, and the co-occurrence of mixed mood features and addictive behaviors seem to raise this risk further.[62]

Similarly, addictive urges and craving are often associated with arousal and motor restlessness that may resemble tension and anxiety usually occurring in depressive mixed states. Hence, craving and/or addictive urges may constitute a differential diagnostic challenge in BD-SUD comorbidity, and it has to be ruled out in the assessment of possible depressive mixed recurrences.

TREATMENT IMPLICATIONS

According to current guidelines, treatment of mixed features arising during both manic and depressive episodes frequently require combination pharmacotherapy.[63] In fact, treating mixed states turns out to be particularly challenging because of intertwined opposite symptoms that may affect both acute and prophylactic efficacy of currently available compounds.[64]

Comorbid SUD are more prevalent in mixed than non-mixed bipolar episodes and are associated with poor outcome, including less favorable response to pharmaco-therapeutic treatment.[65,66] A recent study reported, in fact, that both mixed features and comorbid alcohol misuse were associated with poor response to lithium.[67,68] It is possible that substances of abuse interact, to some extent, with medications, leading to reduced efficacy of therapies, more adverse effects and, ultimately, treatment non-adherence. Moreover, patients with substance abuse tend to have inadequate insight, denying the need for treatments. Impatience, restlessness, and impulsivity, commonly found during mixed states and often exacerbated by substance use, might also favor dropouts. Related socioeconomic factors, such as disorganized lifestyle, unemployment, and difficulties in personal relationships, further contribute to detrimental outcomes.

In such cases, shared therapeutic goals generally rely on the treatment of AD-related symptoms (ie, craving and withdrawal), as well as on prolonged mood stabilization, possibly through multiple steps.[54] In clinical management, treatment engagement, drug detoxification, and acute mood stabilization are the first therapeutic aims. Consolidating remission and reinforcing abstinence, through personal and lifestyle changes, represent the subsequent therapeutic steps. The final maintenance phase should target the risk of both AD and affective recurrences, aiming to reduce both.[68]

Psychopharmacological treatments investigated in mixed bipolar states and SUD include anticonvulsants/mood stabilizers, lithium, and second-generation antipsychotics (SGA), both in monotherapy and in combination. Anticonvulsants, possibly via anti-kindling and gamma-aminobutyric acid (GABA)-mimetic properties, may effectively reduce neuronal hyperexcitability and substance-induced behavioral sensitization, which could, in turn, alleviate craving, as well as some core features of manic mixed symptomatology (eg, impulsivity, hyperactivity, irritability).[68,69]

In BD-SUD comorbidity, both valproate and carbamazepine display a more rapid onset of action than other anticonvulsants and mood stabilizers, and valproate proved to be more effective than lithium for treating mixed features.[63]

Further therapeutic strategies, targeting both substance-related symptoms and affective instability, may consist of combining mood stabilizers with specific anticraving medications. Among these, κ-opioid receptor antagonists, such as naltrexone and nalmefene, have shown beneficial effects in ameliorating both impulsivity and mood-related symptomatology throughout different types of AD.[70] Likewise, naltrexone demonstrated to significantly improve substance-related outcomes, including craving and the number of days of abstinence, as well as mood-related symptoms, in patients with BD-SUD.[71]

In clinical practice, the use of SGA, particularly aripiprazole, olanzapine, and quetiapine, has proved to be the most effective choice for treatment of bipolar patients with addictive behaviors.[72,73] Such class of drugs, besides ensuring fewer collateral effects compared with the first-generation antipsychotics (FGA), seems to modulate cognitive salience through the regulation of the mesolimbic/mesocortical dopaminergic activity. Also, because of their pharmacologic profile on dopaminergic transmission (lower D2 receptor affinity than FGA and "fast-dissociation" kinetics), along with 5-HT2A receptor antagonism, SGA only marginally affect reward processes and may prevent craving.[73]

Several SGA have been investigated for the management of mixed episodes in BD. Most of them showed efficacy in both acute and long-term management of mixed episodes, despite generally exerting a higher efficacy on manic than on depressive symptoms.[5,63,74,75] Among SGA, olanzapine has the best evidence in acute mixed hypo/manic/depressive states as well as in the maintenance phase,[76] and, because of its reported efficacy in AD, might be considered a valid therapeutic option in comorbid patients.[77]

SUMMARY

So far, the literature on AD and mixed mood features suggests the existence of an increased co-occurrence of these conditions. History of AD generally predicts greater affective instability in bipolar episodes, possibly contributing to an increased risk for mixed features. Common neurobehavioral underpinnings between AD and mixed mood episodes may involve increased impulsivity, as well as affective instability. However, underlying pathogenetic mechanisms have still to be ascertained and fully understood. Mixed episodes show poor symptomatic and functional outcome, including increased suicide risk and a more severe course of illness. The co-occurring AD may dampen the efficacy of currently available treatments for patients with BD and negatively influence the overall course of mood disorders with mixed features. Therefore, clinicians should carefully consider these patients to be at heightened risk and, consequently, enhance tailored treatment programs bearing in mind those patients' individual features and increased vulnerability.

DISCLOSURE

The authors have nothing to disclose.

REFERENCES

1. Vieta E, Valentí M. Mixed states in DSM-5: implications for clinical care, education, and research. J Affect Disord 2013;148(1):28–36.
2. Maina G. The concept of mixed state in bipolar disorder: from Kraepelin to DSM-5. J Psychopathol 2013;19:287–95.
3. American Psychiatric Association. Diagnostic and statistical manual of mental disorders. 5th edition. Arlington, VA: American Psychiatric Association; 2013.
4. Shim IH, Woo YS, Bahk WM. Prevalence rates and clinical implications of bipolar disorder "with mixed features" as defined by DSM-5. J Affect Disord 2015;173:120–5.
5. Fagiolini A, Coluccia A, Maina G, et al. Diagnosis, epidemiology and management of mixed states in bipolar disorder. CNS Drugs 2015;29(9):725–40.
6. Muneer A. Mixed states in bipolar disorder: etiology, pathogenesis and treatment. Chonnam Med J 2017;53(1):1–13.
7. McIntyre RS, Ng-Mak D, Chuang CC, et al. Major depressive disorder with subthreshold hypomanic (mixed) features: a real-world assessment of treatment patterns and economic burden. J Affect Disord 2017;210:332–7.
8. Winokur G, Clayton PJ, Reich T. Manic depressive illness. St Louis (MO): C.V. Mosby; 1969.
9. Himmelhoch JM, Mulla D, Neil JF, et al. Incidence and significance of mixed affective states in a bipolar population. Arch Gen Psychiatry 1976;33(9):1062–6.

10. Himmelhoch JM, Garfinkel ME. Sources of lithium resistance in mixed mania. Psychopharmacol Bull 1986;22(3):613–20.

11. Goldberg JF, Garno JL, Leon AC, et al. A history of substance abuse complicates remission from acute mania in bipolar disorder. J Clin Psychiatry 1999;60(11): 733–40.

12. Cassidy F, Ahearn EP, Carroll BJ. Substance abuse in bipolar disorder. Bipolar Disord 2001;3(4):181–8.

13. Winokur G, Coryell W, Akiskal HS, et al. Alcoholism in manic-depressive (bipolar) illness: familial illness, course of illness, and the primary-secondary distinction. Am J Psychiatry 1995;152(3):365–72.

14. Winokur G, Turvey C, Akiskal H, et al. Alcoholism and drug abuse in three groups—bipolar I, unipolars and their acquaintances. J Affect Disord 1998; 50(2–3):81–9.

15. Sonne SC, Brady KT. Substance abuse and bipolar comorbidity. Psychiatr Clin North Am 1999;22(3):609–27, ix.

16. Weiss RD, Greenfield SF, Najavits LM, et al. Medication compliance among patients with bipolar disorder and substance use disorder. J Clin Psychiatry 1998; 59(4):172–4.

17. Stein DJ, Horn N, Ramesar R, et al. Bipolar disorder: emotional dysregulation and neuronal vulnerability. CNS Spectr 2009;14(3):122–6.

18. Kalivas PW, Volkow N, Seamans J. Unmanageable motivation in addiction: a pathology in prefrontal-accumbens glutamate transmission. Neuron 2005;45(5): 647–50.

19. Oliva F, Coppola M, Mondola R, et al. Blood homocysteine concentration and mood disorders with mixed features among patients with alcohol use disorder. BMC Psychiatry 2017;17(1):181.

20. Fraguas R, Papakostas GI, Mischoulon D, et al. Anger attacks in major depressive disorder and serum levels of homocysteine. Biol Psychiatry 2006;60(3): 270–4.

21. McClung CA. Circadian rhythms, the mesolimbic dopaminergic circuit, and drug addiction. ScientificWorldJournal 2007;7:194–202.

22. Becker-Krail D, McClung C. Implications of circadian rhythm and stress in addiction vulnerability. F1000Res 2016;5:59.

23. Pettorruso M, De Risio L, Di Nicola M, et al. Allostasis as a conceptual framework linking bipolar disorder and addiction. Front Psychiatry 2014;5:173.

24. Koob GF, Le Moal M. Drug addiction, dysregulation of reward, and allostasis. Neuropsychopharmacology 2001;24(2):97–129.

25. Karkhanis A, Holleran KM, Jones SR. Dynorphin/Kappa opioid receptor signaling in preclinical models of alcohol, drug, and food addiction. Int Rev Neurobiol 2017;136:53–88.

26. Sinha R, Talih M, Malison R, et al. Hypothalamic-pituitary-adrenal axis and sympatho-adreno-medullary responses during stress-induced and drug cue-induced cocaine craving states. Psychopharmacology (Berl) 2003;170(1):62–72.

27. Olff M, Langeland W, Gersons BP. Effects of appraisal and coping on the neuro-endocrine response to extreme stress. Neurosci Biobehav Rev 2005;29(3): 457–67.

28. Brietzke E, Mansur RB, Soczynska J, et al. A theoretical framework informing research about the role of stress in the pathophysiology of bipolar disorder. Prog Neuropsychopharmacol Biol Psychiatry 2012;39(1):1–8.

29. George O, Le Moal M, Koob GF. Allostasis and addiction: role of the dopamine and corticotropin-releasing factor systems. Physiol Behav 2012;106(1):58–64.

30. Chavkin C, Koob GF. Dynorphin, dysphoria, and dependence: the stress of addiction. Neuropsychopharmacology 2016;41(1):373–4.

31. Moccia L, Mazza M, Di Nicola M, et al. The experience of pleasure: a perspective between neuroscience and psychoanalysis. Front Hum Neurosci 2018;12:359.

32. Shippenberg TS, Zapata A, Chefer VI. Dynorphin and the pathophysiology of drug addiction. Pharmacol Ther 2007;116(2):306–21.

33. Northoff G, Heinzel A, de Greck M, et al. Self-referential processing in our brain–a meta-analysis of imaging studies on the self. Neuroimage 2006;31(1):440–57.

34. Syan SK, Smith M, Frey BN, et al. Resting-state functional connectivity in individuals with bipolar disorder during clinical remission: a systematic review. J Psychiatry Neurosci 2018;43(5):298–316.

35. Wilson SJ, Sayette MA. Neuroimaging craving: urge intensity matters. Addiction 2015;110(2):195–203.

36. Fleck DE, Kotwal R, Eliassen JC, et al. Preliminary evidence for increased fronto-subcortical activation on a motor impulsivity task in mixed episode bipolar disorder. J affective Disord 2011;133(1–2):333–9.

37. Strakowski SM, Adler CM, Almeida J, et al. The functional neuroanatomy of bipolar disorder: a consensus model. Bipolar Disord 2012;14(4):313–25.

38. Phillips ML, Ladouceur CD, Drevets WC. A neural model of voluntary and automatic emotion regulation: implications for understanding the pathophysiology and neurodevelopment of bipolar disorder. Mol Psychiatry 2008;13(9):829, 833-857.

39. Phillips ML, Swartz HA. A critical appraisal of neuroimaging studies of bipolar disorder: toward a new conceptualization of underlying neural circuitry and a road map for future research. Am J Psychiatry 2014;171(8):829–43.

40. Bartra O, McGuire JT, Kable JW. The valuation system: a coordinate-based meta-analysis of BOLD fMRI experiments examining neural correlates of subjective value. Neuroimage 2013;76:412–27.

41. Milton AL, Everitt BJ. The persistence of maladaptive memory: addiction, drug memories and anti-relapse treatments. Neurosci Biobehav Rev 2012;36(4):1119–39.

42. Menon V. Large-scale brain networks and psychopathology: a unifying triple network model. Trends Cogn Sci 2011;15(10):483–506.

43. Sutherland MT, McHugh MJ, Pariyadath V, et al. Resting state functional connectivity in addiction: Lessons learned and a road ahead. Neuroimage 2012;62(4):2281–95.

44. Liang X, He Y, Salmeron BJ, et al. Interactions between the salience and default-mode networks are disrupted in cocaine addiction. J Neurosci 2015;35(21):8081–90.

45. Wang L, Shen H, Lei Y, et al. Altered default mode, fronto-parietal and salience networks in adolescents with Internet addiction. Addict behaviors 2017;70:1–6.

46. Moeller SJ, Fleming SM, Gan G, et al. Metacognitive impairment in active cocaine use disorder is associated with individual differences in brain structure. Eur Neuropsychopharmacol 2016;26(4):653–62.

47. Ambrosi E, Arciniegas DB, Madan A, et al. Insula and amygdala resting-state functional connectivity differentiate bipolar from unipolar depression. Acta Psychiatr Scand 2017;136(1):129–39.

48. Everitt BJ, Robbins TW. Drug addiction: updating actions to habits to compulsions ten years on. Annu Rev Psychol 2016;67:23–50.

49. Healey C, Peters S, Kinderman P, et al. Reasons for substance use in dual diagnosis bipolar disorder and substance use disorders: a qualitative study. J Affect Disord 2009;113(1–2):118–26.
50. McDonald JL, Meyer TD. Self-report reasons for alcohol use in bipolar disorders: why drink despite the potential risks. Clin Psychol Psychother 2011;18(5):418–25.
51. Weiss RD, Mirin SM. Substance abuse as an attempt at self-medication. Psychiatr Med 1985;3(4):357–67.
52. Liskow B, Mayfield D, Thiele J. Alcohol and affective disorder: assessment and treatment. J Clin Psychiatry 1982;43(4):144–7.
53. Di Nicola M, Tedeschi D, Mazza M, et al. Behavioural addictions in bipolar disorder patients: role of impulsivity and personality dimensions. J Affect Disord 2010; 125(1–3):82–8.
54. Varo C, Murru A, Salagre E, et al. Behavioral addictions in bipolar disorders: a systematic review. Eur Neuropsychopharmacol 2019;29(1):76–97.
55. Wölfling K, Beutel ME, Dreier M, et al. Bipolar spectrum disorders in a clinical sample of patients with Internet addiction: hidden comorbidity or differential diagnosis. J Behav Addict 2015;4(2):101–5.
56. Pettersen H, Ruud T, Ravndal E, et al. Walking the fine line: self-reported reasons for substance use in persons with severe mental illness. Int J Qual Stud Health Well-being 2013;8:21968.
57. Janiri D, Di Nicola M, Martinotti G, et al. Who's the leader, mania or depression? Predominant polarity and alcohol/polysubstance use in bipolar disorders. Curr Neuropharmacol 2017;15(3):409–16.
58. Marwaha S, He Z, Broome M, et al. How is affective instability defined and measured? A systematic review. Psychol Med 2014;44(9):1793–808.
59. Lagerberg TV, Aminoff SR, Aas M, et al. Alcohol use disorders are associated with increased affective lability in bipolar disorder. J Affect Disord 2017;208: 316–24.
60. Kathleen Holmes M, Bearden CE, Barguil M, et al. Conceptualizing impulsivity and risk taking in bipolar disorder: importance of history of alcohol abuse. Bipolar Disord 2009;11(1):33–40.
61. Swann AC, Dougherty DM, Pazzaglia PJ, et al. Increased impulsivity associated with severity of suicide attempt history in patients with bipolar disorder. Am J Psychiatry 2005;162:1680–7.
62. Maina G. Management and care of mixed states. J Psychopathol 2013;19: 262–71.
63. Verdolini N, Hidalgo-Mazzei D, Murru A, et al. Mixed states in bipolar and major depressive disorders: systematic review and quality appraisal of guidelines. Acta Psychiatr Scand 2018;138(3):196–222.
64. Mazza M, Mandelli L, Di Nicola M, et al. Clinical features, response to treatment and functional outcome of bipolar disorder patients with and without co-occurring substance use disorder: 1-year follow-up. J Affect Disord 2009;115(1–2):27–35.
65. Messer T, Lammers G, Müller-Siecheneder F, et al. Substance abuse in patients with bipolar disorder: a systematic review and meta-analysis. Psychiatry Res 2017;253:338–50.
66. Etain B, Lajnef M, Brichant-Petitjean C, et al. Childhood trauma and mixed episodes are associated with poor response to lithium in bipolar disorders. Acta Psychiatr Scand 2017;135(4):319–27.
67. Hunt GE, Malhi GS, Cleary M, et al. Comorbidity of bipolar and substance use disorders in national surveys of general populations, 1990-2015: Systematic review and meta-analysis. J Affect Disord 2016;206:321–30.

68. Salloum IM, Thase ME. Impact of substance abuse on the course and treatment of bipolar disorder. Bipolar Disord 2000;2(3 Pt 2):269–80.
69. Di Nicola M, De Risio L, Pettorruso M, et al. Bipolar disorder and gambling disorder comorbidity: current evidence and implications for pharmacological treatment. J Affect Disord 2014;167:285–98.
70. Di Nicola M, De Filippis S, Martinotti G, et al. Nalmefene in alcohol use disorder subjects with psychiatric comorbidity: a naturalistic study. Adv Ther 2017;34(7): 1636–49.
71. Brown ES, Beard L, Dobbs L, et al. Naltrexone in patients with bipolar disorder and alcohol dependence. Depress Anxiety 2006;23(8):492–5.
72. Di Nicola M, Martinotti G, Mazza M, et al. Quetiapine as add-on treatment for bipolar I disorder with comorbid compulsive buying and physical exercise addiction. Prog Neuropsychopharmacol Biol Psychiatry 2010;34(4):713–4.
73. Janiri L, Martinotti G, Di Nicola M. Aripiprazole for relapse prevention and craving in alcohol-dependent subjects: results from a pilot study. J Clin Psychopharmacol 2007;27:519–20.
74. McIntyre RS, Masand PS, Earley W, et al. Cariprazine for the treatment of bipolar mania with mixed features: A post hoc pooled analysis of 3 trials. J Affect Disord 2019;257:600–6.
75. Yatham LN, Kennedy SH, Parikh SV, et al. Canadian Network for Mood and Anxiety Treatments (CANMAT) and International Society for Bipolar Disorders (ISBD) 2018 guidelines for the management of patients with bipolar disorder. Bipolar Disord 2018;20(2):97–170.
76. Takeshima M. Treating mixed mania/hypomania: a review and synthesis of the evidence. CNS Spectr 2017;22(2):177–85.
77. Sani G, Kotzalidis GD, Vöhringer P, et al. Effectiveness of short-term olanzapine in patients with bipolar I disorder, with or without comorbidity with substance use disorder. J Clin Psychopharmacol 2013;33(2):231–5.

Mechanisms

Mechanisms

The Neurobiology of Mixed States

Alessio Simonetti, MD[a,b,c,*], Marijn Lijffijt, PhD[a,d], Alan C. Swann, MD[a,d]

KEYWORDS

- Bipolar disorder • Mixed states • Biology • Monoamines • Circadian rhythms
- Inflammation • Hypothalamic-pituitary-adrenal axis

KEY POINTS

- Mixed mania and mixed depression are characterized by alterations involving multiple biological systems, including monoamines, hypothalamic-pituitary-adrenal axis, inflammatory components, and circadian rhythms.
- Pathophysiologic processes in mixed mania and mixed depression are more severe than in corresponding processes in the respective nonmixed forms.
- Biological alterations suggest that hyperactivation and hyperarousal are the core pathophysiologic mechanisms involved in both mixed mania and mixed depression.

INTRODUCTION

The neurobiology underlying mixes states, or mood phases characterized by combined symptoms of depression and mania, has provoked strong interest since the pre-scientific era.[1] Aretaeus of Cappadocia,[2] following Empedocles' (490–430 BCE) design of illness as an imbalance of 4 elements with corresponding qualities, firstly hypothesized a possible coexistence of melancholia-related and mania-related fluid substances. Furthermore, he conceptualized mixed states, and affective illnesses in general, as systemic, rather than as disorders of the "head," a concept that was followed by Hippocrates[3] and Galen.[4] In the early twentieth century, emphasizing clinical description rather than pathobiological processes, Emil Kraepelin[5] conceptualized mixed states as a more severe forms of both depression and mania and hypothesized hyperarousal and activation as core characteristics. In the early twentieth century, general interest in concepts of mixed states waned. Instead, interest in neurobiological bases of affective disorders focused on dichotomic, nonoverlapping models of mania and depression.[6] A resurgence of interest on mixed states in recent decades,

---

[a] Menninger Department of Psychiatry and Behavioral Sciences, Baylor College of Medicine, 1977 Butler Boulevard, Houston, TX 77030, USA; [b] Department of Neurology and Psychiatry, Sapienza University of Rome, Rome, Italy; [c] Centro Lucio Bini, Rome, Italy; [d] Michael E. DeBakey VA Medical Center, Houston, TX, USA
* Corresponding author.
E-mail addresses: Alessio.simo@gmail.com; alessio.simonetti@bcm.edu

Psychiatr Clin N Am 43 (2020) 139–151
https://doi.org/10.1016/j.psc.2019.10.013
0193-953X/20/© 2019 Elsevier Inc. All rights reserved.

however, has fostered increased research on biological characteristics of combined states and their relationship with those of the respective nonmixed forms. Such alterations have been reported in different, interacting, and partially overlapping systems, including monoamines,[7] hormones,[8] inflammatory markers,[9] circadian regulators,[10] and frontal-subcortical networks.[11] A comprehensive description of the biological systems involved in mixed states relative to nonmixed affective states, however, is lacking. The aim of this article is to review studies that compared neurobiological mechanisms between mixed and nonmixed affective states. Because diagnostic criteria of mixed states vary across studies and are continuously evolving, for initial orientation, the several diagnostic criteria used to define mixed states are discussed. For the same reason, an additional paragraph describing biological findings in manic and depressive phases is provided. Mechanisms mentioned are limited to those that have been investigated in mixed states.

Definition of Mixed States

Across studies, mixed mania has been defined as subsyndromal depression in the context of a manic episode (broad definition),[12] or, in accordance with the *Diagnostic and Statistical Manual of Mental Disorders* (DSM) (Third Edition) and *DSM* (Fourth Edition) criteria, the simultaneous presence of a manic and depressive episode (narrow definition).[13,14] Mixed depression has been described as inner tension, racing/crowded thoughts, irritability, talkativeness, mood lability and emotional reactivity, or early insomnia in the context of a depressive episode,[15] or as depression plus inner or motor agitation, known as agitated depression.[16] The *DSM* (Fifth Edition) introduced the mixed specifier for both manic and depressive (belonging either to unipolar disorder [UD] or bipolar disorder [BD]) episodes, defined as a depressive and manic episode with at least 2 nonoverlapping symptoms of the opposite polarity.[17]

Neurobiological Findings Related to Mania and Depression

Early pharmacologic treatments for depression and mania were found to have effects on monoamine function, and the study of monoamines was facilitated by discovery of stable metabolites for these transmitters. Therefore, early hypotheses on the pathophysiologic processes underlying BD focused on monoamine dysregulation.[18] To this extent, manic states have been related to high plasma levels, cerebrospinal fluid (CSF) levels, and excretion rates of norepinephrine (NE) principle metabolite 3-methoxy-4-hydroxyphenylglycol (MHPG) and of dopamine (DA) principal metabolites vanillymandelic acid (VMA) and homovanillic acid (HVA), whereas depressive states were related to low levels of such metabolites. Severity of mania correlated with MHPG in CSF fluid,[19] whereas a quantitative relationship to depression was less clear.[20]

Patients with mania or with depression had elevated cortisol and higher rates of dexamethasone suppression test (DST) nonsuppression after oral cortisol ingestion, suggesting dysregulation of the hypothalamic-pituitary-adrenal (HPA) axis and a possible related immune system imbalance.[21] Findings of higher proinflammatory cytokine levels and other proinflammatory markers in euthymic, depressive, and manic states[22] support this hypothesis.

Furthermore, both manic and depressive states have been related to altered biological circadian regulators, with opposite patterns of melatonin and cortisol excretion peaks and Circadian Locomotor Output Cycles Kaput (CLOCK) gene expression, that is, phase advance in manic and phase delay in depressive states[10,23] (**Fig. 1**). Therefore, data related to monoamine and circadian regulation seemed to support

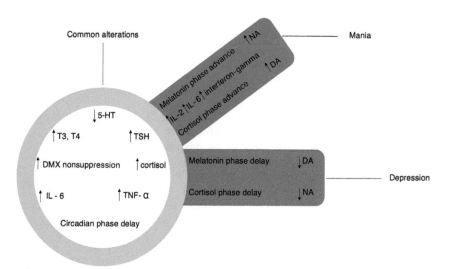

Fig. 1. Specific and common biological alterations in depression and mania. 5HT, serotonin; DA, dopamine; DMX, dexamethasone; IFN, interferon; IL, interleukin; NA, noradrenaline; TNF, tumor necrosis factor; TSH, thyroid releasing hormone.

depression and mania as opposites, but the situation with HPA axis and inflammatory function was less clear.

METHODS

The authors searched MEDLINE/PubMed/Index Medicus, EMBASE, and Cochrane Library databases from inception until May 30, 2019. The search was conducted by 2 independent researchers, using the following search terms: (1) for MEDLINE/ Pubmed/Index Medicus: mixed state* OR mixed depress* OR mixed mani* OR mixed hypomani* OR mixed feature* OR agitated depressi* OR agitated mania OR agitated manic OR agitated hypomani* OR dysphoric mania OR dysphoric manic; (2) for Cochrane Library: mixed state* OR mixed depress* OR mixed mani*; and (3) for EMBASE: mixed state; mixed mania; mixed depression. Clinical and preclinical studies were included. The search generated 2279 articles. The authors screened abstracts (2015) to select articles that report on any biological measure reflecting neurobiological functions in human populations with or animal models of mixed states. Specifically, studies had to address (1) measures derived from human blood, urine, or CSF, (2) human biological rhythms using specific machine-related techniques, such as the electrocardiogram or actigraphy, (3) biological experiments in animal models of mixed states. Articles were grouped as (1) of interest, (2) duplicate, and (3) of no interest. After selection, full articles were retrieved and studied.

RESULTS

The global search returned 2279 results. A small proportion of duplicates or irrelevant records (214) were excluded, so that 2015 underwent title and abstract examination. Of the 2015 articles, 341 were excluded because they were opinions, case reports, or reviews, resulting in 1684 articles that were deemed eligible for further assessment. The final selection resulted in the inclusion of 42 studies that focused on monoamines,

HPA axis functioning, thyroid function, circadian rhythms, inflammatory markers, and neuroimaging. Therefore, this article is divided into distinct sections that address each of those topics. Remaining articles were classified as "other."

ANIMAL MODELS OF MIXED STATES

Mixed symptoms were classically evaluated in mice with the surgical removal of bilateral olfactive bulbs, an area with extensive connections with limbic and prefrontal structures.[24] Olfactory bulbectomy (OB) results in a cascade of modulatory downstream adaptations considered to be associated with behavioral changes resembling mixed states, such as reduced copulation and lower locomotion associated with depression, and exploration, hyperactivity in a forced swim task, aggressiveness, predatory behavior, and nocturnal hyperactivity associated with mania.[25,26] These OB-associated behaviors have been related to increased levels of serotonin (5H-T) in the frontal cortex, striatum, and hippocampus; decreased levels of its metabolite, 5-hydroxyindoleacetic acid (5-HIAA) in the nucleus accumbens[25]; and increased levels of the protein kinase A regulatory subunit RIα in the amygdala.[26] These findings suggest that behaviors resulting from OB are associated with altered neural transmission in pivotal areas related to emotion regulation and neurogenesis.[26] Heath and colleagues[27] found that some aspects of behavioral alterations induced by the OB, such as hyperactivity on a forced swim task, were attenuated by repetitive transcranial magnetic stimulation, possibly through balancing the down-regulation of α-aminobutyric acid and up-regulation of 3-methylhistidine.[27]

Mixed symptoms also were associated with abnormal genetic regulation of circadian rhythms, such as CLOCK genes and their downstream targets: period genes (Per1, Per2, and Per3) and cryptochrome genes (Cry1 and Cry2). Mice with selective CLOCK knockdown in the ventral tegmental area (VTA) showed manic-like symptoms, increased locomotor activity, alteration in circadian rhythms, and disinhibition but also depression-like symptoms, shorter immobility in the forced swim test, and greater latency to escape in the learned helplessness task. Such behavior was related to increased firing rate of dopaminergic cells and up-regulation of cholinergic and glutamatergic channels in the VTA, suggesting the involvement of CLOCK genes in regulating dopaminergic activity in this area.[28] Cry1 knockdown mice also showed behavior resembling mixed states, which was irresponsive to lithium treatment.[29] In these mice, ineffectiveness of lithium also was demonstrated by the lack of effect in increasing hippocampal neurogenesis as well as high levels of striatal glycogen synthase kinase 3β (GSK3β)—a serine-protein kinase specifically inhibited by lithium. Based on these results, the authors hypothesized a specific effect of Cry1 genes in mediating the effect of lithium. Alteration of genes in upstream regulatory processes of CLOCK, namely SHARP1 and SHARP2, also showed symptoms resembling mixed states.[30] These alterations were also related to disruption of rapid eye movement response and theta oscillations due to sleep deprivation.

STUDIES IN HUMANS
Monoamines

Tandon and colleagues[7] found no differences between mixed and nonmixed mania and between mixed and nonmixed depression in CSF levels of HVA and 5-HIAA. Mixed mania was associated, however, with higher levels of VMA compared with nonmixed depression, whereas mixed depression showed lower levels of HVA and

5-HIAA than mania. On the other hand, Swann and colleagues[31] found that mixed mania did not differ from the other 3 aforementioned groups on CSF HVA and 5-HIAA levels, but mixed mania was associated with higher CSF MHPG than mixed depression and with greater urinary NE excretion than nonmixed mania. The latter finding was replicated in another work in which mixed mania was associated with 50% to 100% greater levels of urinary NE excretion compared with nonmixed mania.[32] That same study showed that ratings of anxiety, hostility, and agitation were positively correlated with epinephrine release or excretion, even though the relationship between agitation and epinephrine excretion was less specific than was the case with anxiety and hostility. The relationship between NE transmission and agitation was further demonstrated by Redmond,[20] who found a positive correlation between agitation and CSF MHPG in depression but not in mania (possibly reflecting greater variance in agitation among depressed compared with manic patients, the latter being all highly agitated). Maas and colleagues[33] found a positive correlation between agitation and levels of urinary VMA in subjects with UD. Furthermore, Catalano and colleagues[34] found that mixed dysthymia and nonmixed mania had significantly greater urinary excretion of VMA than both endogenous depressed patients or healthy controls (HCs), with nonmixed mana having higher excretion levels than mixed dysthymia.

Hypothalamus-Pituitary-Adrenal Axis

Krishnan and colleagues[35] reported a 100% rate of DST nonsuppressors in a sample of 10 subjects with mixed mania. Such finding was replicated by Evans and Nemeroff,[36] who showed that lithium treatment was effective in restoring normal DST suppression. Swann and colleagues[37] and Arana and colleagues[38] reported higher rates of DST nonsuppressors in mixed than nonmixed mania, even though in the work of Arana and colleagues,[38] differences do not reach statistical significance. Subjects with mixed mania also showed the highest rates of nonsuppressors (62.5%) than subjects with different diagnoses, namely, schizophrenia (25%), depression (34%), and nonmixed mania (50%).[39] Higher levels of DST nonsuppressors in mixed mania compared with depression (mixed and nonmixed forms) also were reported by Swann and colleagues.[31] Furthermore, in this work, mixed depression was characterized by rates of DST nonsuppression that were equal to or higher than those in nonmixed depression.

Mixed mania showed greater CSF cortisol levels than nonmixed mania[31,37] and nonmixed depression,[37] and blood and CSF cortisol levels correlated significantly with depressed mood, whereas 24-hour cortisol excretion correlated with anxiety.[37] Changes in cortisol levels in mixed depressives with BD type II correlates with changes in verbal fluency, problem solving, and disinhibition.[40] In summary, HPA axis function was increased and disinhibited in mixed compared with nonmixed mania, whereas the relationship in depression was less clear.

Thyroid

Results regarding thyroid function are largely inconsistent. Chang and colleagues[41] found greater thyroid-stimulating hormone (TSH) and lower T4 serum levels in mixed versus nonmixed mania. These result partially corroborated findings from Zarate and colleagues[8] of greater TSH levels in acutely first-episode mixed mania compared with nonmixed mania. Conversely, Kirkegaard and colleagues,[42] Joffe and colleagues,[43] and Cassidy and colleagues[44] did not find any significant differences between mixed and nonmixed mania.

Circadian Rhythms

Salvatore and colleagues[45] found that patients in a manic or mixed state showed reduced nocturnal sleep, greater nocturnal activity, greater daytime sleep and overall less variation between night and day than those during euthymia. This study, however, did not investigate differences between those in manic or mixed state and considered subjects with manic/mixed patients as a whole. Scott and colleagues[46] used a discriminant function analysis and applied actigraphy to classify subjects based on affective state (mania, depression, and mixed mania). Using this model, 42% of manics were misclassified as depressed, whereas the percentage of misclassification between mixed manics and nonmixed manics or depressives was low. This finding suggests that circadian patterns in mixed mania are substantially different from those of nonmixed mania and depression. Krane-Gartiser and colleagues[47] found that mixed mania displayed activity patterns that were similar to nonmixed mania, that is, low variability, high entropy value, and increasing level of activity from morning to evening, but also similar characteristics to nonmixed depression, such as intraindividual activity fluctuations that increased from morning to evening. In another study,[10] subjects with mixed mania showed a 7-hour phase delay in cortisol acrophase and Per1/ARLTN clock genes expression compared with HCs. This phase delay was greater than that observed in subjects with depression and opposite from that observed in subjects with nonmixed mania, who showed 7-hour phase advance in cortisol acrophase and Per1/ARLTN expression. Interestingly, manics experienced a phase delay, whereas mixed and depressed patients experienced phase advance as they reached euthymia. Such findings contrast with those of Sit and colleagues,[48] who reported the occurrence of mixed symptoms in 3 of 4 depressed women with BD after applying morning light therapy. The investigators suggested that endogenous circadian rhythm phase advance, possibly induced by light therapy, might have resulted in the development of manic symptoms rather than be related to recovery from depression. Light intensity and duration of therapy also might play a role in the development of mixed states and might explain the discrepancy between the aforementioned findings.

Inflammatory Markers and Immune System

Cassidy and colleagues[9] investigated levels of albumin and leukocyte count in non-mixed versus mixed mania using both (DSM) (Third Edition Revised) (narrower) and receiver operating characteristics (broader) sample selection criteria. They found lower levels of albumin and greater levels of neutrophil and monocytes in mixed mania versus nonmixed mania. The investigators, therefore, hypothesized that mixed mania is related to a greater inflammatory state than nonmixed mania. This was not corroborated by Luo and colleagues,[49] who reported no differences in levels of tumor necrosis factor (TNF)-α, Il-6, and IL-18, among mixed mania, nonmixed mania, and depression, all of whom had higher levels of these inflammatory markers than HCs. In mixed and manic patients, however, levels of TNF-α and IL-18 correlated with severity of mania.[49]

Haggerty and colleagues[50] investigated levels of thyroid antibodies in affective and nonaffective psychiatric patients and found that only bipolar depressed and mixed manic subjects had greater levels of thyroid antibodies than the other groups, but those results did not survive multiple comparison correction. These findings subsequently were confirmed in a larger sample of affective patients, where, again, post hoc analyses did not show between-subjects differences.[51] In summary, results suggest that inflammation may be increased in mixed states, but are clouded by small sample sizes and variably increased inflammatory function across mood disorders.

Neuroimaging

Research on the structural and functional underpinnings of mixed states is underdeveloped. Nevertheless, Fleck and colleagues[11] reported progressive alteration in the ventrolateral–prefrontal cortex–subcortical network in a sample of manic or mixed patients performing a task assessing sustained attention. Mixed manic patients also showed hyperactivation in this network—specifically in the left thalamus, left cerebellum, and right inferior frontal gyrus—compared with depressed patients during a task assessing impulsivity.[52] These findings suggest poorer sustained attention and impulse control in subjects with mixed mania, possibly because of altered prefrontal constrained of primary emotional brain centers resulting in greater emotional interference. This hypothesis is consistent with findings from Tolmunen and colleagues,[53] who used single-photon emission computed tomography to demonstrate greater serotonin transporter availability in the brain of a 25-year-old woman with BD type II and mixed depression compared with 6 depressed women, which normalized after 1 year of psychotherapy. Unlike the aforementioned studies, Baxter[54] found that subjects with mixed mania showed lower rates of cerebral glucose level than those with nonmixed mania and similar rates to subjects with UD and HCs.

Other

A few studies documented alterations in fat metabolism in mixed depressives and manics. Ghaemi and colleagues[55] reported higher levels of blood cholesterol in mixed mania compared with both UP/BD nonmixed mania and depression. Conversely Cassidy and Carrol[56] reported that the 47.5% of subjects with mixed mania had cholesterol levels in the lowest tenth percentile, in contrast to 26.9% of those with nonmixed mania. Regarding potentially mixed features in depression, Fava and colleagues[57] found that higher levels of anger weakly correlated with lower cholesterol. Piccinni and colleagues[58] measured blood levels of brain-derived neurotrophic factor, a neurotrophin involved in neurogenesis and neuroplasticity, and found no differences between mixed mania and nonmixed depression; both groups had lower levels than HCs. Nardelli and colleagues[59] found that subjects with nonmixed depression and mixed mania had lower heart rate variability than controls, which increased after reaching euthymia. This finding supports the hypothesis that pathology—psychiatric and nonpsychiatric—is related by low heart rate variability.

DISCUSSION

Evidence from studies investigating the neurobiological underpinnings of mixed states, summarized in **Table 1**, includes that mixed mania and mixed depression could be characterized by similar or higher levels of catecholamines and could be characterized by dysregulated HPA axis functioning compared with the respective nonmixed forms. Furthermore, mixed mania could be associated with circadian rhythm patterns that differ from those related to nonmixed depression or mania. Interestingly, endogenous circadian patterns, such as cortisol excretion and CLOCK gene expression, are consistent with a more severe form of phase delay than the one seen in depression or a more severe form of phase advance than the one seen in mania. Mixed mania may be associated with a greater inflammatory state than nonmixed mania, although evidence is weak. Findings on alteration in brain networks and thyroid function are still insufficient or inconsistent.

These findings suggest the involvement of specific pathologic mechanisms in mixed states: (1) altered monoaminergic function, (2) HPA axis dysfunction and hyperinflammation, and (3) circadian dysregulation. Similar mechanisms have been already

Table 1
Biological alterations in manic, depressive, mixed manic, and mixed depressive states

Measure	Mania	Mixed Mania	Depression	Mixed Depression
Monoamnines				
NA	++	+++	−	+
DA	++	++/+++	−	+
Serotonin	−/−−	−	−/−−	−
HPA axis				
Cortisol	+/−	+++	++	+++
DMX nonsuppression	+/−	+++	++	++/+++
Thyroid				
TSH	+	+/−	+	NR
T3, T4	+	+/−	+	NR
Inflammatory components	+	+/++	+	NR
Circadian rhythms*	+/−	−	+	++

Note: *− indicates phase advance, whereas + indicates phase delay.
Abbreviations: DA, dopamine; DMX, desamethasone; NA, noradrenaline; NR, not reported.

hypothesized to be involved in the pathophysiology of manic and depressive episodes.[60] In mixed states, their magnitude appears to be greater than those present in nonmixed mania and depression (see **Table 1**).

Therefore, monoaminergic dysfunction in mixed mania and depression appear not to be simply more severe alterations than those seen in the nonmixed mood phases, that is, greater monoamine levels in mixed than nonmixed mania, and lower monoamine levels in mixed than nonmixed depression.[6] Instead, both mixed depression and mania are characterized by greater or similar, but not lower, levels of monoamines that their nonmixed forms. Excessive monoamine transmission—specifically NE but also DA—have been classically related to hyperactivation and arousal: broad noradrenergic outputs starting from the locus coeruleus mediate the increase of activation and arousal through astrocyte-dependent CA^{2+} release.[61] Dopaminergic activation in the ventral tegmental area, substantia nigra, and dorsal raphe nuclei increases wake states and motivational arousal toward salient stimuli.[62] Similarly, monoamine hyperactivity also has been related to behavioral symptoms of hyperarousal, such as irritability,[63] agitation,[20,33] and insomnia.[64] Such symptoms have been considered as the core features of both mixed depressives and mixed manic states,[1] therefore suggesting that hyperactivation and hyperarousal represent common driving characteristics of both mixed mania and mixed depression.

In accordance with this hypothesis, greater alterations in other systems involved in mixed states, such as HPA, inflammatory components, and circadian rhythms, have been related to a greater level of monoamine release and a higher level of arousal.[40,65–67] Evidence from treatment effects partially support this hypothesis. Drugs that decrease arousal and directly or indirectly modulate catecholamine function in the brain, such as antipsychotics, lithium, and anticonvulsants, are potentially effective in reducing both mixed manic and mixed depressive episodes.[68–70] There are exceptions, however: lithium monotherapy appears less effective in mixed than in nonmixed manic states,[19,71] and no anticonvulsant other than valproate, carbamazepine, and oxcarbazepine has been shown to be effective in mania.[72] Conversely, drugs that generally increase attention and alertness, as well as monoamine levels, like antidepressants, have been associated with higher risk to induce or worsen mixed symptoms.[15,73]

Several questions on the underlying neurobiology and treatment of mixed states remain open. First, the vast majority of the studies on neurobiological alterations in mixed states focused on mixed mania, so the nature of mixed depression, in particular as related to major depressive disorder, is far less understood and the applicability of the aforementioned pathophysiologic mechanisms to this mixed mood phase is speculative. Second, recent advances in neuroimaging techniques unveiled that for both manic and depressive states, monoaminergic transmission alterations are subtle, rather than global, and might be enhanced in some areas and blunted in others.[72] The lack of recent studies, however, assessing regional differences in monoaminergic transmission alterations in samples with mixed states impedes the formulation of more detailed hypotheses. Third, the lack of effectiveness of certain antipsychotics on mixed states,[74] or the greater effectiveness of valproate compared with lithium in mixed mania,[1,71] confirms that the current knowledge on the pathophysiology of such states is incomplete. Differences between lithium and valproate effects may be instructive. Although both lithium and valproate decrease calcium levels via inositol monophosphate inactivation, lithium acts through direct inhibition, whereas valproate through reduced synthesis.[75] Furthermore, compared with valproate, lithium regulates the expression of a smaller number of genes in serotonergic cell lines,[76] and its efficacy seems to be affected by knockdown of Cry1, which also has been shown to induce mixed symptoms in mice.[29] All such evidence suggests that other possible mechanisms might play an important role in the pathophysiology of mixed states and might account for the aforementioned treatment differences.

SUMMARY

Both manic and depressive mixed states could be related to greater monoamine levels, higher levels of HPA dysregulation and inflammation, and circadian rhythms alteration than their nonmixed forms. These findings contradict the dichotomous view of mania and depression and corroborate Kraepelin's view of mixed states as result of a pathologic drive state due to activation and hyperarousal.

DISCLOSURE

The authors have nothing to disclose.

REFERENCES

1. Swann AC, Perugi G, Frye MA, et al. Bipolar mixed states: an International Society for bipolar disorders task force report of symptom structure, course of illness, and diagnosis. Am J Psychiatry 2013;170:31–42.
2. Aretaeus. On the causes and symptoms of chronic disease. Boston: Milford House; 1972.
3. Hippocrates. The genuine works of hippocrates. New York: Dover; 1868.
4. Galen. On the natural faculties. Cambridge (England): Harvard University Press; 1916.
5. Kraepelin E. Manic-depressive illness and paranoia. Edinburgh (Scotland): Livingstone; 1921.
6. Schildkraut JJ. The catecholamine hypothesis of affective disorders: a review of supporting evidence. Am J Psychiatry 1965;122:509–22.

7. Tandon R, Channabasavanna SM, Greden JF. CSF biochemical correlates of mixed affective states. Acta Psychiatr Scand 1978;78:289–97.

8. Zarate CA, Tohen M, Zarate SB. Thyroid function tests in first-episode bipolar disorder manic and mixed types. Biol Psychiatry 1997;42:302–4.

9. Cassidy F, Wilson WH, Carrol BJ. Leukocytosis and hypoalbuminemia in mixed bipolar states: evidence for immune activation. Leukocytosis hypoalbuminemia mixed Bipolar states : Evid immune activation 2002;105:60–4.

10. Moon JH, Cho CH, Son GH, et al. Advanced circadian phase in mania and delayed circadian phase in mixed mania and depression returned to normal after treatment of bipolar disorder. EBioMedicine 2016;11:285–95.

11. Fleck DE, Eliassen JC, Durling M, et al. Functional MRI of sustained attention in bipolar mania. Mol Psychiatry 2012;17:325–36.

12. McElroy SL, Keck PE, Pope HG, et al. Clinical and research implications of the diagnosis of dysphoric or mixed mania or hypomania. Am J Psychiatry 1992; 149:1633–44.

13. American Psychiatric Association. Diagnostic and statistical manual of mental disorders, fourth edition, text revision. Washington, DC: American Psychiatric Association; 2000.

14. American Psychiatric Association. Diagnostic and statistical manual of mental, third edition, Revised. Washington, DC: American Psychiatric Association; 1987.

15. Sani G, Napoletano F, Vöhringer PA, et al. Mixed depression: clinical features and predictors of its onset associated with antidepressant use. Psychother Psychosom 2014;83:213–21.

16. Koukopoulos A, Sani G, Koukopoulos AE, et al. Melancholia agitata and mixed depression. Acta Psychiatr Scand 2007;115:50–7.

17. American Psychiatric Association. Diagnostic and statistical manual of mental disorders. 5th Edition. Arlington (VA): American Psychiatric Publishing; 2013.

18. Manji HK, Quiroz JA, Payne JL, et al. The underlying neurobiology of bipolar disorder. World Psychiatry 2003;2:136–46.

19. Swann AC, Koslow SH, Katz MM, et al. Lithium carbonate treatment of mania: cerebrospinal fluid and urinary monoamine metabolites and treatment outcome. Arch Gen Psychiatry 1987;44:345–54.

20. Redmond DE. Cerebrospinal fluid amine metabolites. Arch Gen Psychiatry 2011; 43:938–47.

21. Daban C, Vieta E, Mackin P, et al. Hypothalamic-pituitary-adrenal axis and bipolar disorder. Psychiatr Clin North Am 2005;28:469–80.

22. Berk M. Neuroprogression: pathways to progressive brain changes in bipolar disorder. Int J Neuropsychopharmacol 2009;12:441–5.

23. Alloy LB, Ng TH, Titone MK, et al. Circadian rhythm dysregulation in bipolar spectrum disorders. Curr Psychiatry Rep 2017;19:21.

24. Kelly JP, Wrynn AS, Leonard BE. The olfactory bulbectomized rat as a model of depression: an update. Pharmacol Ther 1997;74:299–316.

25. Lumia AR, Teicher MH, Salchli F, et al. Olfactory bulbectomy as a model for agitated hyposerotonergic depression. Brain Res 1992;587:181–5.

26. Mucignat-Caretta C, Bondi' M, Caretta A. Animal models of depression: olfactory lesions affect amygdala, subventricular zone, and aggression. Neurobiol Dis 2004;16:386–95.

27. Heath A, Lindberg DR, Makowiecki K, et al. Medium- and high-intensity rTMS reduces psychomotor agitation with distinct neurobiologic mechanisms. Transl Psychiatry 2018;8:126.

28. Mukherjee S, Coque L, Cao J, et al. Knock-down of CLOCK in the VTA through RNAi results in a mixed state of mania and depression-like behavior. Biol Psychiatry 2010;68:503–11.

29. Schnell A, Sandrelli F, Ranc V, et al. Mice lacking circadian clock components display different mood-related behaviors and do not respond uniformly to chronic lithium treatment. Chronobiol Int 2015;32:1075–89.

30. Baier PC, Brzózka MM, Shahmoradi A, et al. Mice lacking the circadian modulators SHARP1 and SHARP2 display altered sleep and mixed state endophenotypes of psychiatric disorders. PLoS One 2014;9:e110310.

31. Swann AC, Stokes PE, Secunda SK, et al. Depressive mania versus agitated depression: Biogenic amine and hypothalamic-pituitary-adrenocortical function. Biol Psychiatry 1994;35:803–13.

32. Swann AC, Secunda SK, Koslow SH, et al. Mania: sympathoadrenal function and clinical state. Psychiatry Res 1991;37:195–205.

33. Maas JW, Katz MM, Koslow, et al. Adrenomedullary function in depressed patients. J Psychiatr Res 1994;28:357–67.

34. Catalano A, Campanini T, De Risio C, et al. Study of the urinary excretion of vanillylmandelic acid during depressive syndromes, maniacal states and mixed states. Sist Nerv 1966;18:100–23.

35. Krishnan RR, Maltbie AA, Davidson JRT. Abnormal cortisol suppression in bipolar patients with simultaneous manic and depressive symptoms. Am J Psychiatry 1983;140:203–5.

36. Evans DL, Nemeroff CB. The dexamethasone suppression test in mixed bipolar disorder. Am J Psychiatry 1983;140:615–7.

37. Swann AC, Stokes PE, Casper R, et al. Hypothalamic-pituitary-adrenocortical function in mixed and pure mania. Acta Psychiatr Scand 1992;85:270–4.

38. Arana GW, Baldessarini RJ, Ornsteen M. The dexamethasone suppression test for diagnosis and prognosis in psychiatry. Commentary and review. Arch Gen Psychiatry 1985;42:1193–204.

39. Stokes PE, Stoll PM, Koslow SH, et al. Pretreatment DST and hypothalamic-pituitary-adrenocortical function in depressed patients and comparison groups: a multicenter study. Arch Gen Psychiatry 1984;41:257–67.

40. Lee HH, Chang CH, Wang LJ, et al. The correlation between longitudinal changes in hypothalamic–pituitary–adrenal (HPA)-axis activity and changes in neurocognitive function in mixed-state bipolar II disorder. Neuropsychiatr Dis Treat 2018;14:2703–13.

41. Chang KD, Keck PE, Stanton SP, et al. Differences in thyroid function between bipolar manic and mixed states. Biol Psychiatry 1998;43:730–3.

42. Kirkegaard C, Bjørum N, Cohn D, et al. Thyrotrophin-Releasing Hormone (TRH) stimulation test in manic-depressive illness. Arch Gen Psychiatry 1978;35:1017–21.

43. Joffe RT, Young LT, Cooke RG, et al. The thyroid and mixed affective states. Acta Psychiatr Scand 1994;90:131–2.

44. Cassidy F, Ahearn EP, Carroll BJ. Thyroid function in mixed and pure manic episodes. Bipolar Disord 2002;4:393–7.

45. Salvatore P, Baldessarini RJ, De Panfilis C, et al. Circadian activity rhythm abnormalities in ill and recovered bipolar I disorder patients. Bipolar Disord 2008;10:256–65.

46. Scott J, Vaaler AE, Fasmer OB, et al. A pilot study to determine whether combinations of objectively measured activity parameters can be used to differentiate

between mixed states, mania, and bipolar depression. Int J Bipolar Disord 2017; 5:5.

47. Krane-Gartiser K, Vaaler AE, Fasmer OB, et al. Variability of activity patterns across mood disorders and time of day. BMC Psychiatry 2017;17:1–8.

48. Sit D, Wisner KL, Hanusa BH, et al. Light therapy for bipolar disorder: a case series in women. Bipolar Disord. Bipolar Disord 2007;9:918–27.

49. Luo Y, He H, Zhang M, et al. Altered serum levels of TNF-α, IL-6 and IL-18 in manic, depressive, mixed state of bipolar disorder patients. Psychiatry Res 2016;244:19–23.

50. Haggerty JJ, Evans DL, Golden RN, et al. The presence of antithyroid antibodies in patients with affective and nonaffective psychiatric disorders. Biol Psychiatry 1990;27:51–60.

51. Haggerty JJ Jr, Silva SG, Mason GA, et al. Prevalence of antithyroid antibodies in mood disorders. Depress Anxiety 1997;5:91–6.

52. Fleck DE, Kotwal R, Eliassen JC, et al. Preliminary evidence for increased fronto-subcortical activation on a motor impulsivity task in mixed episode bipolar disorder. J Affect Disord 2011;133(1–2):333–9.

53. Tolmunen T, Joensuu M, Saarinen PI, et al. Elevated midbrain serotonin transporter availability in mixed mania: A case report. BMC Psychiatry 2004;4:1–6.

54. Baxter LR. Cerebral metabolic rates for glucose in mood disorders. Arch Gen Psychiatry 2011;42:441–7.

55. Ghaemi SN, Shields GS, Hegarty JD, et al. Cholesterol levels in mood disorders: high or low? Bipolar Disord 2000;2:60–4.

56. Cassidy F, Carroll BJ. Hypocholesterolemia during mixed manic episodes. Eur Arch Psychiatry Clin Neurosci 2002;252:110–4.

57. Fava M, Abraham M, Pava J, et al. Cardiovascular risk factors in depression: the role of anxiety and anger. Psychosomatics 1996;37:31–7.

58. Piccinni A, Veltri A, Costanzo D, et al. Decreased plasma levels of brain-derived neurotrophic factor (BDNF) during mixed episodes of bipolar disorder. J Affect Disord 2015;171:167–70.

59. Nardelli M, Valenza G, Gentili C, et al. Temporal trends of neuro-autonomic complexity during severe episodes of bipolar disorders. Conf Proc IEEE Eng Med Biol Soc 2014;2014:2948–51.

60. Lee HJ, Son GH, Geum D. Circadian rhythm hypotheses of mixed features, anti-depressant treatment resistance, and manic switching in bipolar disorder. Psychiatry Investig 2013;10:225–32.

61. Duffy S, MacVicar B. Adrenergic calcium signaling in astrocyte networks within the hippocampal slice. J Neurosci 1995;15:5535–50.

62. Pfaff D, Ribeiro A, Matthews J, et al. Concepts and mechanisms of generalized central nervous system arousal. Ann N Y Acad Sci 2008;1129:11–25.

63. Yamamoto KI, Shinba T, Yoshii M. Psychiatric symptoms of noradrenergic dysfunction: a pathophysiological view. Psychiatry Clin Neurosci 2014;68:1–20.

64. Wang ZJ, Liu JF. The molecular basis of insomnia: implication for therapeutic approaches. Drug Dev Res 2016;77:427–36.

65. Raison CL, Miller AH. When not enough is too much: The role of insufficient glucocorticoid signaling in the pathophysiology of stress-related disorders. Am J Psychiatry 2003;160:1554–65.

66. Michopoulos V, Powers A, Gillespie CF, et al. Inflammation in fear-and anxiety-based disorders: PTSD, GAD, and beyond. Neuropsychopharmacology 2017; 42:254–70.

67. Baglioni C, Spiegelhalder K, Regen W, et al. Insomnia disorder is associated with increased amygdala reactivity to insomnia-related stimuli. Sleep 2014;37:1907–17.
68. Krystal AD, Goforth HW, Roth T. Effects of antipsychotic medications on sleep in schizophrenia. Int Clin Psychopharmacol 2008;23:150–60.
69. Marneros A, Goodwin FK. Bipolar disorders: mixed states, rapid-cycling, and atypical forms. New York: Cambridge University Press; 2005.
70. Viktorin A, Lichtenstein P, Thase ME, et al. The risk of switch to mania in patients with bipolar disorder during treatment with an antidepressant alone and in combination with a mood stabilizer. Am J Psychiatry 2014;171:1067–73.
71. Swann AC, Bowden CL, Morris D, et al. Depression during mania: treatment response to lithium or divalproex. Arch Gen Psychiatry 1997;54:37–42.
72. Nikolaus S, Müller H-W, Hautzel H. Different patterns of dopaminergic and serotonergic dysfunction in manic, depressive and euthymic phases of bipolar disorder. Nuklearmedizin 2017;56:191–200.
73. Reinhard DL, Whyte J, Sandel ME. Improved arousal and initiation following tricyclic antidepressant use in severe brain injury. Arch Phys Med Rehabil 1996;77:80–3.
74. Grunze H, Vieta E, Goodwin GM, et al. The World Federation of Societies of Biological Psychiatry (WFSBP) guidelines for the biological treatment of bipolar disorders: update 2009 on the treatment of acute mania. World J Biol Psychiatry 2009;10:85–116.
75. Vaden DL, Ding D, Peterson B, et al. Lithium and valproate decrease inositol mass and increase expression of the yeast INO1 and INO2 genes for inositol biosynthesis. J Biol Chem 2001;276:15466–71.
76. Balasubramanian D, Pearson JF, Kennedy MA. Gene expression effects of lithium and valproic acid in a serotonergic cell line. Physiol Genomics 2018;51:43–50.

Temporal Structure of Mixed States

Does Sensitization Link Life Course to Episodes?

Alan C. Swann, MD[a,b,*], Marijn Lijffijt, PhD[a],
Alessio Simonetti, MD[a,c]

KEYWORDS

- Bipolar disorder • Mixed states • Arousal • Impulsive behavior • Recurrence
- Behavioral sensitization • Depression • Mania

KEY POINTS

- A continuum of mixed features spans depressive and manic states. Regardless of preponderance of depressive or manic affect, they are characterized by hyperarousal, including impulsivity, anxiety, and agitation.
- Mixed states are associated with illness course characteristics, including severe recurrence and traumatic and/or addictive stimuli.
- These characteristics, along with elevated catecholamine and hypothalamic-pituitary-adrenocortical function, are consistent with susceptibility to behavioral sensitization, which links long-term illness course to short-term behavior regulation.

INTRODUCTION

The terms "bipolar disorder" and "manic-depressive illness" imply an illness characterized by 2 opposing "poles" or mood states. This discussion of underlying mechanisms of mixed states will approach bipolar disorder as a condition of long-term behavior dysregulation in which symptomatic states, such as depression, mania, or anxiety, are complications of the underlying illness. Understanding mixed states, as well as bipolar disorder itself, may be hampered by our insistence on seeing the illness through the lens of apparently opposite mood states rather than from the perspective of mechanisms driving susceptibility to these states.

Manic and depressive symptoms are not mutually exclusive.[1] They are not generally negatively correlated—whether subjects are mainly depressed,[2] manic,[3] or either.[4,5]

[a] Department of Psychiatry, Baylor College of Medicine, 1977 Butler Boulevard, Suite E4.400, Houston, TX 77030, USA; [b] Mental Health Care Line, Michael E. DeBakey VAMC, 2002 East Holcombe Boulevard, Houston, TX 77030, USA; [c] Department of Psychiatry and Neurology, Sapienza University of Rome, Rome, Italy
* Corresponding author. Department of Psychiatry, Baylor College of Medicine, 1977 Butler Boulevard, Suite E4.400, Houston, TX 77030.
E-mail address: Alan.Swann@bcm.edu

Psychiatr Clin N Am 43 (2020) 153–165
https://doi.org/10.1016/j.psc.2019.10.005
0193-953X/20/Published by Elsevier Inc.

Over centuries, there have been 2 predominate models of mixed states. Combinatorial models posit essentially linear combinations of depressive and manic features. Kraepelin[1] proposed combinations of elements, each of which could be considered depressed or manic. A second, noncombinatorial model, from the Vienna School,[6] invokes biological mechanisms governing drive and emotions. The Vienna criteria delineate a mixed affective subtype with sustained instability, the "persistent presence of a drive state contradictory to the mood state and/or the emotional resonance"[7(p164)]. Kraepelin proposed that mixed states were driven by a mechanism resembling hyperarousal and represented a more severe form of bipolar disorder.[1] The original classical descriptions of the illness by Hippocrates, Aretaeus, and others[8] (see Gabriele Sani and Alan C. Swann's article, "Mixed States: Historical Impact and Evolution of the Concept," in this issue) had already proposed a lifelong, recurrent, potentially progressive condition predisposing to combinations of manic, depressive, psychotic, or agitated states, with state-related potential for suicidal and/or aggressive behavior, and associated with arousal and stress.[8]

We focus on potential physiologic mechanisms driving mixed states. First, we discuss symptomatic structure, its relationship to hyperarousal, and its convergence between depressive and manic mixed states. We then address the longer term course of mixed states, including predisposing factors and course of illness. We propose that susceptibility to mixed states is related to arousal stemming from early sensitization to highly salient stressful or rewarding stimuli.[9]

SYMPTOMATIC STRUCTURE OF MIXED EPISODES

Kraepelin formulated mixed states as free-standing or transitional episodes, rather than depressive or manic subtypes.[1] Aretaeus and his contemporaries described mixed states as the basis for what we call affective disorders.[8] However, mixed states have recently been studied as subtypes of manic or depressive episodes. We review the properties of predominately manic or depressive mixed states, because that is the manner in which they have generally been studied, and their potential convergence. We emphasize anxiety because of its strong connection to mixed features regardless of affective state, combined activation and depression, and the manner in which these are driven by hyperarousal.[9]

Manic Episodes

Manic episodes with 2 or more nonoverlapping depressive symptoms had poorer response to lithium than those with fewer depressive symptoms.[10] Increased anxiety emerged with 2 depressive symptoms; suicidal behavior and early onset of illness, with 3 or more symptoms.[5]

Anxiety

In describing what he considered the commonest mixed state, Kraepelin used "depressive" and "anxious" mania interchangeably, describing patients as "frantically anxious," reflecting general hyperarousal.[1] In mania, high anxiety scores are associated with lithium resistance.[11] Anxiety scores are correlated with depression scores in mania[5] and are minimal in nonmixed mania.[5,11,12] Anxiety seems to be a core symptom of manic mixed episodes.[13]

Depressive Episodes

Characteristics distinguishing depressive mixed episodes emerge at low mania symptom scores.[2] Depressive episodes with 2 or 3 manic symptoms have properties associated with bipolar disorder (a history of free-standing mania or hypomania, a family history of bipolar disorder) and mixed states (severe course, co-occurring ill-nesses).[14,15] Manic symptoms in depressive episodes were related to severe illness-course; receiver operating characteristic analysis revealed a threshold at modest manic symptom scores (score of 6) for early onset, suicide attempt, or trau-matic brain injury.[2] Some patients may experience hypomanic or manic symptoms only during depression,[14,15] especially early in the course of illness, because depres-sion is usually the first episode in bipolar disorder.[16] In patients originally diagnosed with major depressive disorder, a decreased need for sleep, increased energy, and increased goal-directed activity during depressive episodes predicted "diagnostic change" to bipolar disorder.[17] The illness course seems to be related to diagnosis: pa-tients with early onset, frequent episodes, a family history of bipolar disorder, and mania-related symptoms limited to depressive episodes eventually met diagnostic criteria for bipolar disorder.[15,17] Our requirement for free-standing mania or hypoma-nia to diagnose bipolar disorder may delay diagnosis and appropriate treatment.

Anxiety
Unlike mania, where anxiety is basically limited to mixed episodes, anxiety is pervasive in depression, mixed or not.[15,17] Sato and colleagues[18] wrote that it is "unlikely to play a major role in the core phenomenological features of mixed depression." Yet, in bipo-lar depressive episodes, severity of anxiety correlates with mania[5] as well as with depression scores.[2] Therefore, anxiety is strongly related to depressive mixed states. Its diagnostic usefulness may be limited because anxiety is prominent in nonmixed depression, but it is an important clinical expression of hyperarousal underlying mixed states.

Symptoms Across Depressive and Manic Episodes

Depressive or manic features can exist independently or in combination.[5] Factor an-alyses of affective episodes show that manic and depressive symptoms are generally not correlated,[4,5] identifying constructs that may be useful in recognizing mixed states regardless of polarity.[19] We developed a measure of the extent to which symptoms were mixed independent of dominant affect, the Mixed State Index, essentially the product of normalized depression and mania scores.[5] High Mixed State Index score was related to severe course of illness, trait- and action-impulsivity, and suicidal behavior. Discriminant function analysis identified worry, negative self-evaluation, increased energy, visible hyperactivity, and racing thoughts as associated with mixed states, regardless of nominal polarity.[5]

Anxiety across episodes
Increased anxiety was predicted by at least 2 depressive symptoms in mania, or at least 1 manic symptom in depression. Anxiety correlated with depressive symptoms in manic episodes, with manic symptoms in depressive episodes, and with the degree to which symptoms were mixed across all episodes.[5] This pervasive role is consistent with mixed states driven by hyperarousal, with anxiety as a core feature.[1,19]

Agitation

Agitation, prominent in depressive, manic, and mixed states, includes 2 basic distur-bances[20]: painful inner tension, with driven non–goal-directed motor activity (pacing, tension, wringing hands) and often prominent in depression, regardless of manic symptoms[12,20]; and increased, poorly regulated, driven goal-directed activity, often with irritability and impatience, prominent in mania, regardless of depressive symp-toms.[12,20] Mixed episodes, whether predominately depressive or manic, generally include both aspects of agitation.[1,12]

EPISODE PHENOMENOLOGY: SUMMARY

During mixed states, depressive and manic symptoms can cover the full range of severity, each potentially varying, negatively, positively, or independently, over time.[21] Characteristics of depressive and manic mixed states converge[5] and occur with relatively mild symptoms of the "opposite" type. A subgroup of patients with bipolar disorder seems to be susceptible to mixed states. This susceptibility is characterized by hyperarousal symptoms during episodes, whose mechanism may be reflected by course of illness. It is also associated with illness course characteristics that may precede the first mixed episode and may exist between episodes.

MIXED STATES AND COURSE OF ILLNESS
Recurrence

Age of onset
In mixed mania, data on age of onset are inconsistent.[22,23] Interpretation is limited by variable definitions of age of onset and of mixed states. In general, subjects were considered mixed if any manic episode was mixed, but one negative study focused on mixed first episodes.[24] Onset was earlier in patients with at least 1 mixed episode over 10 years.[25] Specificity of early onset for mixed states versus stronger genetic liability to bipolarity is unclear. Studies of mixed depressive patients found consistently earlier age of onset than nonmixed depressions.[2,26,27] Mixed features across polarities were related to early onset independent of episode type.[5] This was only partially accounted for by severity of early onset bipolar disorder in general.[28]

Episode recurrence
Patients with mixed manic or depressive states have more lifetime episodes of illness than those without mixed states.[25,29–33] Mixed states can also occur as fewer episodes of longer duration.[31] Regardless, individuals with mixed states experience longer periods of mood instability.

Time to syndrome resolution is longer for mixed than for depressive or manic episodes.[27,31,34] One study of 143 mixed and 118 manic episodes found mixed episodes were longer, with lower rates of interepisode remission,[31] and earlier relapse after remission.[35] Accordingly, course and prognosis of mixed mania are worse than for nonmixed mania.[22,23]

Consistency of mixed episodes
The possibility of a subtype of bipolar disorder characterized by susceptibility to mixed states has been addressed prospectively and retrospectively.

Prospective studies In 247 manic patients (97 mixed) followed for 24 months after hospitalization, index mixed states were followed by a 12-fold excess of subsequent mixed states, and 6.5 times more depressive episodes, than patients presenting in mania. In contrast, manic index episodes were followed by 10 times more mania and 6 times more hypomania than were mixed states.[36] Prospective comparison of subjects with 2 discrete manic or mixed episodes found that recurrence was consistent with the index episode, regardless of criteria.[37] In bipolar depression, mixed depressive states were largely stable over 2 years.[38] These studies show that mixed and nonmixed bipolar presentations are stable, at least over 12 to 24 months.

Retrospective studies Retrospective studies, regardless of the specific mixed state criteria used, consistently found increased histories of mixed episodes in patients with currently mixed episodes.[31,39] Patients whose manic episodes were exclusively mixed had more previous mixed episodes than those with both mixed and nonmixed manic episodes.[33]

Conclusions Prospective studies, with the advantage of directly observed episodes, and retrospective studies, with the advantage of longer periods of observation, concur that susceptibility to mixed states seems to be essentially stable within individuals, regardless of index episode type.

Complications and Co-occurring Illnesses

Suicidality

Predominately manic mixed states combine depression with the impulsivity and hyperactivity of mania, resulting in suicidal ideation higher than nonmixed mania[30,39–43] and correlating with depressive symptoms during manic episodes.[5,43] Among 184 inpatients with bipolar I disorder, past suicidality was increased in manic episodes with at least 3 depressive symptoms.[42] Prospectively studied patients with mixed episodes had a higher rate of suicide attempts than those without mixed states, although this finding may have been influenced by age of onset.[32] Patients with exclusively mixed manic episodes had higher risk for suicide than those with both mixed and nonmixed episodes.[33]

Predominately depressed Mixed depressive episodes combine the hopelessness of depression with the impulsivity and hyperactivity of mania,[2,5,44] leading to increased suicide attempt rate over those without concomitant manic features.[2,5,26] Increased anxiety in mixed states may exacerbate suicide risk.[45] Suicidal behavior was increased with "subsyndromal hypomania" during depression compared with purely depressive episodes.[15]

   Unlike nonmixed manic episodes, risk of suicide is already increased in nonmixed depression. Manic symptoms adds to risk. Noneuphoric hypomanic symptoms were associated with increased suicidality in depressed patients who had never experienced free-standing hypomania or mania.[16] In bipolar depression, receiver operating curve analysis showed increased suicide attempt history with Mania Rating Scale score of 8, parallel to increased impulsivity.[2]

Conclusions Suicidal behavior is associated with sensitizing features related to illness recurrence, early stress, and addictions.[9] Mixed states, depressive or manic, combine hopelessness with impulsivity and activation, leading to high potential suicide risk. Knowledge that an individual was susceptible to mixed states would aid in anticipating emergence of mixed features, with attendant risk for suicide.

Co-occurring conditions

Stress-related disorders Individuals with mixed manic or depressive episodes are more likely to have experienced early-life stressors and to have stress-related disorders.[46]

Anxiety disorders Co-occurring anxiety disorders are more common in patients with mixed than nonmixed manic[40] or depressive[47] episodes. This was confirmed by 2 large longitudinal studies: NESARC[48] and the Zurich study.[49] Co-occurring anxiety disorders are associated with a more severe course of illness and increased service use.[50] Anxiety susceptibility in people with mixed states may extend beyond the mixed episodes.

Substance use disorders Alcohol and substance abuse seem to be more prevalent in mixed than nonmixed manic episodes,[2,34,51] with poor outcome and less favorable response to lithium.[34,52] Differences in lifetime alcohol abuse, however, were not always confirmed.[39] History of substance use disorder predicted greater mood instability in bipolar depressive episodes,[53] possibly contributing to increased risk for mixed features and suicidal behavior.

Secondary mixed states Mixed states may be more likely than other episodes to be associated with substance-related, nonpsychiatric medical, or neurologic disorders, even more than manic or depressive episodes in general.[34] Even with clear previous primary affective episodes, any mixed episode may be related to another medical condition requiring treatment, episode-related trauma, or neglect of health.[54]

Course of Illness: Summary

Patients who are susceptible to mixed states differ from those who are not, with more episodes, increased suicidality, higher rates of co-occurring stress- or addiction-related conditions, and poorer response to treatments.

Patients with a more unstable form of bipolar disorder, including susceptibility to mixed states, are likely to be lithium resistant,[52] although lithium remains a valuable treatment component. Mixed episodes increase the likelihood of subsequent mixed states.[31,33,36–39] **Fig. 1** summarizes the structure of mixed states. Episode symptoms are related to illness course, with central roles of arousal/activation and reward dysregulation. These illness-course characteristics, like the episode characteristics described elsewhere in this article, seem to be consistent across mixed depression and mixed mania, raising questions of (1) mechanisms underlying mixed episodes and associated course of illness, and (2) how, because they have important potential clinical and treatment consequences, susceptibility to mixed states can be identified efficiently.

MECHANISMS AND RECOMMENDATIONS
Potential Mechanisms of Mixed States

Both Kraepelin[1] and the Vienna school[7] proposed that mixed episodes resulted from a driven state, related to emotional lability and activation.[8,9] Consistent with clinical

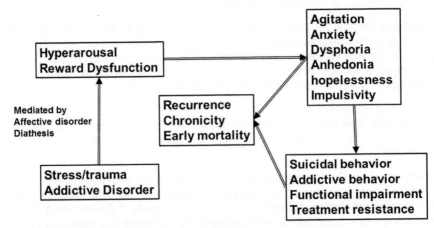

Fig. 1. Structure of mixed states. Mixed states are a manifestation of long-term illness course in affective disorders. The susceptibility to hyperarousal and reward dysfunction that generally characterizes affective disorders is exaggerated, possibly related to individual variation and exposure to salient stimuli. This predisposes to combined activation and negative affect, with their clinical consequences.

studies, catecholaminergic and hypothalamic-pituitary-adrenocortical function in mixed states is increased beyond nonmixed manic or depressive episodes.[32,55] These results, from more than nearly 100 years, converge to suggest that hyperarousal underlies mixed episodes.

Mixed states occur in the context of early onset, frequent episodes and/or prolonged affective instability, with increased stress-related[47] and substance use[51,53] disorders. Mechanisms underlying this relationship between susceptibility to episode-related behavioral instability and a long-term unfavorable illness course are a potential target for diagnosis and treatment.

Bipolar disorders have high heritability but specific genetic bases have been elusive, raising the question of environmental or epigenetic mechanisms. Like other long-term psychiatric and nonpsychiatric illnesses,[56] bipolar disorder may have a sequential course with a prodrome (high genetic or environmental risk without overt illness), progressing through early symptoms, syndromal episodes, and progressively increasing risk of recurrence, severity, and related complications like addictions and severe behavioral disturbances.[56-58] The trajectory of illness varies[57]; mechanisms underlying neuroprogression, whether genetic, environmental, or interactions between the two, affect a substantial number of individuals, with wide-ranging severity.[57,59] Basic manifestations of this progression may include episodic-stable (or "classic) and complicated or unstable-progressive episodes, as well as episode sensitization.[57]

Episodic-stable (or classic)[57] episodes, although potentially severe, are infrequent and time limited, without prominent comorbidities, either depressive or manic without combining or rapidly alternating between the two, and with strong short-term[52] and long-term[58] response to lithium.

Complicated or unstable-progressive episodes have earlier onset and greater frequency, with partial or transient recovery, and common sensitization-related problems including substance use and trauma history.[60,61] Across mood disorders, long-term impairment is more strongly related to episode frequency than affective symptom severity.[62] These characteristics of neuroprogression resemble sensitization[9] and mixed states.[53]

Characteristics of neuroprogression seem to be persistent and familial,[52] although trauma or addiction can convert a classic to a complicated course.[63] A complicated course is associated with impulsive behavior, including suicidality,[40,43] and sensitizing events, including frequent episodes,[64-66] substance use,[62] and traumas.[63,66] Mixed states seem to be a hallmark of complicated illness course, with sensitization-related characteristics including substance use disorders, early stressors, and severe recurrence.[2,5,9,60,61,67] Impulsivity[2,5,67] and cerebrospinal fluid norepinephrine or its metabolites[32,55] are higher in episodes with mixed characteristics than in more exclusively manic or depressive episodes.

Episode sensitization may be a component of illness progression,[57,61] with sensitivity to stressors and/or addictions, accelerating episode frequency and treatment resistance.[52,53,60,61] An increased number of episodes was associated with accelerated recurrence and delayed recovery in bipolar disorder.[67] This could result from relationships between episodes and substance-abuse or stressors,[60] or results of episodes themselves like increased norepinephrine and/or dopamine.[9,55,68] Rather than progressive increases in episode frequency, recurrence could have a presensitized course, with increased episode frequency from the outset or developing early, perhaps related to early trauma.[65] Recurrence is predicted more strongly by the interaction between early trauma and number of previous episodes than number of episodes alone, consistent with sensitization.[61]

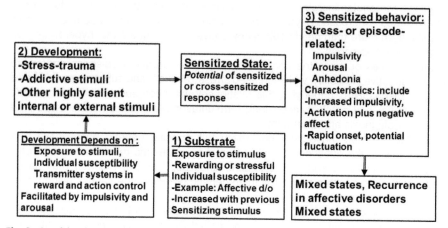

Fig. 2. Sensitization to addictive or stressful stimuli. The diagram summarizes the manner in which, in susceptible individuals, exposure to highly salient stimuli, such as stress perceived as inescapable or highly rewarding addictive stimuli, can lead to development of behavioral sensitization, which generalizes across rewarding and addictive stimuli.[9] Many characteristics of affective episodes, including the potential for increased arousal and catecholaminergic function,[12,32,53,55] can potentiate sensitization. Characteristics of sensitized behavior resemble mixed states.[9]

Childhood trauma is associated with interepisode functional impairment and suicidal behavior in bipolar disorder.[69] Previous abuse magnified momentary effects of stress on negative affect,[70] predisposing to stress-related impulsivity. Childhood trauma questionnaire scores correlated significantly with Affective Lability Scale scores in bipolar disorder, in contrast with healthy controls.[71] Characteristics of mixed states and their consequences are related to effects of early exposure to traumatic[72] and/or addictive[73] stimuli, which are partially mediated by norepinephrine.[74] Arousal[75,76] and affective lability[72] have been reported to mediate relationships among negative affect, affective instability, and stress.[73]

Fig. 2 summarizes the characteristics of behavioral sensitization. Susceptibility to sensitization varies, but is increased in recurrent-progressive psychiatric disorders, especially bipolar disorder.[9] However, within bipolar disorder it also seems to vary widely.[59] Sensitization and impulsivity are responses to salient stimuli that involve increased arousal[75,77] and require dopamine,[78] glutamate,[78] and norepinephrine,[79,80] with inhibition by gamma-aminobutyric acid[81] and serotonin.[81,82] Sensitization requires norepinephrine-serotonin uncoupling[83] with decreased limbic serotonin.[84] This increases noradrenergic locus coeruleus activity directly and through glutamate receptors,[78,82] leading to a potential cycle of increasing locus coeruleus disinhibition, resulting in increased impulsivity and arousal. Stress-induced arousal is an important potential consequence of sensitized behavior[9,77,85] and mixed states.

SUMMARY

Mixed episodes are characterized by combined or rapidly alternating behavioral states, possibly driven by hyperarousal with increased catecholaminergic function.[32,55] They are associated with early onset, recurrent course (or prolonged mood instability), early stressors, and substance use disorders.[53] These characteristics suggest that mixed states are an expression of behavioral sensitization in bipolar disorder.[9] Susceptibility to behavioral sensitization could result from interacting genetic susceptibilities and environmental or pharmacologic sensitizing stimuli. Treatment would involve pharmacologic and behavioral therapies aimed at minimizing or managing potentially sensitizing stimuli and preventing expression of sensitized behavior. Educational and community measures addressing early substance use and adaptation to stressors would have great practical value.

DISCLOSURE

A.C. Swann: Grant support from American Foundation for Suicide Prevention, National Institutes of Health; Veterans Administration Cooperative Studies Program; Department of Defense. M. Lijffijt: Grant support from National Institutes of Health; Department of Defense.

REFERENCES

1. Kraepelin E. Mixed States. In Kraepelin E, Manic-depressive insanity and paranoia. Robertson GM, editor; Barclay RM, translator. Edinburgh (Scotland): E & S Livingstone; 1921. p. 99-117.
2. Swann AC, Moeller FG, Steinberg JL, et al. Manic symptoms and impulsivity during bipolar depressive episodes. Bipolar Disord 2007;9(3):206–12.
3. Dilsaver SC, Chen YR, Shoaib AM, et al. Phenomenology of mania: evidence for distinct depressed, dysphoric, and euphoric presentations. Am J Psychiatry 1999;156(3):426–30.
4. Johnson SL, Morriss R, Scott J, et al. Depressive and manic symptoms are not opposite poles in bipolar disorder. Acta Psychiatr Scand 2011;123(3):206–10.
5. Swann AC, Steinberg JL, Lijffijt M, et al. Continuum of depressive and manic mixed states in patients with bipolar disorder: quantitative measurement and clinical features. World Psychiatry 2009;8(3):166–72.
6. Berner P, Gabriel E, Katschnig H, et al. Diagnostic criteria for schizophrenia and affective psychoses (world psychiatric association). Washington, DC: American Psychiatric Association; 1983.
7. Janzarik W. Dynamische Grundkonstellationen in endogenen psychosen. Berlin: Springer; 1959.
8. Swann AC. Mixed features: evolution of the concept, past and current definitions, and future prospects. CNS Spectr 2017;22:161–9.
9. Lijffijt M, O'Brien B, Salas R, et al. Interactions of immediate and long-term action regulation in the course and complications of bipolar disorder. Philos Trans R Soc Lond B Biol Sci 2018. https://doi.org/10.1098/RSTB.2018.0132.
10. Swann AC, Bowden CL, Morris D, et al. Depression during mania: treatment response to lithium or divalproex. Arch Gen Psychiatry 1997;54:37–42.
11. Swann AC, Secunda SK, Katz MM, et al. Lithium treatment of mania: clinical characteristics, specificity of symptom change, and outcome. Psychiatry Res 1986; 18:127–41.
12. Swann AC, Secunda SK, Katz MM, et al. Specificity of mixed affective states: clinical comparison of mixed mania and agitated depression. J Affect Disord 1993; 28:81–9.
13. Cassidy F. Anxiety as a symptom of mixed mania: implications for DSM-5. Bipolar Disord 2010;12(4):437–9.
14. Benazzi F, Akiskal HS. Delineating bipolar II mixed states in the Ravenna-San Diego collaborative study: the relative prevalence and diagnostic significance

of hypomanic features during major depressive episodes. J Affect Disord 2001; 67(1–3):115–22.

15. Zimmermann P, Bruckl T, Nocon A, et al. Heterogeneity of DSM-IV major depressive disorder as a consequence of subthreshold bipolarity. Arch Gen Psychiatry 2009;66(12):1341–52.

16. Akiskal HS, Benazzi F, Perugi G, et al. Agitated "unipolar" depression reconceptualized as a depressive mixed state: implications for the antidepressant-suicide controversy. J Affect Disord 2005;85(3):245–58.

17. Fiedorowicz JG, Endicott J, Leon AC, et al. Subthreshold hypomanic symptoms in progression from unipolar major depression to bipolar disorder. Am J Psychiatry 2011;168(1):40–8.

18. Sato T, Bottlender R, Kleindienst N, et al. Irritable psychomotor elation in depressed inpatients: a factor validation of mixed depression. J Affect Disord 2005;84(2–3):187–96.

19. Bertschy G, Gervasoni N, Favre S, et al. Frequency of dysphoria and mixed states. Psychopathology 2008;41(3):187–93.

20. Katz MM, Secunda SK, Koslow SH, et al. A multivantaged approach to measurement of behavioral and affect states for clinical and psychobiological research. Psychol Rep 1984;55:619–71.

21. Kotin J, Goodwin FK. Depression during mania: clinical observations and theoretical implications. Am J Psychiatry 1971;129:55–62.

22. McElroy SL, Keck PE, Pope HG, et al. Clinical and research implications of the diagnosis of dysphoric or mixed mania or hypomania. Am J Psychiatry 1992; 149:1633–44.

23. Cassidy F, Yatham LN, Berk M, et al. Pure and mixed manic subtypes: a review of diagnostic classification and validation. Bipolar Disord 2008;10(1 Pt 2):131–43.

24. Baldessarini RJ, Bolzani L, Cruz N, et al. Onset-age of bipolar disorders at six international sites. J Affect Disord 2010;121(1–2):143–6.

25. Gonzalez-Pinto A, Barbeito S, Alonso M, et al. Poor long-term prognosis in mixed bipolar patients: 10-year outcomes in the vitoria prospective naturalistic study in Spain. J Clin Psychiatry 2010;72(671):676.

26. Goldberg JF, Perlis RH, Bowden CL, et al. Manic symptoms during depressive episodes in 1,380 patients with bipolar disorder: findings from the STEP-BD. Am J Psychiatry 2009;166(2):173–81.

27. Benazzi F. Bipolar disorder–focus on bipolar II disorder and mixed depression. Lancet 2007;369(9565):935–45.

28. Suppes T, Leverich GS, Keck PE, et al. The Stanley Foundation Bipolar Treatment Outcome Network. II. Demographics and illness characteristics of the first 261 patients. J Affect Disord 2001;67(1–3):45–59.

29. Swann AC, Janicak PL, Calabrese JR, et al. Structure of mania: depressive, irritable, and psychotic clusters with different retrospectively-assessed course patterns of illness in randomized clinical trial participants. J Affect Disord 2001; 67(1–3):123–32.

30. Hantouche EG, Akiskal HS, Azorin JM, et al. Clinical and psychometric characterization of depression in mixed mania: a report from the French National Cohort of 1090 manic patients. J Affect Disord 2006;96:225–32.

31. Perugi G, Akiskal HS, Micheli C, et al. Clinical subtypes of bipolar mixed states: validating a broader European definition in 143 cases. J Affect Disord 1997;43(3): 169–80.

32. Post RM, Rubinow DR, Uhde TW, et al. Dysphoric mania. Clinical and biological correlates. Arch Gen Psychiatry 1989;46:353–8.

33. Pacchiarotti I, Mazzarini L, Kotzalidis GD, et al. Mania and depression. Mixed, not stirred. J Affect Disord 2011;133:105–13.
34. Himmelhoch JM, Garfinkel ME. Sources of lithium resistance in mixed mania. Psychopharmacol Bull 1986;22:613–20.
35. Tohen M, Waternaux CM, Tsuang MT. Outcome in Mania. A 4-year prospective follow-up of 75 patients utilizing survival analysis. Arch Gen Psychiatry 1990; 47:1106–11.
36. Baldessarini RJ, Salvatore P, Khalsa HM, et al. Dissimilar morbidity following initial mania versus mixed-states in type-I bipolar disorder. J Affect Disord 2010; 126(1–2):299–302.
37. Cassidy F, Ahearn E, Carroll BJ. A prospective study of inter-episode consistency of manic and mixed subtypes of bipolar disorder. J Affect Disord 2001;67(1–3): 181–5.
38. Sato T, Bottlender R, Sievers M, et al. Evaluating the inter-episode stability of depressive mixed states. J Affect Disord 2004;81(2):103–13.
39. Akiskal HS, Hantouche EG, Bourgeois ML, et al. Gender, temperament, and the clinical picture in dysphoric mixed mania: findings from a French national study (EPIMAN). J Affect Disord 1998;50(2–3):175–86.
40. Dilsaver SC, Chen YR, Swann AC, et al. Suicidality, panic disorder, and psychosis in bipolar depression, depressive-mania, and pure mania. Psychiatry Res 1997; 73:47–56.
41. Strakowski SM, McElroy SL, Keck PE Jr, et al. Suicidality among patients with mixed and manic bipolar disorder. Am J Psychiatry 1996;153(5):674–6.
42. Goldberg JF, Garno JL, Leon AC, et al. Association of recurrent suicidal ideation with nonremission from acute mixed mania. Am J Psychiatry 1998;155(12): 1753–5.
43. Goldberg JF, Garno JL, Portera L, et al. Correlates of suicidal ideation in dysphoric mania. J Affect Disord 1999;56(1):75–81.
44. Balazs J, Benazzi F, Rihmer Z, et al. The close link between suicide attempts and mixed (bipolar) depression: implications for suicide prevention. J Affect Disord 2006;91(2–3):133–8.
45. Diefenbach GJ, Woolley SB, Goethe JW. The association between self-reported anxiety symptoms and suicidality. J Nerv Ment Dis 2009;197(2):92–7.
46. Garno JL, Goldberg JF, Ramirez PM, et al. Impact of childhood abuse on the clinical course of bipolar disorder. Br J Psychiatry 2005;186:121–5.
47. Akiskal HS. The dark side of bipolarity: detecting bipolar depression in its pleomorphic expressions. J Affect Disord 2005;84(2–3):107–15.
48. Agosti V, Stewart JW. Hypomania with and without Dysphoria: comparison of comorbidity and clinical characteristics of respondents from a national community sample. J Affect Disord 2008;108(1–2):177–82.
49. Angst J, Gamma A, Benazzi F, et al. Does psychomotor agitation in major depressive episodes indicate bipolarity? Evidence from the Zurich Study. Eur Arch Psychiatry Clin Neurosci 2009;259(1):55–63.
50. Goldstein BI, Levitt AJ. The specific burden of comorbid anxiety disorders and of substance use disorders in bipolar I disorder. Bipolar Disord 2008;10(1):67–78.
51. Strakowski SM, Tohen M, Stoll AL, et al. Comorbidity in mania at first hospitalization. Am J Psychiatry 1992;149:554–6.
52. Duffy A, Alda M, Kutcher S, et al. A prospective study of the offspring of bipolar parents responsive and nonresponsive to lithium treatment. J Clin Psychiatry 2002;63(12):1171–8.

53. Swann AC, Stokes PE, Secunda SK, et al. Depressive mania vs agitated depression: biogenic amine and hypothalamic-pituitary-adrenocortical function. Biol Psychiatry 1994;35:803–13.
54. Swann AC, Lafer B, Perugi G, et al. Bipolar mixed states: an international society for bipolar disorders task force report of symptom structure, course of illness, and diagnosis. Am J Psychiatry 2013;170:31–42.
55. Swann AC. Mania and mixed states. In: Glick RL, Berlin JS, Fishkind A, et al, editors. Emergency psychiatry, principles and practice. Philadelphia: Lippincott, Williams & Wilkins; 2008. p. 189–200.
56. Muneer A. Staging models in bipolar disorder: a systematic review of the literature. Clin Psychopharmacol Neurosci 2016;14(2):117–30.
57. Duffy A, Vandeleur C, Heffer N, et al. The clinical trajectory of emerging bipolar disorder among the high-risk offspring of bipolar parents: current understanding and future considerations. Int J Bipolar Disord 2017;5:37.
58. Greil W, Kleindienst N, Erazo N, et al. Differential response to lithium and carbamazepine in the prophylaxis of bipolar disorder. J Clin Psychopharmacol 1998; 18(6):455–60.
59. Passos IC, Mwangi B, Vieta E, et al. Areas of controversy in neuroprogression in bipolar disorder. Acta Psychiatr Scand 2016;134(2):91–103.
60. Post RM, Kalivas P. Bipolar disorder and substance abuse: pathological and therapeutic implications of their comorbidity and cross-sensitization. Br J Psychiatry 2013;202(3):172–6.
61. Weiss RB, Stange JP, Boland EM, et al. Kindling of life stress in bipolar disorder: comparison of sensitization and autonomy models. J Abnorm Psychol 2015; 124(1):4–16.
62. Goldberg JF, Harrow M, Grossman LS. Recurrence of affective episodes in bipolar and unipolar mood disorders at follow-up. Br J Psychiatry 1995;166:382–5.
63. Post RM. Epigenetic basis of sensitization to stress, affective episodes, and stimulants: implications for illness progression and prevention. Bipolar Disord 2016; 18:315–24.
64. Kessing LV, Andersen PK. Evidence for clinical progression of unipolar and bipolar disorders. Acta Psychiatr Scand 2016;135:51–64.
65. Anderson SF, Monroe SM, Rohde P, et al. Questioning kindling: an analysis of cycle acceleration in unipolar depression. Clin Psychol Sci 2015;4:229–38.
66. Swann AC, Secunda SK, Stokes PE, et al. Stress, depression, and mania: relationship between perceived role of stressful events and clinical and biochemical characteristics. Acta Psychiatr Scand 1990;81:389–97.
67. Park DY, Do D, Chang L, et al. Episode accumulation associated with hastened recurrence and delayed recovery in bipolar disorder. J Affect Disord 2018;227(2): 657–64.
68. Swann AC, Koslow SH, Katz MM, et al. Lithium treatment of mania: CSF and urinary monoamine metabolites and treatment outcome. Arch Gen Psychiatry 1987; 44:345–54.
69. Etain B, Henry C, Bellivier F, et al. Beyond genetics: childhood affective trauma in bipolar disorders. Bipolar Disord 2008;10:867–76.
70. Rauschenberg C, van Os J, Cremers D, et al. Stress sensitivity as a putative mechanism linking childhood trauma and psychopathology in youth's daily life. Acta Psychiatr Scand 2017;136(4):373–88.
71. Aas M, Aminoff SR, Lagerberg TV, et al. Affective lability in bipolar disorders is associated with high levels of childhood trauma. J Psychiatr Res 2014; 218(1–2):252–5.

72. Aas M, Henry C, Bellivier F, et al. Affective lability mediates the association between childhood trauma and suicide attempts, mixed episodes, and co-morbid anxiety disorders in bipolar disorders. Psychol Med 2017;47(5):902–12.
73. Hellberg SN, Russlee TI, Robinson MJF. Cued for risk: evidence for an incentive sensitization framework to explain the interplay between stress and anxiety, substance abuse, and reward uncertainty in disordered gambling behavior. Cogn Aff Behav Neurosci 2019;19(3):737–58.
74. Song AH, Kucyi A, Napadow V, et al. Pharmacological modulation of noradrenergic arousal circuitry disrupts functional connectivity of the locus coeruleus in humans. J Neurosci 2017;37(29):6938–45.
75. Pearlstein JG, Johnson SL, Modavi K, et al. Neurocognitive mechanisms of emotion-related impulsivity: the role of arousal. Psychophysiology 2019;56(2): e13293.
76. Zhang S, Hu S, Hu J, et al. Barratt Impulsivity and Neural Regulation of Physiological Arousal. PLoS One 2015;10(6):e0129139.
77. Kandel ER. Cellular Insights into the multivariant nature of arousal. In: McFadden D, editor. Neural mechanisms in behavior. New York: Springer-Verlag; 1980. p. 260–91.
78. Malmo RB. Activation: a neuropsychological dimension. Psychol Rev 1959;66: 367–86.
79. Kalivas PW. Interactions between dopamine and excitatory amino acids in behavioral sensitization to psychostimulants. Drug Alcohol Depend 1995;37:95–100.
80. Vanderschuren LJ, Beemster P, Schoffelmeer AN. On the role of noradrenaline in psychostimulant-induced psychomotor activity and sensitization. Psychopharmacology 2003;169(2):176–85.
81. Alttoa A, Eller M, Herm L, et al. Amphetamine-induced locomotion, behavioral sensitization to amphetamine, and striatal D2 receptor function in rats with high or low spontaneous exploratory activity: differences in the role of locus coeruleus. Brain Res 2007;1131:138–48.
82. Thayer JF, Friedman BH. Stop that! Inhibition, sensitization, and their neurovisceral concomitants. Scand J Psychol 2002;43:123–30.
83. Aston-Jones G, Akaoka H, Charlety P, et al. Serotonin selectively attenuates glutamate-induced activation of noradrenergic locus coeruleus neurons. J Neurosci 2001;11(3):760–9.
84. Salomon L, Lanteri C, Glowinski J, et al. Behavioral sensitization to amphetamine results from an uncoupling between noradrenergic and serotonergic neurons. Proc Natl Acad Sci U S A 2006;103:7476–81.
85. Heidbreder CA, Oertle T, Feldon J. Dopamine and serotonin imbalances in the left anterior cingulate and pyriform cortices following the repeated intermittent administration of cocaine. Neuroscience 1999;89:701–15.

Treatment

Pharmacologic Treatment of Mixed States

Maurizio Pompili, MD, PhD[a],*, Gustavo H. Vazquez, MD, PhD, FRCPC[b,c],
Alberto Forte, MD[c,d,1], Debbi Ann Morrissette, PhD[e],
Stephen M. Stahl, MD, PhD[f,g,2]

KEYWORDS

- Lithium • Mixed features • Mixed depression • Mood stabilizers
- Pharmacologic treatment • Second-generation antipsychotics

KEY POINTS

- The current literature supporting the efficacy of second-generation antipsychotics (SGAs) and mood stabilizers (MS) for the treatment of mixed symptoms is scarce.
- SGAs in the acute phase, particularly olanzapine, showed some efficacy. Valproate was found to be effective in the prevention of new affective episodes after dysphoric mania. Lithium is considered as a first-line treatment in the prevention of episodes of any polarity after a mixed episode.
- Antidepressants should not be used in the absence of a mood stabilizer or one of the SGAs with mood stabilizing properties in the treatment of mixed states.

INTRODUCTION

Despite the fact that several guidelines are available for clinicians as recommendations for the treatment of any polarity of bipolar disorders (BD),[1–4] there is still a lack of treatment guidelines providing up-to-date recommendations after the release of the relatively recent latest edition of the Diagnostic and Statistical Manual of Mental

[a] Department of Neurosciences, Mental Health and Sensory Organs, Suicide Prevention Center, Sant'Andrea Hospital, Sapienza University of Rome, Rome, Italy; [b] Department of Psychiatry, Queen's University, 752 King Street West, Kingston, Ontario K7L 4X3, Canada; [c] International Consortium for Research on Mood & Psychotic Disorders, McLean Hospital, Belmont, MA, USA; [d] Department Neurosciences, Mental Health and Sensory Organs, Suicide Prevention Center, Sant'Andrea Hospital, Sapienza University of Rome, Rome, Italy; [e] Neuroscience Education Institute, 5900 La Place Court, Suite 120, Carlsbad, CA 92008, USA; [f] Department of Psychiatry, University of California San Diego, San Diego, CA, USA; [g] University of Cambridge, Cambridge, UK
[1] Present address: Via di Grottarossa, 1035, 00189 Rome, Italy.
[2] Present address: 1917 Palomar Oaks Way, Suite 200, Carlsbad, CA 92008.
* Corresponding author. Department of Psychiatry, Sant'Andrea Hospital, Sapienza University of Rome, Via di Grottarossa, 1035, 00189 Rome, Italy
E-mail address: maurizio.pompili@uniroma1.it

Psychiatr Clin N Am 43 (2020) 167–186
https://doi.org/10.1016/j.psc.2019.10.015
0193-953X/20/© 2019 Elsevier Inc. All rights reserved.

Disorders (DSM-5).[5–7] DSM-5 introduced a new nosologic entity characterized by subthreshold hypomanic or manic symptoms occurring during depressive episodes of either major depressive disorder (MDD) or BD I or II.[6] As previously noted, each treatment guideline developed before the new DSM-5 specifier on mixed features is based on the previous conceptualization of DSM-IV criteria and is related to co-occurring full-blown, threshold-level depression with full-blown, threshold-level mania (mixed mania).[7] Consequently, treatment recommendations for mixed states overlapped with those for bipolar mania, and studies designed to address the efficacy of medications in mixed affective symptoms still remain an unmet need of current research on mood disorders treatment.[8]

Despite the relatively high prevalence of mixed symptoms among patients suffering from mood disorders[9–11] and the significant number of studies exploring the effectiveness of atypical antipsychotics (SGAs) and mood stabilizers (MS) as pharmacologic treatment of major depression MDD and BD,[1,2] the current published literature supporting the specific efficacy of SGAs and MS for the treatment of mixed symptoms is scarce.

Given the clinical and epidemiologic relevance of mixed features both in BD and unipolar disorder, the existing gaps between the updated diagnostic criteria, and the latest research findings in the treatment of mood disorders, the aim of the present paper is to develop an overview on the treatment of both mania and depression with mixed features.

ATYPICAL ANTIPSYCHOTICS IN THE TREATMENT OF MIXED STATES

In a comprehensive electronic literature search through June 2019, the authors identified 16 randomized controlled trials (RCTs) evaluating the efficacy of SGAs in the treatment of mood episodes with mixed symptoms and/or features (**Table 1**), although all of the studies applied the DSM-IV or DSM-IV-TR diagnostic criteria for MDD and BD. Several studies have compared the responses to SGAs and placebo in patients with manic or mixed episodes associated with BD I.[12–20] Five studies investigated the clinical effect of SGAs and placebo on patients with an acute episode of major depression with mixed features in either MDD[21,22] or BD,[23–25] and one RCT study explored the efficacy of quetiapine for patients suffering from a BD type II hypomanic episode with mixed features.[26]

Aripiprazole

In a 3-week randomized, double-blind, placebo-controlled trial, Sachs and colleagues (2006) studied the efficacy of aripiprazole for the treatment of acute or mixed episodes in patients with BD type I. The investigators reported a significant improvement in patients receiving aripiprazole versus placebo in the Young Mania Rating Scale (YMRS), Clinical Global Improvement-Bipolar Version Severity of Illness scale (CGI-BP-S), and Positive and Negative Syndrome Scale (PANSS) total scores at the endpoint. There were no statistically significant differences in the Montgomery–Asberg Depression Rating Scale (MADRS) total scores between aripiprazole and placebo arms at the end of the trial.

Asenapine

Asenapine 5 and 10 mg BID significantly improved manic symptoms, according to the change on the YMRS and CGI-BP-S total scores, versus placebo in the subset of patients with mixed episodes in two 3-week RCTs studies.[12,13] However, in only 1 of the 2 studies asenapine demonstrated efficacy versus placebo for significantly improving depressive symptoms measured by MADRS by the end of the third week.[12]

Table 1
Overview of studies reporting pharmacologic treatment of mixed states

Study	N	Study Population	Meds	Study Design	Results	Primary Measure	Notes
Tohen et al,[16] 1999	139	DSM-IV criteria for acute manic or mixed episodes in patients with BD I	Olanzapine vs placebo	3-wk randomized, double-blind, placebo-controlled study	YMRS: −4.88 points (placebo) vs −10.26 (olanzapine) $P = .02$ CGI-BP-S: −0.59 (placebo) vs −0.89 (olanzapine) Not statistically significant PANSS: −3.09 (placebo) vs −11.06 (olanzapine) $P = .02$ HAMD 21: −3.00 (placebo) vs −2.9 (olanzapine) Not statistically significant	YMRS HAMD 21 CGI-BP-S PANSS	
Tohen et al,[20] 2000	115	DSM-IV criteria for acute mania or mixed episode in patients with BD I	Olanzapine vs placebo	4-wk randomized, double-blind, placebo-controlled study	YMRS: −14.8 (olanzapine) vs −8.1 (placebo); $P < .001$	YMRS HAMD-21 CGI-BP PANSS	Similar improvement in HAMD-21 total score between olanzapine vs placebo ($P = .09$) No worsening on depressive symptoms
Keck et al,[19] 2003	210	DSM-IV criteria for acute mania or mixed episode in patients with BD I	Ziprasidone vs placebo	3-wk randomized, double-blind, placebo-controlled study	YMRS: −12.4 (ziprasidone) vs −7.8 (placebo); $P = .005$ CGI-BP-S: −1.3 (ziprasidone) vs −0.9 (placebo); $P < .01$	YMRS CGI-BP-S	Randomization was done at a 2:1 ratio for the 3-wk double-blind treatment with ziprasidone (40–80 mg twice daily) or placebo

(continued on next page)

Table 1
(continued)

Study	N	Study Population	Meds	Study Design	Results	Primary Measure	Notes
Sachs et al,[15] 2006	272	DSM-IV criteria for acute manic or mixed episodes in patients with BD I	Aripiprazole vs placebo	3-wk randomized, double-blind, placebo-controlled study	YMRS: −7.2 points (placebo) vs −12.5 (aripiprazole); $P < .001$ CGI-BP-S: −0.97 (placebo) vs −1.42 (aripiprazole); $P < .01$ PANSS: −5.33 (placebo) vs −10.08 (aripiprazole); $P < .05$ MADRS: −3.02 (placebo) vs −4.33 (aripiprazole) Not statistically significant	YMRS MADRS CGI-BP-S PANSS	Mean baseline MADRS score at start of the study was low (15)
McIntyre et al,[13] 2009	488	Manic or mixed episode associated with BD I (DSM-IV)	Asenapine vs placebo vs olanzapine	3-wk, randomized, double-blind, placebo-controlled, parallel-group study, with olanzapine used to assess assay sensitivity	Improved YMRS: Asenapine vs placebo: −3.7; $P < .007$ Olanzapine vs placebo: −6.8; $P < .0001$ Improved CGI-BP-S: Asenapine vs placebo: −0.4; $P = .012$ Olanzapine vs placebo: −0.7; $P < .0001$ Improved MADRS:	YMRS CGI-BP-S MADRS	Completion rate with olanzapine was higher than those of placebo ($P = .01$) and asenapine ($P \leq .001$) Two deaths by suicide occurred during the study. One was deemed possibly related to treatment (asenapine) and the other unlikely to be related to treatment

Study	N	Criteria	Intervention	Study design	Measures	Results	Comments
						Asenapine vs placebo: −1.1; P=NS Olanzapine vs placebo: −2.2; P < .003	(olanzapine) by the investigator
Vieta et al,[17] 2010	493	DSM-IV criteria for acute manic or mixed episodes in patients with BD I	Paliperidone ER vs placebo, with quetiapine as control	3-wk (acute phase) + 9-wk (maintenance phase) randomized, double-blind, placebo-controlled study	YMRS GAF	3-wk endpoint: YMRS: Paliperidone ER superior to placebo: −5.5; P < .001 Quetiapine superior to placebo was −4.2; P < .001) Quetiapine to paliperidone ER was 1.5; P = .099 GAF (change from baseline): 6.7 (placebo), 12.2 (paliperidone ER), and 11.6 (quetiapine) group. P < .001 for both the paliperidone ER and quetiapine. 12-wk endpoint: YMRS: Paliperidone ER was noninferior to quetiapine GAF (change from baseline): 14.9 (paliperidone ER), 15.8 (quetiapine): (P = .525)	Patients randomized to a ratio of 2:2:1 for paliperidone ER, quetiapine, placebo in the acute phase. Patients on placebo were switched to paliperidone ER in the maintenance phase PANSS and CGI-BP-S scores showed no difference between the paliperidone ER and quetiapine groups at the 12-wk endpoint No statistically significant change in improvement of YMRS at 3-wk endpoint between paliperidone ER and placebo in respect to diagnoses subsets (mania/mixed episodes)

(continued on next page)

Table 1
(continued)

Study	N	Study Population	Meds	Study Design	Results	Primary Measure	Notes
Cutler et al,[18] 2011	316	DSM-IVcriteria for acute mania or mixed episode in patients with BD I	Quetiapine XR vs placebo	3-wk randomized, double-blind, placebo-controlled study	YMRS: For patients with mania:]quetiapine XR) −16.34 vs (placebo) −11.32; P < .001 For patients with mixed mania: (quetiapine XR) −13.79 vs (placebo) −11.45; P = .107 MADRS: For patients with mania: change between quetiapine XR and placebo: −2.42; P = .005	YMRS MADRS	In terms of YMRS and MADRS improvement: quetiapine XR = placebo in mixed episodes group, but superior in pure manic episodes

Study	N	Diagnosis	Treatment	Design	Results	Outcomes
Berwaerts et al,[14] 2012	766	Most recent manic or mixed episode of BD I (DSM-IV)	Acute phase: paliperidone vs olanzapine Continuation phase: paliperidone vs olanzapine vs placebo	3-wk acute phase + 12-wk continuation phase, randomized double-blind, parallel group study	For patients with mixed mania: change between quetiapine XR and placebo: -3.01; $P = .188$ Median time to recurrence of manic symptoms: 558 d on paliperidone ER vs 283 d on placebo; $P = .017$ Was not observed on olanzapine, as <50% of patients (23%). Post-hoc pairwise comparisons of olanzapine with placebo and olanzapine with paliperidone ER showed that time to recurrence of any mood symptoms was significantly longer with olanzapine ($P \leq .001$ vs either treatment group) Median time to recurrence of depressive symptoms: lower in the placebo group than that in the paliperidone ER group; however, the difference	Time to recurrence of mood symptoms YMRS MADRS Recurrence of mood symptoms was defined as any one of the following: • YMRS≥15 and CGI-BP-S for mania≥4 • YMRS<15, MADRS≥16, and CGI-BP-S for depression≥4 • Voluntary or involuntary hospitalization for any mood symptoms • Therapeutic intervention to prevent or treat an impending mood episode (ie, use of benzodiazepines for >3 consecutive days; supplementation with another medication. • Any other clinically relevant event that suggests a recurrent mood episode

(continued on next page)

Table 1
(continued)

Study	N	Study Population	Meds	Study Design	Results	Primary Measure	Notes
					was not statistically significant		
Patkar et al,[25] 2012	73	DSM-IV criteria for major depressive episode with mixed features in BD	Ziprasidone vs placebo	6 wk Randomized, Double-Blind, Placebo-Controlled Study	MADRS: -5.4; $P < .05$	MADRS	
Suppes et al,[26] 2013	55	BD II experiencing hypomania with mixed symptoms	Quetiapine vs placebo, as adjunctive treatment	8-wk, randomized, double-blind, placebo-controlled trial	YMRS, CGI-BP-S: No statistically significant improvement between the 2 groups. MADRS: Statistically significant improvement in the quetiapine group over placebo of -6.93; $P = .0445$; however, this difference diminished between weeks 6 and 8. GAF:	YMRS CGI-BP-S MADRS GAF	Mixed symptoms defined as scores of more than or equal to 12 on YMRS and more than or equal to 15 on MADRS

Study	N	Diagnostic criteria	Comparison	Study design	Outcome	Results	Notes
						Statistically significant improvement in the quetiapine group over placebo of 4.40; $P = .0445$	
Tohen et al,[23] 2014	1214	DSM-IV criteria for major depressive episode with mixed features in BD	Olanzapine vs placebo	6-wk randomized, double-blind, placebo-controlled study	MADRS	MADRS: -3.76 ($P = .002$) vs -3.20 ($P < .001$) vs -3.44 ($P = .002$) for 0, 1, or 2, ≥ 3 manic symptoms	n = 690 on olanzapine, n = 524 on placebo. Pooled analysis from Tohen et al. 2003 and Tohen et al. 2012
McIntyre et al,[24] 2015	272	DSM-IV criteria for major depressive episode with mixed features in BD	Lurasidone vs placebo	6-wk randomized, double-blind, placebo-controlled study	MADRS	MADRS: -4.8; $P = .001$	n = 182 on lurasidone, n = 90 on placebo
Patkar et al,[21] 2015	49	DSM-IV criteria for major depressive disorder with mixed features	Ziprasidone vs placebo	13-wk randomized, double-blind, placebo-controlled study	MADRS	MADRS: -1.57; $P = .48$, not statistically significant	Crossover study

(continued on next page)

Table 1
(continued)

Study	N	Study Population	Meds	Study Design	Results	Primary Measure	Notes
Landbloom et al,[12] 2016	367 (108 with mixed episodes)	Manic or mixed episode associated with BD I (DSM-IV)	Asenapine vs Placebo	3-wk, randomized, double-blind, placebo-controlled trial	Improved YMRS: asenapine, 5 mg, bid vs placebo −3.5; P = .0136, and asenapine, 10 mg, bid vs placebo −4.0; P = .0100 Improved CGI-BP-S: asenapine, 5 mg, bid vs placebo −0.5; P = .0100, and asenapine, 10 mg, bid vs placebo −0.5; P = .0052 Improved PANSS: asenapine, 5 mg, bid vs placebo −3.8; P = .0081, and asenapine, 10 mg, bid vs placebo −3.2; P = .0247 Improve MADRS: asenapine, 5 mg, bid vs placebo −5.8; P = .0066, and asenapine, 10 mg, bid vs placebo −5.9; P = .0059	YMRS CGI-BP-S PANSS MADRS	No statistically significant change in reduction of YMRS or CGI from placebo group in respect to diagnoses subsets (mania/mixed episodes)
Suppes et al,[22] 2016	209	DSM-IV criteria for major depressive disorder with mixed features	Lurasidone vs placebo	A randomized, double-blind, placebo-controlled study	YMRS: −7.0 compared with −4.9; P < .001 MADRS: −20.5 compared with −13.0; P < .001 CGI-S: −1.8 compared with −1.2; P < .001	YMRS CGI-BP-S MADRS	

Cariprazine

The most recent SGA to be added to the clinicians' armamentarium is cariprazine. Cariprazine has demonstrated efficacy in the treatment of both depression and mania in the context of BD. A retrospective post hoc analysis of 3 trials of cariprazine (1.5–3 mg/d) for the treatment of bipolar depression investigated the efficacy of cariprazine for the treatment of depression with mixed features in the context of BD type I.[27] It should be noted that this study did not use the DSM-5 criteria for mixed features (at least 3 [hypo]manic symptoms excluding psychomotor agitation, irritability, and distractibility); rather, this study looked at patients with BD I with 4 or more items on the YMRS. Of the 1383 patients with BD, 58.4% were experiencing concomitant manic symptoms (YMRS score ≥4 but <10 (1 study) or 12 [2 studies]). Both patients with and without manic symptoms showed significant improvement in MADRS, Hamilton Depression Rating Scale (HAMD)-17, and CGI total scores from baseline to week 6 compared with placebo.[27]

Lurasidone

Most recently, the efficacy of lurasidone for the treatment of patients with unipolar and bipolar depressive disorders with mixed features was studied in 2 different clinical trials. In a randomized, double-blind, placebo-controlled study, patients with a major depressive episode with mixed features receiving lurasidone, 20 to 60 mg, daily versus placebo showed a statistically significant clinical improvement according to the changes in the YMRS, CGI-BP-S, and MADRS total scores between baseline and endpoint at week 6.[22] In another 6-week, randomized, double-blind, placebo-controlled study of lurasidone versus placebo for the treatment of patients suffering from a major depressive episode with mixed features in BD, the clinical improvement according to the MADRS total scores resulted in a statistically significant difference in favor of the active arm.[24]

Olanzapine

Olanzapine efficacy was tested in 2 different randomized, double-blind, placebo-controlled studies among patients with DSM-IV criteria for BDI acute manic or mixed episode.[16,20] Although the improvement in the YMRS total scores was statistically significantly different for olanzapine versus placebo, both active and placebo arms demonstrated a similar HAMD-21 total score changes at the endpoint. In a pooled analysis from 2 RCT studies on olanzapine for the treatment of major depressive episode with mixed features in BD, MADRS total scores in subjects receiving olanzapine were significantly improved versus placebo among patients displaying acute depression plus either 0, 1, 2, or 3 or more hypo/manic symptoms.[23]

Paliperidone

Paliperidone extended-release (ER) versus olanzapine versus placebo was studied in an acute (3 weeks) and continuation (12 weeks) phase in a randomized, double-blind, parallel-group trial.[14] Paliperidone and olanzapine demonstrated significantly greater improvements on manic symptom total scores, although the median time to recurrence of depressive symptoms in the paliperidone ER group was not statistically significantly different from the placebo arm. In a similarly designed randomized, double-blind, placebo-controlled 3-week acute phase and 9-week maintenance phase study, with quetiapine as control active arm, paliperidone ER was superior to placebo and noninferior to quetiapine for the improvement YMRS, PANSS, Global Assessment of Functioning (GAF), and CGI-BP-S total scores at the endpoint.[17]

Quetiapine

In the only double-blind, placebo-controlled RCT study in patients with BD II experiencing hypomania with mixed symptoms,[26] the adjunctive treatment of quetiapine did not produce a statistically significant improvement in the YMRS and CGI-BP-S total scores when compared with placebo at endpoint (8 weeks). Even though there was a significant initial improvement among those subjects receiving quetiapine versus placebo in the depressive symptoms according to the MADRS total scores change, the clinical difference disappeared by weeks 6 and 8. The investigators of the study reported a significant improvement in the GAF total scores at endpoint only for the patients receiving quetiapine as an add-on therapeutic. In a 3-week double-blind RCT study, the efficacy of quetiapine XR versus placebo was evaluated for the treatment of acute mania or mixed episode in patients with BD I.[18] By the end of the trial, and according to YMRS and MADRS total scores improvement, quetiapine XR performed statistically similar to placebo for the treatment of the patients suffering from a mixed episode but was significantly superior to placebo at endpoint for those patients with a pure manic episode.

Ziprasidone

We have identified 3 different randomized, double-blind, placebo-controlled trials studying the efficacy of ziprasidone for the treatment of mixed features among patients with mood disorders. In a 3-week RCT study, subjects suffering from a BD I manic or mixed episode receiving ziprasidone, 40 to 80 mg, twice daily versus placebo demonstrated a significantly superior improvement on the YMRS and CGI-BP-S total scores at the endpoint.[19] In a 6-week RCT study in bipolar patients with a diagnosis of a major depressive episode with mixed features, ziprasidone was statistically superior to placebo for improving depressive symptoms as measured by MADRS total scores.[25] However, in a crossover 13-week RCT, placebo-controlled study with patients diagnosed with MDD with mixed features, the MADRS total scores in the subjects receiving ziprasidone did not separate from those in the placebo arm at endpoint.[21]

MOOD STABILIZERS IN THE TREATMENT OF MIXED STATES
Lithium

The role of lithium in the treatment of mixed states still requires clarification, and it is receiving increasing attention from clinicians and researchers.[28] Despite a lack of specific reports on lithium as monotherapy in the treatment of both mixed mania and depression, lithium is considered as a first-line treatment in the prevention of episodes of any polarity after a mixed episode.[29–32] However, several studies suggested lithium as adjunctive therapy in the treatment of acute mania, also with mixed features.[33–35] In a retrospective analysis of the relationship between depressive symptoms and treatment response in acute manic episodes, lithium was found to be ineffective in the treatment of acute mania with pretreatment-reported depressive symptoms.[36,37] Given the suicide preventative properties of lithium,[38] its neuroprotective effects, and its long-term preventive efficacy, lithium might be a valuable option, and more studies are needed to test its efficacy in mixed states.[28]

Valproate

Valproate was found to be effective in the prevention of new affective episodes after dysphoric mania, notably more effective than lithium in a 12-month maintenance study (n = 123) comparing valproate, lithium, and placebo.[39] However, another study did not confirm the superiority of valproate compared with lithium in the prevention of new episodes in patients with BD.[30]

Limited evidence is available for the efficacy of valproate in the treatment of acute mixed states. One study, back in 1992, already suggested a possible use of divalproex in mixed states, despite the lack of an adequate population to perform a subgroup analysis in mixed patients.[40] Other RCTs showed the efficacy of valproate compared with placebo in acute mania, but limited evidence on a mixed subgroup of patients were available.[36,37,41] Some reports recommended the use of valproate in combination with SGAs, such as aripirazole[42] and quetiapine.[43–45]

A limited amount of evidence exists regarding the use of intravenous valproate in acute mixed episodes, such as small samples showing a reduction of agitation in patients showing mixed features,[46] as recently suggested in adolescent patients with suspected substance abuse.[47] Of note, valproate was found to be not as effective as risperidone in early age (6–15 years) mixed mania.[48] Despite the limited available studies, valproate was recommended as a second-line monotherapy treatment according to the International College of Neuropsychopharmacology[49] and the World Federation of Societies of Biological Psychiatry.[5] Moreover, it is clinically relevant that valproate does not interfere with the pharmacokinetics of asenapine,[50] so that clinicians may consider the combination of both in the treatment of acute mixed states.

Carbamazepine and Oxcarbazepine

Evidence suggests that carbamazepine could be an option for the treatment of mixed features in both manic and depressive episodes. Two large, 3-week, randomized, double-blind, placebo-controlled trials tested the efficacy of ER carbamazepine versus placebo for manic or depressive symptoms in mixed states.[51,52] By pooling data from the 2 RCT, the investigators concluded that carbamazepine is effective in the treatment of patients with BD I with either acute manic or depressive symptoms in mixed episodes.[53] As stated earlier, carbamazepine monotherapy is the only mood stabilizer considered as a second-line choice by 2 different international guidelines in the acute phase.[5,49] However, carbamazepine was poorly studied as a maintenance treatment of patients with mixed states.[10]

Also oxcarbamazepine was found to be effective in patients who did not respond to lithium as adjunctive therapy.[54]

Lamotrigine

Lamotrigine is only approved for the maintenance treatment of BD, especially for preventing episodes of depression in BD I.[4,55] However, there is not enough evidence to support the use of lamotrigine for the management of mania or mixed mania in either acute or maintenance treatment.[10]

Topiramate

Some evidence also exists for the use of topiramate in the treatment of acute mixed mania. Despite that no RCT has confirmed the effectiveness of topiramate in mixed states; a retrospective chart review, including 44 patients resistant to previous treatments, suggested some effect of topiramate in reducing manic symptoms.[56] Two open studies suggested some partial improvement in manic and mixed states but only as adjunctive treatment.[57]

ANTIDEPRESSANTS AND THE TREATMENT OF DEPRESSIVE MIXED STATES

As stated by Stahl and colleagues,[7] antidepressant monotherapy should not be an option for the treatment of patients with mixed depression of any type (unipolar, BP II, or BP I), given persisting evidence that raise concerns about the efficacy of antidepressants in treating any kind of BD and their potential for mood dysregulation.[3,4,58,59]

Among antidepressants, tricyclic antidepressants and serotonin–norepinephrine reuptake inhibitors showed the highest risk of affective switch, whereas bupropion and some selective serotonin reuptake inhibitors showed a lower risk.[3,60–63]

The role of antidepressants in maintenance treatment is controversial and not established by controlled trials in mixed depression, but in a small minority of patients they might be useful in the long term.[4] In particular, continuation might be recommended after an initial positive or partial response to antidepressants.[64] However, antidepressants should not be used in the absence of a mood stabilizer or one of the SGAs with mood-stabilizing properties in the treatment of mixed states.

DISCUSSION OF EVIDENCE AND CLINICAL RECOMMENDATIONS

Although there is limited evidence in terms of treating DSM-5–defined mixed features, there are a variety of SGAs and MS that have shown efficacy in treating both manic and depressive symptoms as well as DSM-IV–defined mixed states. There is clearly a need for clinical trials specifically designed to include patients with DSM-5–based diagnoses in order to determine the best course of action in terms of treating patients with mixed features and aid in the further development of novel agents specifically designed to ameliorate both depressive and manic symptoms as well as their concomitant presentation.

As reviewed earlier, prospective, retrospective, and naturalistic studies demonstrated that mixed states are challenging to treat for clinicians, suggesting that acute affective episodes with mixed symptoms or features tend to respond poorly to treatments that are usually more effective for other phases of BD (such as lithium and other pharmacotherapies). Despite the efficacy of SGAs in the acute phase, patients with mixed states have a poorer long-term prophylactic response to treatment in general.[65] One question raised by experts in the field, given the high risk for suicidal behavior in mixed states, is the role of prophylactic lithium in patients susceptible to present with mixed states.[66] Of note, lithium seems to reduce suicidal behavior even when it is not effective in preventing affective episodes so that it might be a valid option in case of suicide risk in mixed states.[67] Moreover, clinicians must be aware that antidepressants without mood-stabilizing treatments have limited efficacy and they carry the potential for harm in mixed depressive episodes.[7]

The difficulties of the pharmacologic treatment of mixed state reside in the presence of depressive symptomatology during acute mania and mania symptoms during the depression, as it has been reported for centuries.

Since Kraepelin (1921),[68] the mood cycling up and down has also been put in connection with the thought processes and volition (will). Pharmacologic treatment of mixed states is, therefore, most challenging for clinicians, as they have to face the various clinical presentation of these patients as categorized by Kraepelin with the recognition of depressive or anxious mania (depressed mood but elevated will and thought); excited depression (depressed mood and will but elevated thought); mania with thought poverty (elevated mood and will but decreased thought); manic stupor (elevated mood but decreased will and thought); depression with flight of ideas (depressed mood and thought but elevated will); and inhibited mania (elevated mood and thought but decreased will).

Psychic anxiety is also another major issue in the treatment of mixed states. Recent studies confirmed that psychic anxiety, with feelings of tenseness and irritability, is a core symptom of mania with depressive symptoms. Most dimensional studies report high anxiety scores associated with depression.[69] Furthermore, agitation is common in patients with depressive or anxious mania as having "high levels of excitement." Agitation is prominent in all mood states but with different components, with the experience of painful inner tension, which produces increased nongoal-directed motor activity, typical of agitation during depressive episodes.[66] Also, irritability was observed as a core symptom in patients with the presence of depressive symptoms during mania. Irritable temperament should be considered as a possible indicator of mania with depressive symptoms.[70]

From such consideration emerges the need to provide a dimensional approach when assessing mixed states and provide treatment accordingly. In conclusion, despite being challenging, mixed states have now been reconducted to the original classification, which opens new therapeutic perspectives. Thanks to available treatment, a patient can encounter beneficial pharmacologic treatment of core symptoms of their conditions. However, future studies should provide a more homogenous classification of mixed states and therefore observe the impact of specific pharmacologic treatment of this peculiar disorder.

DISCLOSURE

S.M. Stahl is an Adjunct Professor of Psychiatry at the University of California San Diego; Honorary Visiting Senior Fellow at the University of Cambridge, UK; and Director of Psychopharmacology for California Department of State Hospitals. Over the past 36 months (January 2016–December 2018) Dr S.M. Stahl has served as a *consultant* to Acadia, Adamas, Alkermes, Allergan, Arbor Pharmaceutcials, AstraZeneca, Avanir, Axovant, Axsome, Biogen, Biomarin, Biopharma, Celgene, Concert, Clear-View, DepoMed, Dey, EnVivo, EMD Serono, Ferring, Forest, Forum, Genomind, Innovative Science Solutions, Intra-Cellular Therapies, Janssen, Jazz, Lilly, Lundbeck, Merck, Neos, Novartis, Noveida, Orexigen, Otsuka, PamLabs, Perrigo, Pfizer, Pierre Fabre, Reviva, Servier, Shire, Sprout, Sunovion, Taisho, Takeda, Taliaz, Teva, Tonix, Trius, Vanda, Vertex, and Viforpharma; he has been a *board member* of RCT Logic and Genomind; he has served on *speakers bureaus* for Acadia, Astra Zeneca, Dey Pharma, EnVivo, Eli Lilly, Forum, Genentech, Janssen, Lundbeck, Merck, Otsuka, PamLabs, Pfizer Israel, Servier, Sunovion, and Takeda, and he has received *research and/or grant support* from Acadia, Alkermes, AssureX, AstraZeneca, Arbor Pharmaceuticals, Avanir, Axovant, Biogen, Braeburn Pharmaceuticals, BristolMyer Squibb, Celgene, CeNeRx, Cephalon, Dey, Eli Lilly, EnVivo, Forest, Forum, GenOmind, GlaxoSmithKline, Intra-Cellular Therapies, ISSWSH, Janssen, JayMac, Jazz, Lundbeck, Merck, Mylan, Neurocrine, Neuronetics, Novartis, Otsuka, PamLabs, Pfizer, Reviva, Roche, Sepracor, Servier, Shire, Sprout, Sunovion, TMS NeuroHealth Centers, Takeda, Teva, Tonix, Vanda, Valeant, and Wyeth (updated 1-23-2018). M. Pompili: Advisory Boards: Janssen, Ferrer, Italfarmaco; Lectures: FB Health, Lundbeck, Angelini, Otsuka, Allergan. Other authors: nothing to declare.

REFERENCES

1. Yatham LN, Kennedy SH, Parikh SV, et al. Canadian Network for Mood and Anxiety Treatments (CANMAT) and International Society for Bipolar Disorders (ISBD) 2018 guidelines for the management of patients with bipolar disorder. Bipolar Disord 2018;20(2):97–170.

2. Kennedy SH, Lam RW, McIntyre RS, et al. Canadian Network for Mood and Anxiety Treatments (CANMAT) 2016 clinical guidelines for the management of adults with major depressive disorder. Can J Psychiatry 2016;61(9):540–60.

3. Grunze H, Vieta E, Goodwin GM, et al. The World Federation of Societies of Biological Psychiatry (WFSBP) guidelines for the biological treatment of bipolar disorders: update 2010 on the treatment of acute bipolar depression. World J Biol Psychiatry 2010;11(2):81–109.

4. Goodwin GM, Consensus Group of the British Association for Psychopharmacology. Evidence-based guidelines for treating bipolar disorder: revised second edition–recommendations from the British Association for Psychopharmacology. J Psychopharmacol 2009;23(4):346–88.

5. Grunze H, Vieta E, Goodwin GM, et al. The World Federation of Societies of Biological Psychiatry (WFSBP) guidelines for the biological treatment of bipolar disorders: acute and long-term treatment of mixed states in bipolar disorder. World J Biol Psychiatry 2018;19(1):2–58.

6. American Psychiatric Association. Diagnostic and statistical manual of mental disorders, 5th edition (DSM-5). 4th edition. Diagnostic Stat Man Ment Disord; 2013. p. 280. TR.

7. Stahl SM, Morrissette DA, Faedda G, et al. Guidelines for the recognition and management of mixed depression. CNS Spectr 2017;22(2):203–19.

8. Grunze H, Azorin JM. Clinical decision making in the treatment of mixed states. World J Biol Psychiatry 2014;15(5):355–68.

9. Tondo L, Vázquez GH, Pinna M, et al. Characteristics of depressive and bipolar disorder patients with mixed features. Acta Psychiatr Scand 2018;138(3): 243–52.

10. Verdolini N, Hidalgo-Mazzei D, Murru A, et al. Mixed states in bipolar and major depressive disorders: systematic review and quality appraisal of guidelines. Acta Psychiatr Scand 2018;138(3):196–222.

11. Vázquez GH, Lolich M, Cabrera C, et al. Mixed symptoms in major depressive and bipolar disorders: a systematic review. J Affect Disord 2018;225:756–60.

12. Landbloom RL, Mackle M, Wu X, et al. Asenapine: efficacy and safety of 5 and 10 mg bid in a 3-week, randomized, double-blind, placebo-controlled trial in adults with a manic or mixed episode associated with bipolar I disorder. J Affect Disord 2016;190:103–10.

13. McIntyre RS, Cohen M, Zhao J, et al. A 3-week, randomized, placebo-controlled trial of asenapine in the treatment of acute mania in bipolar mania and mixed states. Bipolar Disord 2009;11(7):673–86.

14. Berwaerts J, Melkote R, Nuamah I, et al. A randomized, placebo- and active-controlled study of paliperidone extended-release as maintenance treatment in patients with bipolar I disorder after an acute manic or mixed episode. J Affect Disord 2012;138(3):247–58.

15. Sachs G, Sanchez R, Marcus R, et al. Aripiprazole in the treatment of acute manic or mixed episodes in patients with bipolar I disorder: a 3-week placebo-controlled study. J Psychopharmacol 2006;20(4):536–46.

16. Tohen M, Sanger TM, McElroy SL, et al. Olanzapine versus placebo in the treatment of acute mania. Olanzapine HGEH Study Group. Am J Psychiatry 1999; 156(5):702–9.

17. Vieta E, Nuamah IF, Lim P, et al. A randomized, placebo- and active-controlled study of paliperidone extended release for the treatment of acute manic and mixed episodes of bipolar I disorder. Bipolar Disord 2010;12(3):230–43.

18. Cutler AJ, Datto C, Nordenhem A, et al. Extended-release quetiapine as mono-therapy for the treatment of adults with acute mania: a randomized, double-blind, 3-week trial. Clin Ther 2011;33(11):1643–58.
19. Keck PE, Versiani M, Potkin S, et al. Ziprasidone in the treatment of acute bipolar mania: a three-week, placebo-controlled, double-blind, randomized trial. Am J Psychiatry 2003;160(4):741–8.
20. Tohen M, Jacobs TG, Grundy SL, et al. Efficacy of olanzapine in acute bipolar mania: a double-blind, placebo-controlled study. The Olanzipine HGGW Study Group. Arch Gen Psychiatry 2000;57(9):841–9.
21. Patkar AA, Pae C-U, Vöhringer PA, et al. A 13-week, randomized double-blind, placebo-controlled, cross-over trial of ziprasidone in bipolar spectrum disorder. J Clin Psychopharmacol 2015;35(3):319–23.
22. Suppes T, Silva R, Cucchiaro J, et al. Lurasidone for the treatment of major depressive disorder with mixed features: a randomized, double-blind, placebo-controlled study. Am J Psychiatry 2016;173(4):400–7.
23. Tohen M, Kanba S, McIntyre RS, et al. Efficacy of olanzapine monotherapy in the treatment of bipolar depression with mixed features. J Affect Disord 2014;164: 57–62.
24. McIntyre RS, Cucchiaro J, Pikalov A, et al. Lurasidone in the treatment of bipolar depression with mixed (subsyndromal hypomanic) features: post hoc analysis of a randomized placebo-controlled trial. J Clin Psychiatry 2015;76(4):398–405.
25. Patkar A, Gilmer W, Pae C, et al. A 6 week randomized double-blind placebo-controlled trial of ziprasidone for the acute depressive mixed state. Mazza M, ed. PLoS One 2012;7(4):e34757.
26. Suppes T, Ketter TA, Gwizdowski IS, et al. First controlled treatment trial of bipolar II hypomania with mixed symptoms: quetiapine versus placebo. J Affect Disord 2013;150(1):37–43.
27. McIntyre RS, Masand PS, Earley W, et al. Cariprazine for the treatment of bipolar mania with mixed features: A post hoc pooled analysis of 3 trials. J Affect Disord 2019;257:600–6.
28. Sani G, Fiorillo A. The use of lithium in mixed states. CNS Spectr 2019;1–3. https://doi.org/10.1017/S1092852919001184.
29. Backlund L, Ehnvall A, Hetta J, et al. Identifying predictors for good lithium response - a retrospective analysis of 100 patients with bipolar disorder using a life-charting method. Eur Psychiatry 2009;24(3):171–7.
30. Kessing LV, Hellmund G, Geddes JR, et al. Valproate v. lithium in the treatment of bipolar disorder in clinical practice: observational nationwide register-based cohort study. Br J Psychiatry 2011;199(1):57–63.
31. Weisler RH, Nolen WA, Neijber A, et al, Trial 144 Study Investigators. Continuation of quetiapine versus switching to placebo or lithium for maintenance treatment of Bipolar I Disorder. J Clin Psychiatry 2011;72(11):1452–64.
32. Nolen WA, Weisler RH. The association of the effect of lithium in the maintenance treatment of bipolar disorder with lithium plasma levels: a post hoc analysis of a double-blind study comparing switching to lithium or placebo in patients who re-sponded to quetiapine (Trial 144). Bipolar Disord 2013;15(1):100–9.
33. Tohen M, Chengappa KNR, Suppes T, et al. Efficacy of olanzapine in combination with valproate or lithium in the treatment of mania in patients partially nonrespon-sive to valproate or lithium monotherapy. Arch Gen Psychiatry 2002;59(1):62–9.
34. Baker RW, Brown E, Akiskal HS, et al. Efficacy of olanzapine combined with val-proate or lithium in the treatment of dysphoric mania. Br J Psychiatry 2004;185(6): 472–8.

35. Berwaerts J, Lane R, Nuamah IF, et al. Paliperidone extended-release as adjunctive therapy to lithium or valproate in the treatment of acute mania: a randomized, placebo-controlled study. J Affect Disord 2011;129(1–3):252–60.

36. Bowden CL, Brugger AM, Swann AC, et al. Efficacy of divalproex vs lithium and placebo in the treatment of mania. The Depakote Mania Study Group. JAMA 1994;271(12):918–24.

37. Swann AC, Bowden CL, Morris D, et al. Depression during mania. Treatment response to lithium or divalproex. Arch Gen Psychiatry 1997;54(1):37–42.

38. Baldessarini RJ, Tondo L, Davis P, et al. Decreased risk of suicides and attempts during long-term lithium treatment: a meta-analytic review. Bipolar Disord 2006; 8(5 Pt 2):625–39.

39. Bowden CL, Collins MA, McElroy SL, et al. Relationship of mania symptomatology to maintenance treatment response with divalproex, lithium, or placebo. Neuropsychopharmacology 2005;30(10):1932–9.

40. Freeman TW, Clothier JL, Pazzaglia P, et al. A double-blind comparison of valproate and lithium in the treatment of acute mania. Am J Psychiatry 1992; 149(1):108–11.

41. Bowden CL, Swann AC, Calabrese JR, et al. A randomized, placebo-controlled, multicenter study of divalproex sodium extended release in the treatment of acute mania. J Clin Psychiatry 2006;67(10):1501–10.

42. Yatham LN, Fountoulakis KN, Rahman Z, et al. Efficacy of aripiprazole versus placebo as adjuncts to lithium or valproate in relapse prevention of manic or mixed episodes in bipolar I patients stratified by index manic or mixed episode. J Affect Disord 2013;147(1–3):365–72.

43. Vieta E, Suppes T, Ekholm B, et al. Long-term efficacy of quetiapine in combination with lithium or divalproex on mixed symptoms in bipolar I disorder. J Affect Disord 2012;142(1–3):36–44.

44. Vieta E, Suppes T, Eggens I, et al. Efficacy and safety of quetiapine in combination with lithium or divalproex for maintenance of patients with bipolar I disorder (international trial 126). J Affect Disord 2008;109(3):251–63.

45. Suppes T, Vieta E, Liu S, et al, Trial 127 Investigators. Maintenance treatment for patients with bipolar I disorder: results from a north american study of quetiapine in combination with lithium or divalproex (trial 127). Am J Psychiatry 2009;166(4): 476–88.

46. Grunze H, Erfurth A, Amann B, et al. Intravenous valproate loading in acutely manic and depressed bipolar I patients. J Clin Psychopharmacol 1999;19(4): 303–9.

47. Battaglia C, Averna R, Labonia M, et al. Intravenous valproic acid add-on therapy in acute agitation adolescents with suspected substance abuse. Clin Neuropharmacol 2018;41(1):38–42.

48. Geller B, Luby JL, Joshi P, et al. A randomized controlled trial of risperidone, lithium, or divalproex sodium for initial treatment of Bipolar I Disorder, manic or mixed phase, in children and adolescents. Arch Gen Psychiatry 2012;69(5):515.

49. Fountoulakis KN, Grunze H, Vieta E, et al. The International College of Neuro-Psychopharmacology (CINP) treatment guidelines for Bipolar disorder in adults (CINP-BD-2017), part 3: the clinical guidelines. Int J Neuropsychopharmacol 2016;20(2):pyw109.

50. Gerrits MGF, de Greef R, Dogterom P, et al. Valproate reduces the glucuronidation of asenapine without affecting asenapine plasma concentrations. J Clin Pharmacol 2012;52(5):757–65.

51. Weisler RH, Kalali AH, Ketter TA, SPD417 Study Group. A multicenter, randomized, double-blind, placebo-controlled trial of extended-release carbamazepine capsules as monotherapy for bipolar disorder patients with manic or mixed episodes. J Clin Psychiatry 2004;65(4):478–84.

52. Weisler RH, Keck PE, Swann AC, et al. Extended-release carbamazepine capsules as monotherapy for acute mania in bipolar disorder: a multicenter, randomized, double-blind, placebo-controlled trial. J Clin Psychiatry 2005;66(3):323–30.

53. Weisler RH, Hirschfeld R, Cutler AJ, et al. Extended-release carbamazepine capsules as monotherapy in bipolar disorder : pooled results from two randomised, double-blind, placebo-controlled trials. CNS Drugs 2006;20(3):219–31.

54. Benedetti A, Lattanzi L, Pini S, et al. Oxcarbazepine as add-on treatment in patients with bipolar manic, mixed or depressive episode. J Affect Disord 2004;79(1–3):273–7.

55. Connolly KR, Thase ME. The clinical management of bipolar disorder: a review of evidence-based guidelines. Prim Care Companion CNS Disord 2011;13(4). https://doi.org/10.4088/PCC.10R01097.

56. Marcotte D. Use of topiramate, a new anti-epileptic as a mood stabilizer. J Affect Disord 1998;50(2–3):245–51.

57. Chengappa KN, Rathore D, Levine J, et al. Topiramate as add-on treatment for patients with bipolar mania. Bipolar Disord 1999;1(1):42–53.

58. Cerullo MA, Strakowski SM. A systematic review of the evidence for the treatment of acute depression in bipolar I disorder. CNS Spectr 2013;18(4):199–208.

59. Cleare A, Pariante C, Young A, et al. Evidence-based guidelines for treating depressive disorders with antidepressants: a revision of the 2008 British Association for Psychopharmacology guidelines. Nutt DJ, Blier P, eds. J Psychopharmacol 2015;29(5):459–525.

60. Sani G, Napoletano F, Vöhringer PA, et al. Mixed depression: clinical features and predictors of its onset associated with antidepressant use. Psychother Psychosom 2014;83(4):213–21.

61. Bjørklund L, Horsdal HT, Mors O, et al. Trends in the psychopharmacological treatment of bipolar disorder: a nationwide register-based study. Acta Neuropsychiatr 2016;28(2):75–84.

62. Gijsman HJ, Geddes JR, Rendell JM, et al. Antidepressants for bipolar depression: a systematic review of randomized, controlled trials. Am J Psychiatry 2004;161(9):1537–47.

63. Patel R, Reiss P, Shetty H, et al. Do antidepressants increase the risk of mania and bipolar disorder in people with depression? A retrospective electronic case register cohort study. BMJ Open 2015;5(12):e008341.

64. Altshuler LL, Post RM, Hellemann G, et al. Impact of antidepressant continuation after acute positive or partial treatment response for bipolar depression: a blinded, randomized study. J Clin Psychiatry 2009;70(4):450–7.

65. González-Pinto A, Barbeito S, Alonso M, et al. Poor long-term prognosis in mixed bipolar patients: 10-year outcomes in the Vitoria prospective naturalistic study in Spain. J Clin Psychiatry 2011;72(5):671–6.

66. Swann AC, Lafer B, Perugi G, et al. Bipolar mixed states: an international society for bipolar disorders task force report of symptom structure, course of illness, and diagnosis. Am J Psychiatry 2013;170(1):31–42.

67. Müller-Oerlinghausen B. Arguments for the specificity of the antisuicidal effect of lithium. Eur Arch Psychiatry Clin Neurosci 2001;251(Suppl 2):II72–5.

68. Kraepelin E. Manic-depressive insanity and paranoia. Edinburgh (Scotland): E. & S. Livingstone; 1921.
69. Gonzalez-Pinto A, Aldama A, Mosquera F, et al. Epidemiology, diagnosis and management of mixed mania. CNS Drugs 2007;21(8):611–26.
70. Akiskal HS, Hantouche EG, Bourgeois ML, et al. Gender, temperament, and the clinical picture in dysphoric mixed mania: findings from a French national study (EPIMAN). J Affect Disord 1998;50(2–3):175–86.

The Role of Electroconvulsive Therapy in the Treatment of Severe Bipolar Mixed State

Giulio Perugi, MD[a,b,*], Pierpaolo Medda, MD[a],
Margherita Barbuti, MD[a], Martina Novi, MD[a],
Beniamino Tripodi, MD[a]

KEYWORDS

- Mixed states • Electroconvulsive therapy • Bipolar disorder

KEY POINTS

- Electroconvulsive therapy (ECT) is an effective treatment of severe mixed state (MS), resistant or nonresponsive to pharmacotherapy.
- Because of inadequate diagnostic delimitation, many patients with severe MS are misdiagnosed and not referred to ECT.
- Considering ECT as a "last resort" may decrease the chance of recovery in many patients, who could have potentially responded if timely treated.
- The duration of the mixed episode seems to be one of the predictors of nonresponse.
- Because of the very low incidence of serious adverse events and no mood-destabilizing effect, ECT should be considered a valid option also in a long-term perspective.

INTRODUCTION

Mixed state (MS) is one of the major phases of bipolar disorder (BD). Compared with manic and depressive states, it is characterized by a more complex clinical presentation[1,2] and a less favorable response to conventional pharmacologic treatments.[3,4]

The treatment of MS is a therapeutic challenge, mostly because it has been associated with a reduced response to mood stabilizers and a frequent need for drug combinations.[4] However, the use of antidepressants in MS has been reported to worsen

The authors declare no funding sources for this study and no previous data presentation or particular disclaimer statements.
[a] Department of Clinical and Experimental Medicine, University of Pisa, Via Roma 67, Pisa 56100, Italy; [b] Psychiatry Unit 2, Azienda Ospedaliero-Universitaria Pisana, Pisa, Italy
* Corresponding author. Department of Clinical and Experimental Medicine, University of Pisa, Via Roma 67, Pisa 56100, Italy.
E-mail address: giulio.perugi@med.unipi.it

short-term intraepisodic mood instability and mixed symptomatology,[5-7] whereas the use of antipsychotics may aggravate or induce severe depressive symptoms.[8,9]

Clinical research has shown the limitations of lithium salts in the treatment of MS.[3,10] Valproate and carbamazepine, as well as second-generation antipsychotics (SGAs)[11-13] resulted more efficacious than lithium in the treatment of mixed mania. Nevertheless, most of the evidence is derived from clinical trials enrolling manic patients with few depressive symptoms (dysphoric mania) rather than severe MS with psychotic, catatonic, and delirious features.[3]

Although electroconvulsive therapy (ECT) has been used for the first time with outstanding outcome in a patient with mixed, delirious and psychotic features,[14] its effectiveness in MS has not been extensively studied for different reasons. In particular, the development of pharmacotherapy shifted the attention of the clinical research on the more drug-responsive depressive and manic states. With the aim of defining syndromes typically responsive to pharmacologic treatment, the international diagnostic systems (from Diagnostic and Statistical Manual of Mental Disorders Third Edition [DSM-III] to DSM-5 and from International Classification of Diseases, Ninth Revision [ICD-9] to ICD-11) started to consider depression and mania as the core manifestations of depressive and BDs, respectively. Actually, in the original definition of manic-depressive illness,[15] based on the accurate description of the clinical presentation and the natural outcome of the syndrome, MS was not just a complication, but the most common clinical manifestation and the most important unifying core feature of manic-depressive insanity. On the contrary, pure mania and depression were considered as uncommon extreme variants.

Because of inadequate diagnostic delimitation and because of its pleomorphic clinical presentation, MS is still often underdiagnosed and misdiagnosed.[1,16-19] Since DSM-III, mixed episode has not received specific criteria characterization and has been basically defined as the combination of mania and major depression co-occurring or rapidly alternating in the same period. This combinatory model has shaped the clinical research conducted in recent years and has led to considering MS mainly as a subtype of manic or depressive episodes, rather than in Kraepelinian terms of specific features or episode components.

By taking this view to the extreme, DSM-5 removed the diagnosis of mixed episode and proposed a "with mixed features" specifier to be applied to manic, hypomanic, and major depressive episodes. This approach is in part data driven and overcomes the problems derived from the extremely narrow definition of the previous editions of the manual. The possibility of classifying depression "with mixed features" represents another major improvement. Fortunately, in the ICD-11 a specific diagnostic category for mixed episode has been preferred to a "specifier." A diagnostic category is obviously more likely to improve diagnostic sensitivity and ensure specific treatment strategy in comparison to a simple specifier. Unfortunately, however, as regards the definition of mixed episodes, ICD-11 is very similar to DSM-5, and the essential feature is "the presence of several prominent manic and depressive symptoms consistent with those observed in Manic Episodes and Depressive Episodes, which either occur simultaneously or alternate very rapidly...".

This narrowly combinatory model could be applied to the less severe mixed forms, with prominent and clear mood symptoms.[3] Conversely, in severe MS the sustained protracted affective instability is invariably associated with nonmood symptoms such as anxiety, cognitive and motor indecisiveness, emotional perplexity, perceptual disturbances, sense of external interference, depersonalization, and grossly disorganized behavior.[2,18] In most of these cases the symptomatology cannot be captured in terms of superposition of depressive and manic symptomatology. As a result, many patients with severe MS are considered schizophrenic or neurocognitive disorders and never treated with ECT.

CLINICAL STUDIES OF ELECTROCONVULSIVE THERAPY IN MIXED STATES

Clinical trials focused on the treatment of MS are disappointingly limited, and the use of ECT has not been specifically described by most of the clinical practice guidelines for the treatment of BD.[20] However, case series and several prospective and retrospective naturalistic studies strongly supported the effectiveness of ECT in severe MS, with response rates ranging from 56% to 93% of the cases (**Table 1**).

In the literature, the first data reported on the use of ECT in MS is from a retrospective study from the Aarhus Psychiatric Hospital.[21] This investigator observed a high response rate (70%) to unilateral ECT course in a sample of 19 treatment-resistant mixed patients. In a prospective study, Devanand and colleagues[22] compared the clinical course and the treatment response after ECT in 3 groups of patients: depressed (n = 38), manic (n = 5), and mixed (n = 10). Using the Clinical Global Impression-Severity scale (CGI-S) score as response criterion (<2), the response rate was 76.3% in depressed, 100% in manic, and 80% in mixed group. Mixed patients showed a longer period of hospitalization and a higher number of ECT sessions in comparison to the depressed ones. These results suggest that MS are more difficult to treat and may take longer to respond than "pure" bipolar depressive or manic episodes.

In a case-series study, Gruber and colleagues[23] showed the efficacy of ECT in 41 patients presenting a manic episode, according to the research diagnostic criteria. All patients were monitored using the Schedule for Affective Disorders and Schizophrenia-Change (SADS-C). Eight patients, who satisfied the criteria both for mania and depression, did not improve after pharmacologic treatment and were further considered for ECT. One of the medication-refractory patients did not consent to the procedure, whereas the other 7 underwent to the ECT and remitted.

A prospective study compared ECT response in 41 mixed-manic and 23 bipolar depressed patients refractory to pharmacotherapy.[24] Both groups underwent the same number of ECT sessions and were screened using the Montgomery–Asberg Depression Rating Scale, the Brief Psychiatric Rating Scale (BPRS), and the CGI-S scale, showing a significant decrease in all the posttreatment scores. The response rates at the end point were 56% for the mixed-manic patients and 26% for the bipolar depressive ones. In this study, the number of responses among patients exhibiting depression was particularly low, and the investigators did not clearly report the ECT dosing method they used. Hence, it is possible that the efficacy of ECT may have been compromised by an inadequate procedure.

In contrast with this observation, Medda and colleagues[25] found a high response rate (CGI ≤ 2) after a course of bilateral ECT in patients with both MS (n = 50) and depressed bipolar I (n = 46) (67.4% vs 76.0%). In this study, no difference in the remission rate of MS (34.8%) and depression (41.3%) was reported either. However, the final scores on Young Mania Rating Scale (YMRS), BPRS total, and BPRS psychotic cluster were higher in the MS than in the depression group. The only other difference was that MS reported more residual agitation and psychotic features compared with the "purely" depressive patients.

The same investigators examined the efficacy of ECT in a large sample of 197 MS patients, focusing on possible predictors of response. Eighty-two patients (41.6%) were considered responders, 60 (30.5%) remitters, whereas less than 30%

Table 1
Studies examining the efficacy and tolerability of electroconvulsive therapy in patients with bipolar mixed episodes

Authors	Study Design	Diagnostic Criteria	Outcome Measures	N° of Patients	N° of ECT (mean ± SD)	Response Rate	Adverse Events
Strömgren,[21] 1988	Retrospective	ICD-9	Clinical judgment	19	11 (range 2–20)	68%	Not reported
Davanand et al,[22] 2000	Chart review	DSM-IV	CGI-I	10	9.3 ± 4.0	80%	Not reported
Gruber et al,[23] 2000	Case series	RDC	SADS-C	7	13.57 ± 4.3	100%	Not reported
Ciapparelli et al,[24] 2001	Prospective	DSM-IV	BPRS, CGI-S MADRS	41	7.2 ± 1.7	56%	Not reported
Medda et al,[25] 2010	Prospective	DSM-IV	BPRS CGI-I HDRS-17 YMRS	50	7.4 ± 2.4	76%	Prolonged apnea (2 pt.) Prolonged seizure (1 pt.) Postcritical delirium (1 pt)
Medda et al,[18] 2014	Prospective	DSM-IV	BPRS CGI-I HDRS-17 YMRS	197	7.48 ± 2.2	72%	Severe confusion (1 pt.) Severe headache (1 pt.) Cardiac arrhythmia (2 pt.) Respiratory complications (1 pt.)
Palma et al,[27] 2016	Retrospective	DSM-IV-TR McElroy's [12] Akiskal's [14]	CGI-I	15	5.1 ± 2.2	93%	Not reported

Abbreviations: BPRS, brief psychiatric rating scale; CGI-I, Clinical Global Impression-Improvement scale; CGI-S, Clinical Global Impression-Severity scale; HDRS-17, Hamilton Depression Rating Scale-17 items; pt, patients; RDC, research diagnostic criteria; YMRS, young mania rating scale.

(n = 55; 27.9%) were considered nonresponders. The lifetime comorbidity with obsessive-compulsive disorder, the severity of YMRS baseline score, as well as the length of the current episode were significantly associated with absence of response.[26]

More recently, Palma and colleagues[27] reported retrospective data concerning patients with BD who underwent ECT few years before in 3 different polarity episodes (4 manic, 28 depressed, and 18 mixed). Retrospective rating was made using CGI scores and all the episodes recovered, except for a single patient with MS.

Catatonic features have consistently been observed in patients with severe MS.[28] Catatonia is a neuropsychiatric syndrome characterized by motor dysregulation, associated with changes in thought, mood, and vigilance. Immobility, stupor, mutism, negativism, and rigidity are the most typical symptoms.[28] A large body of evidence supports the view of catatonia as an independent neuropsychiatric syndrome.[29] However, in a systematic study, the presence of catatonia was evaluated in patients with BD with manic or mixed episode[30]: 24 of 39 patients with mixed mania (61%) and only 3 of 60 patients with pure mania (5%) were considered catatonic. Patients with catatonic symptoms require specific therapeutic interventions, particularly benzodiazepines or ECT, avoiding antipsychotic drugs.[31] The remarkable efficacy of ECT in catatonic patients is generally acknowledged, but it is based on open and retrospective studies with limited samples. Furthermore, most of these studies were carried out in heterogeneous samples. Patients were diagnosed with schizophrenia (20%–100%) or mood disorders (0%–63%), and the large diagnostic variability depended on the selected populations and on the diagnostic attitudes of the investigators.[32–34] In these studies, ECT resulted very effective with response rates ranging from 80% to 90%. Only one report showed a response rate of 59%.[35]

All these observations provide strong evidence of the safety and efficacy of ECT in patients with severe MS, refractory to pharmacotherapy. The methodologies used in these studies were very different and in none of them a comparison treatment or placebo was used. However, most of the patients described in these observational, naturalistic studies were obviously not eligible for randomized controlled trials and they were so compromised from a psychopathological and physical point of view that the chances of a placebo or a drug response were truly negligible. Based on this evidence, ECT should be considered the treatment of choice in patients with severe, drug-refractory MS with psychotic, catatonic, or delirious features, although clinicians should be vigilant for residual symptoms requiring further management.

THE ROLE OF ELECTROCONVULSIVE THERAPY IN THE MANAGEMENT OF MIXED STATES

Despite a growing armamentarium of antidepressant, antipsychotic, and mood stabilizer drugs, BD poses many treatment challenges. Many patients remain refractory to pharmacologic treatment, and chronicity, functional impairment, and mortality remain elevated.[7,36–39]

Over the years, the high rate of treatment nonresponse has favored dramatically the use of complex polypharmacy.[22] Although several examples of "rational polypharmacy"[40,41] and the anecdotal evidence that some patients with BD may benefit from certain complex regimens, the effectiveness of combined treatment consisting of 3 or more medications is not demonstrated.[42] Whether "rational" or "irrational," the increased use of complex polypharmacy raises several concerns about the long-term outcome of BD including increased switches rate and the possible induction of rapid cycling and chronic MS.[40,43]

Concerns about the efficacy of current pharmacologic treatments are particularly relevant for bipolar depression and MS. In particular, MS resulted frequently refractory to SGAs and mood stabilizers.[2,18] In other words, many severe MS should be considered nonresponsive to the currently available pharmacologic options more than "drug resistant." The intrinsic limitations of the pharmacotherapy increase the importance of a more accurate definition of the role of ECT in these conditions.

ECT has a unique place in the therapeutic options available for BD, and it has been shown highly effective in severe and drug refractory depressive, manic, and MS in highly suicidal patients and in those presenting delirium and/or catatonic features.[20,44–49] In the light of these observations, clinical guidelines and treatment algorithms for BD should be modified for patients with severe MS and catatonic features, Unfortunately, in all the treatment guidelines for BD, the role of ECT is minimized and for bipolar MS is proposed as a "second-line" or "third-line" option to be applied as a last resort only in drug-resistant patients.[5,7,50–55]

In this perspective, ECT is almost never conceived as an early option for MS, independently from the severity or the variety of the clinical presentation. Many practitioners do not consider referral for ECT before multiple medications have been tried, a process that may span many months or even years and leave the patient seriously ill and dysfunctional for a prolonged period of time.[56] This occurs despite the evidence that the length of the episode is one of the variables frequently associated with reduced rates of response to all treatments, including ECT.[57] On the contrary, the available literature supports the preferential use of ECT compared with pharmacotherapy when the patient is in a very severe condition and is urgently or emergently ill. In such cases, ECT should be considered at an early stage, perhaps before any medication trial. Situations that compel the use of ECT as a "first-line" intervention are active suicidal ideation and behavior; severe weight loss; malnutrition or dehydration with subsequent worsening of the medical status; psychosis accompanied by agitation; and severe mixed, delirious, and catatonic states[58] (**Fig. 1**). 393010100021951

With an appropriate baseline assessment and a monitoring during the procedure, ECT is very safe with a very low incidence of serious adverse events

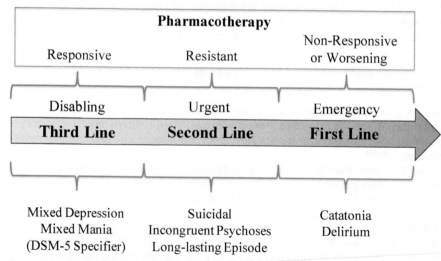

Fig. 1. Role of ECT in mixed states.

(the ECT-related mortality rate was estimated at 2.1 per 100,000 treatments).[59] In patients with MS, the treatment did not cause any serious adverse events and showed a high tolerability. Only less than 5% of the patients interrupt the ECT course prematurely for the onset of side effects.

In the last 2 decades, literature on cognitive effects associated to ECT has produced misleading data perpetuating the stigma surrounding ECT.[60] The fear of cognitive adverse effects continues to be a major limitation to the appropriate prescription of ECT by psychiatrists, even in clinical conditions where it could be very effective.[27]

The cognitive side effect secondary to ECT consists mainly of retrograde amnesia related to personal and public events.[61] Over time, the memory loss diminishes with the most distant events returning first, but some events that occurred during the ECT course can be forgotten forever.[49] In most cases, severe MS has a cognitive impact on memory, attention, and executive functions, leading to severe impairment in academic, occupational, and daily functioning. In these patients impairment memory related to ECT is usually clinically irrelevant.

In addition, consistently with existing literature, ECT-induced mania or depression is virtually nonexistent.[25,62,63] In this perspective, long-term mood destabilization, including cycle induction or acceleration, is very unlikely,[2,20] and ECT may be considered a mood-stabilizing treatment.[64]

Although commonly and widely used, the term "mood stabilizer" is still poorly defined. Some investigators have suggested that an agent is a mood stabilizer if it is efficacious in decreasing the frequency or severity of any type of episode and if it does not worsen the frequency or severity of other types of episodes.[65–67] Others have proposed a more stringent definition that requires that an agent possesses efficacy in treating manic, mixed, and depressive episodes (avoiding the induction of switching into the opposite phase) and in preventing relapses and recurrences (increasing the duration of the "free" intervals).[68]

In the absence of a univocal definition, conventional mood stabilizers such as lithium and anticonvulsants represent the best candidates to achieve the above-mentioned goals but with several disadvantages. They show limited clinical efficacy in severe acute MS, in particular in the presence of psychotic, catatonic, and delirious features. In these patients, adjunctive antidepressant and antipsychotics are routinely used with scarce effectiveness and an increasing risk of chronicity and long-term destabilization. For these patients, ECT may represent an effective and valid alternative also considering a long-term perspective.

SUMMARY

ECT resulted an effective treatment of all the phases of BD, with a clinically significant response in approximately two-thirds of the patients with severe and drug-resistant MS. In patients with delirious and catatonic features, ECT is effective in more than 80% of the cases.

In patients with severe MS, pharmacologic treatments with antipsychotics and antidepressants can be not only ineffective, but can be frequently associated with complications such as chronicity, mood destabilization, and suicidality. The same consideration should be done for MS with catatonic features, where the use of antipsychotics and mood stabilizers may exacerbate the catatonic state.

The duration of the mixed episode seem to be the main predictor of nonresponse, suggesting that chronicity of the symptomatology may contribute to treatment resistance in general, including ECT. Unfortunately, current guidelines and consequent large part of the clinical practice look at ECT as a "last resort." As a consequence, a large proportion of patients with BD are treated for a long period of time with different types of antidepressants and antipsychotics, often in combination, before receiving an appropriate therapy. This worldwide practice may increase the risk of mood destabilization and chronic complications and may decrease the chance of recovery in many patients, who could have potentially responded if timely treated with ECT.

Finally, considering the burden of neurologic and metabolic side effects associated with long-term use of complex pharmacologic regimens with SGAs, antidepressants, and mood stabilizers, ECT should be considered a safe option with a very low incidence of serious adverse events and no long-term mood-destabilizing effect.

DISCLOSURE

G. Perugi has acted as consultant of Lundbeck, Angelini, and FB-Health. He received grant/research support from Lundbeck and Angelini. He is on the speaker/advisory board of Sanofi-Aventis, Lundbeck, FB-Health, and Angelini. All other authors have no conflicts of interest or financial disclosures to report.

REFERENCES

1. Swann AC, Lafer B, Perugi G, et al. Bipolar mixed states: an international society for bipolar disorders task force report of symptom structure, course of illness, and diagnosis. Am J Psychiatry 2013;170(1):31–42.
2. Medda P, Mauri M, Fratta S, et al. Long-term naturalistic follow-up of patients with bipolar depression and mixed state treated with electroconvulsive therapy. J ECT 2013;29(3):179–88.
3. Swann AC, Bowden CL, Morris D, et al. Depression during mania. Treatment response to lithium or divalproex. Arch Gen Psychiatry 1997;54(1):37–42.
4. Kruger S, Trevor Young L, Braunig P. Pharmacotherapy of bipolar mixed states. Bipolar Disord 2005;7(3):205–15.
5. Ghaemi SN, Hsu DJ, Soldani F, et al. Antidepressants in bipolar disorder: the case for caution. Bipolar Disord 2003;5(6):421–33.
6. Goldberg JF, Harrow M, Whiteside JE. Risk for bipolar illness in patients initially hospitalized for unipolar depression. Am J Psychiatry 2001;158(8):1265–70.
7. Post RM, Baldassano CF, Perlis RH, et al. Treatment of bipolar depression. CNS Spectr 2003;8(12):1–10 [quiz: 11].
8. Ahlfors UG, Baastrup PC, Dencker SJ, et al. Flupenthixol decanoate in recurrent manic-depressive illness. A comparison with lithium. Acta Psychiatr Scand 1981; 64(3):226–37.
9. Nelson LA, Swartz CM. Melancholic symptoms during concurrent olanzapine and fluoxetine. Ann Clin Psychiatry 2000;12(3):167–70.
10. Post RM, Ketter TA, Uhde T, et al. Thirty years of clinical experience with carbamazepine in the treatment of bipolar illness: principles and practice. CNS Drugs 2007;21(1):47–71.
11. Calabrese JR, Rapport DJ, Kimmel SE, et al. Rapid cycling bipolar disorder and its treatment with valproate. Can J Psychiatry 1993;38(3 Suppl 2):S57–61.
12. Post RM, Uhde TW, Roy-Byrne PP, et al. Correlates of antimanic response to carbamazepine. Psychiatry Res 1987;21(1):71–83.
13. Khazaal Y, Tapparel S, Chatton A, et al. Quetiapine dosage in bipolar disorder episodes and mixed states. Prog Neuropsychopharmacol Biol Psychiatry 2007; 31(3):727–30.
14. Shorter E. The doctrine of the two depressions in historical perspective. Acta Psychiatr Scand Suppl 2007;(433):5–13.

15. Kraepelin E. Manic-depressive illness and paranoia. Edinburgh (United Kingdom): E & S Livingstone; 1921.

16. Angst J, Azorin JM, Bowden CL, et al. Prevalence and characteristics of undiagnosed bipolar disorders in patients with a major depressive episode: the BRIDGE study. Arch Gen Psychiatry 2011;68(8):791–8.

17. Koukopoulos A, Sani G. DSM-5 criteria for depression with mixed features: a farewell to mixed depression. Acta Psychiatr Scand 2014;129(1):4–16.

18. Medda P, Toni C, Perugi G. The mood-stabilizing effects of electroconvulsive therapy. J ECT 2014;30(4):275–82.

19. Perugi G, Akiskal HS, Micheli C, et al. Clinical characterization of depressive mixed state in bipolar-I patients: Pisa-San Diego collaboration. J Affect Disord 2001;67(1–3):105–14.

20. Loo C, Katalinic N, Mitchell PB, et al. Physical treatments for bipolar disorder: a review of electroconvulsive therapy, stereotactic surgery and other brain stimulation techniques. J Affect Disord 2011;132(1–2):1–13.

21. Stromgren LS. Electroconvulsive Therapy in Aarhus, Denmark, in 1984: Its Application in Nondepressive Disorders. Convuls Ther 1988;4(4):306–13.

22. Devanand DP, Polanco P, Cruz R, et al. The efficacy of ECT in mixed affective states. J ECT 2000;16(1):32–7.

23. Gruber NP, Dilsaver SC, Shoaib AM, et al. ECT in mixed affective states: a case series. J ECT 2000;16(2):183–8.

24. Ciapparelli A, Dell'Osso L, Tundo A, et al. Electroconvulsive therapy in medication-nonresponsive patients with mixed mania and bipolar depression. J Clin Psychiatry 2001;62(7):552–5.

25. Medda P, Perugi G, Zanello S, et al. Comparative response to electroconvulsive therapy in medication-resistant bipolar I patients with depression and mixed state. J ECT 2010;26(2):82–6.

26. Medda P, Toni C, Mariani MG, et al. Electroconvulsive therapy in 197 patients with a severe, drug-resistant bipolar mixed state: treatment outcome and predictors of response. J Clin Psychiatry 2015;76(9):1168–73.

27. Palma M, Ferreira B, Borja-Santos N, et al. Efficacy of Electroconvulsive Therapy in Bipolar Disorder with Mixed Features. Depress Res Treat 2016;2016:8306071.

28. Fink M. Rediscovering catatonia: the biography of a treatable syndrome. Acta Psychiatr Scand Suppl 2013;(441):1–47.

29. Moskowitz AK. "Scared stiff": catatonia as an evolutionary-based fear response. Psychol Rev 2004;111(4):984–1002.

30. Kruger S, Cooke RG, Spegg CC, et al. Relevance of the catatonic syndrome to the mixed manic episode. J Affect Disord 2003;74(3):279–85.

31. Sienaert P, Dhossche DM, Vancampfort D, et al. A clinical review of the treatment of catatonia. Front Psychiatry 2014;5:181.

32. Rohland BM, Carroll BT, Jacoby RG. ECT in the treatment of the catatonic syndrome. J Affect Disord 1993;29(4):255–61.

33. England ML, Ongur D, Konopaske GT, et al. Catatonia in psychotic patients: clinical features and treatment response. J Neuropsychiatry Clin Neurosci 2011; 23(2):223–6.

34. Raveendranathan D, Narayanaswamy JC, Reddi SV. Response rate of catatonia to electroconvulsive therapy and its clinical correlates. Eur Arch Psychiatry Clin Neurosci 2012;262(5):425–30.

35. van Waarde JA, Tuerlings JH, Verwey B, et al. Electroconvulsive therapy for catatonia: treatment characteristics and outcomes in 27 patients. J ECT 2010;26(4): 248–52.

36. Yatham LN, Kennedy SH, Schaffer A, et al. Canadian Network for Mood and Anxiety Treatments (CANMAT) and International Society for Bipolar Disorders (ISBD) collaborative update of CANMAT guidelines for the management of patients with bipolar disorder: update 2009. Bipolar Disord 2009;11(3):225–55.

37. Solomon DA, Keitner GI, Miller IW, et al. Course of illness and maintenance treatments for patients with bipolar disorder. J Clin Psychiatry 1995;56(1):5–13.

38. Judd LL, Akiskal HS, Schettler PJ, et al. The long-term natural history of the weekly symptomatic status of bipolar I disorder. Arch Gen Psychiatry 2002; 59(6):530–7.

39. Weinstock LM, Miller IW. Psychosocial predictors of mood symptoms 1 year after acute phase treatment of bipolar I disorder. Compr Psychiatry 2010;51(5): 497–503.

40. Kingsbury SJ, Yi D, Simpson GM. Psychopharmacology: rational and irrational polypharmacy. Psychiatr Serv 2001;52(8):1033–6.

41. Fraser LM, O'Carroll RE, Ebmeier KP. The effect of electroconvulsive therapy on autobiographical memory: a systematic review. J ECT 2008;24(1):10–7.

42. Sachs GS, Peters AT, Sylvia L, et al. Polypharmacy and bipolar disorder: what's personality got to do with it? Int J Neuropsychopharmacol 2014;17(7):1053–61.

43. Bates JA, Whitehead R, Bolge SC, et al. Correlates of medication adherence among patients with bipolar disorder: results of the bipolar evaluation of satisfaction and tolerability (BEST) study: a nationwide cross-sectional survey. Prim Care companion J Clin Psychiatry 2010;12(5).

44. ValentíM BA, García-Amador M, Molina O, et al. Electroconvulsive therapy in the treatment of mixed states in bipolar disorder. Eur Psychiatry 2008;23:53–6.

45. Kho KH, van Vreeswijk MF, Simpson S, et al. A meta-analysis of electroconvulsive therapy efficacy in depression. J ECT 2003;19(3):139–47.

46. Kellner CH, Ahle GM, Geduldig ET. Electroconvulsive therapy for bipolar disorder: evidence supporting what clinicians have long known. J Clin Psychiatry 2015;76(9):e1151–2.

47. UKECTReviewGroup. Efficacy and safety of electroconvulsive therapy in depressive disorders: a systematic review and meta-analysis. Lancet 2003;361(9360): 799–808.

48. Mukherjee S, Sackeim HA, Schnur DB. Electroconvulsive therapy of acute manic episodes: a review of 50 years' experience. Am J Psychiatry 1994;151(2):169–76.

49. American Psychiatric Association. The practice of electroconvulsive therapy: recommendations for treatment, training and privileging. 2nd edition. Washington, DC: Americam Psichiatic Association; 2001.

50. Nivoli AM, Colom F, Murru A, et al. New treatment guidelines for acute bipolar depression: a systematic review. J Affect Disord 2011;129(1–3):14–26.

51. American Psychiatric Association. Practice guideline for the treatment of patients with bipolar disorder (revision). Am J Psychiatry 2002;159(4 Suppl):1–50.

52. Grunze H, Kasper S, Goodwin G, et al. World Federation of Societies of Biological Psychiatry (WFSBP) guidelines for biological treatment of bipolar disorders. Part I: Treatment of bipolar depression. World J Biol Psychiatry 2002;3(3):115–24.

53. Grunze H, Kasper S, Goodwin G, et al. The world federation of societies of biological psychiatry (WFSBP) guidelines for the biological treatment of bipolar disorders, part II: treatment of mania. World J Biol Psychiatry 2003;4(1):5–13.

54. Kusumakar V, Yatham LN, Haslam DR, et al. Treatment of mania, mixed state, and rapid cycling. Can J Psychiatry 1997;42(Suppl 2):79S–86S.

55. Sachs GS, Printz DJ, Kahn DA, et al. The Expert Consensus guideline series: medication treatment of bipolar disorder 2000. Postgrad Med 2000;(Spec No): 1–104.

56. Beale MD, Kellner CH. ECT in treatment algorithms: no need to save the best for last. J ECT 2000;16(1):1–2.

57. Perugi G, Medda P, Zanello S, et al. Episode length and mixed features as predictors of ECT nonresponse in patients with medication-resistant major depression. Brain Stimul 2012;5(1):18–24.

58. Kellner CH, Greenberg RM, Murrough JW, et al. ECT in treatment-resistant depression. Am J Psychiatry 2012;169(12):1238–44.

59. Torring N, Sanghani SN, Petrides G, et al. The mortality rate of electroconvulsive therapy: a systematic review and pooled analysis. Acta Psychiatr Scand 2017; 135(5):388–97.

60. Semkovska M, McLoughlin DM. Retrograde autobiographical amnesia after electroconvulsive therapy: on the difficulty of finding the baby and clearing murky bathwater. J ECT 2014;30(3):187–8 [discussion: 189–90].

61. Semkovska M, McLoughlin DM. Measuring retrograde autobiographical amnesia following electroconvulsive therapy: historical perspective and current issues. J ECT 2013;29(2):127–33.

62. Andrade C, Gangadhar BN, Swaminath G, et al. Mania as a side effect of electroconvulsive therapy. Convuls Ther 1988;4(1):81–3.

63. Lewis DA, Nasrallah HA. Mania associated with electroconvulsive therapy. J Clin Psychiatry 1986;47(7):366–7.

64. Goodwin FK, Jamison KR. Manic-depressive illness. New York: Oxford University Press; 2007. p. 284–5.

65. Sachs GS. Bipolar mood disorder: practical strategies for acute and maintenance phase treatment. J Clin Psychopharmacol 1996;16(2 Suppl 1):32S–47S.

66. Bowden CL. New concepts in mood stabilization: evidence for the effectiveness of valproate and lamotrigine. Neuropsychopharmacology 1998;19(3):194–9.

67. Ketter TA, Calabrese JR. Stabilization of mood from below versus above baseline in bipolar disorder: a new nomenclature. J Clin Psychiatry 2002;63(2):146–51.

68. Calabrese JR, Rapport DJ. Mood stabilizers and the evolution of maintenance study designs in bipolar I disorder. J Clin Psychiatry 1999;60(Suppl 5):5–13 [discussion: 14–5].

Psychotherapy for Mixed Depression and Mixed Mania

Brittany O'Brien, PhD[a,b,1], Delphine Lee, LCSW[b], Alan C. Swann, MD[a,b],
Sanjay J. Mathew, MD[a,b], Marijn Lijffijt, PhD[a,b,*,1]

KEYWORDS

- Psychotherapy • Mixed features • Patient-centered approach
- Evidence-based treatment • Suicide • Anxiety • Hypomania

KEY POINTS

- Treatment guidelines for mixed depression and for mixed (hypo)mania focus generally on pharmacologic intervention.
- In individuals with major depressive disorder, psychotherapy in conjunction with psychopharmacology has treatment effects almost twice as large compared with single intervention.
- Because of the clinical profile, mixed depression defined as (past) major depressive episode with 2 or more manic symptoms could benefit from psychotherapies for bipolar disorder.
- Psychotherapies for mixed states should incorporate modules for reducing suicide risk and anxiety, characteristics of mixed states, and adapt a person-centered rather than manualized approach.

INTRODUCTION

Worldwide, 11% to 13% of adults have a lifetime history of major depressive disorder (MDD),[1,2] and 1% of adults worldwide have a lifetime history of bipolar disorder (BD)[2]; 23.8% of individuals with MDD and 35.2% of individuals with BD experience at least 3 (hypo)manic symptoms during a major depressive episode (MDE), and 35.1% of individuals with BD experience at least 3 MDE symptoms during a (hypo)manic episode.[3] Irrespective of primary episode, the presence of at least 2 symptoms of the opposite pole is associated with an earlier age onset, rapid cycling, a higher risk of psychosis, a higher risk of a substance use disorder, enhanced anxiety, a higher risk of a suicide

[a] Michael E. DeBakey VA Medical Center, Houston, TX 77030, USA; [b] Menninger Department of Psychiatry and Behavioral Sciences, Baylor College of Medicine, 1977 Butler Boulevard, Houston, TX 77030, USA
[1] Both authors contributed equally to this work.
* Corresponding author. Menninger Department of Psychiatry and Behavioral Sciences, Baylor College of Medicine, 1977 Butler Boulevard, Houston, TX 77030.
E-mail address: marijn.lijffijt@bcm.edu

Psychiatr Clin N Am 43 (2020) 199–211
https://doi.org/10.1016/j.psc.2019.10.014
0193-953X/20/Published by Elsevier Inc.
psych.theclinics.com

Abbreviations	
BD	Bipolar disorder
CBT	Cognitive-behavioral therapy
DBT	Dialectical behavior therapy
MDD	Major depressive disorder
MDE	Major depressive episode

attempt,[4–7] and increased treatment resistance.[7,8] In BD, MDE with irritability is associated with delayed recovery.[9]

Treatment guidelines for mixed states focus almost exclusively on pharmacologic interventions and electroconvulsive therapy.[10] Guidance about psychological interventions is absent, despite evidence of the efficacy and extended benefits of psychological interventions across psychiatric disorders, in particular when combined with pharmacotherapy.[11,12] To our knowledge there is no evidence-based psychotherapy for mixed depression or mixed (hypo)mania.

The presence of mixed states present several challenges for treatment, including:

1. A higher likelihood of a severe illness course, with early onset and frequent and/or prolonged periods of affective and behavioral instability.
2. Increased susceptibility to comorbid addiction, trauma-related disorders, and suicide.
3. Treatment targets that shift, in various combinations, over time.

The approach for any psychotherapy treatment plan for mixed states will benefit from being tailored to the patient given his or her specific clinical profile. The treatment plan needs also to be flexible, accounting for the changing and varying needs of a patient at different stages of the illness course. In this article, we (i) describe the clinical characteristics of mixed depression and/or (hypo)mania, (ii) present evidence-based methods and techniques that we believe should be considered for patients with mixed states, and (iii) present a case report to illustrate a tailored, adaptive psychotherapy treatment plan for a patient with MDD with mixed features.

CLINICAL CHARACTERISTICS OF MIXED STATES

To meet criteria for mixed states, an individual must meet (or have met) clinical criteria for MDE and/or a (hypo)manic episode with at least some symptoms of the opposite pole. The *Diagnostic and Statistical Manual of Mental Disorders*, 5th edition, defines the mixed features specifier as having at least 3 symptoms of the opposite pole excluding irritability and psychomotor agitation.[13] However, these diagnostic criteria will likely misdiagnose a proportion of individuals as having pure MDE or pure (hypo)mania, even though they would benefit from treatment for mixed states. Research has shown a more severe clinical illness course for individual who have MDE or (hypo)mania with at least 2 symptoms of the opposite pole, including irritability and agitation. MDE with at least 2 (hypo)manic symptoms in the context of MDD overlap with clinical characteristics of BD rather than MDD.[14] Mixed MDE in the context of MDD or BD is associated with symptoms of overactivation (irritability, psychic and psychomotor agitation, talkativeness, flight of ideas, or racing thoughts); other symptoms of mania, including expansive mood, rarely occur during mixed depression.[5,15–18] In addition to mania-associated overactivation, mixed MDE is also characterized by mood lability, including anger.[17] Worry and negative self-evaluation cuts across mixed depression and (hypo)mania.[5] Depression and (hypo)mania with at least 2 symptoms of the opposite pole have been associated with increased anxiety. Depression and (hypo)mania with at least 3 symptoms of the opposite pole have been associated with increased suicide risk.[5] These findings suggest 3 things:

1. Individuals with MDE or (hypo)mania are at higher risk of a more severe illness course and premature mortality when at least 2 symptoms of the opposite pole are present, including the presence of irritability and agitation.
2. Mixed MDE in the context of MDD resembles the clinical characteristics of MDE in the context of BD, suggesting that individuals with mixed MDE in the context of MDD may more optimally benefit from treatments designed for BD than for MDD.
3. Interventions of mixed states must address the increased risk of suicide and enhanced anxiety.

CONSIDERATIONS FOR PSYCHOTHERAPY OF MIXED STATES

A literature search in PubMed, Google Scholar, WorldCat, and the Cochrane Library revealed no psychotherapy studies specifically for mixed depression or (hypo)mania. This finding suggests that there are few resources for psychosocial treatments specifically designed to meet the needs of patients with mixed depression or (hypo)mania.

Fortunately, a rich array of psychotherapies already exist for MDD and BD from which interventions can be drawn to create an integrated, evidence-based treatment plan tailored to each patient's clinical profile. Because the clinical characteristics of mixed depression in MDD overlap with the clinical characteristics of BD,[14] clinicians are encouraged to consult evidence-based therapies for BD that address the range of symptoms that may occur in a manic, depressive, or mixed episode of the illness. Given the usual severity of illness for patients with mixed states, psychological interventions have to be adjunctive and complementary to pharmacologic intervention rather than used as a stand-alone treatment.

Evidence-based treatment for BD include cognitive-behavioral therapy (CBT), family-focused therapy, and interpersonal and social rhythms therapy.[19] CBT is based on the premise that mood disturbance is the consequence of maladaptive, dysfunctional thinking and that problematic cognitions can be modified.[19–21] Family-focused therapy is based on the premise that caregiver criticism and hostility contribute to and increase relapse risk, which can be modified by changing communication among family members and increasing problem-solving skills.[19] Interpersonal and social rhythms therapy attributes BD-associated mood episodes as a disturbance to circadian rhythms, which can be modified by regulating daily routines and sleep–wake rhythms.[19]

CBT, family-focused therapy, and interpersonal and social rhythms therapy consist of interventions aimed at teaching of coping skills, social and communication skills, symptom recognition, capitalizing on personal strength and resources, functional thinking, adaptive thinking, relaxation, problem solving, sleep–wake cycles, and mindfulness. Although each therapy is unique in terms of structure and emphasis, all include psychoeducation. Controlled clinical trials have shown immediate and sustained effects of these therapies to attenuate symptoms of depression and of mania, lengthen time to relapse, diminish time ill, improve sleep, and improve medication adherence.[19,22–26] CBT is effective in decreasing suicidal behaviors[27] as well as symptoms of anxiety in the context of anxiety disorders.[28]

Interventions for mixed states should also address suicide risk and anxiety. Dialectical behavior therapy (DBT), developed originally for borderline personality disorder (which clinically resembles mixed states) and suicidality,[29] proposes that overt and covert actions are learned behaviors and are amendable through cognitive modification, training of new skills, exposure, and dealing with unexpected situations. DBT reduces self-directed violent behaviors[30,31] by increasing mindfulness, emotion regulation, and distress tolerance.[25]

In this article, we propose a person-centered treatment approach that integrates evidence-based psychological interventions to address common challenges and symptoms that present in episodes of MDD or BD with mixed states. Treatment addresses (i) illness-related safety, (ii) therapy participation, (iii) current symptoms and difficulties, and (iv) relapse prevention. Many of the techniques that we refer to have been used in psychotherapy trials for BD. **Fig. 1** and **Table 1** display the breakdown and the proposed interventions for psychotherapy for a patient with mixed states. We conclude with a case example of Laura to illustrate a tailored, adaptive psychotherapy treatment plan for a patient with MDD with mixed features.

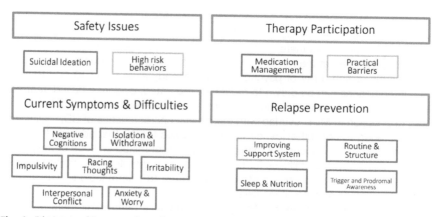

Fig. 1. Diagram of interventions for mixed depression or mixed (hypo)mania.

PHARMACOLOGIC TREATMENT

Treatment guidelines of mixed states recommend pharmacologic interventions and/or electroconvulsive therapy.[10] Communication between the health care providers providing medication management and providing psychotherapy is vital to align treatment goals and manage issues related to potential noncompliance.

Assessment of Mixed States and Symptoms

The Schedule for Affective Disorders and Schizophrenia (SADS) is a clinical interview that assesses severity of symptoms of depression, mania, suicidality, anxiety, and psychosis associated with mixed states that would otherwise require various separate forms;[32-34] the SADS has a change version, which can be used at follow-up. Treatment providers can also assess each disorder and problem area independently (see **Table 1**).

ILLNESS-RELATED SAFETY ISSUES AND TREATMENT PARTICIPATION
Suicide Risk Management

Development of a safety plan, approached in a collaborative and constructive fashion, can provide an early opportunity in therapy for alliance building between patient and therapist.[35] It also creates a model for adaptive, active, and collaborative coping. Suicide risk interventions commonly teach cognitive reframing techniques and problem-

Table 1
Symptoms of mixed states and interventions

Symptom	Assessment Tool	Interventions
Suicide risk	Collaborative Assessment and Management of Suicidality (CAMS)	Collaborative assessment and management of suicidality
	Beck Scale for Suicide Ideation (BSSI)	Crisis response plan (CRP)
	Sheehan Suicide Tracking Scale (S-STS)	Distress tolerance skills (DBT)
	Concise Health Risk Tracking Scales (CHRT-SR; CHRT-C)	Cognitive-behavioral therapy (CBT)
Impulsivity	Barratt Impulsiveness Scale (BIS-11)	Mindfulness (DBT)
		Emotional regulation skills (DBT)
	UPPS Impulsivity Behavior Scale (UPPS)	Distress tolerance skills (DBT)
		Coping ahead (DBT)
Irritability/agitation	Irritability, Depression, Anxiety (IDA) Scale	Emotion regulation skills (DBT)
		Interpersonal and social rhythms therapy (IPSRT)
Low mood	Beck Depression Inventory (BDI)	Accumulating positives (DBT)
Worry and anxiety	Penn State Worry Questionnaire (PSWQ)	Cognitive Restructuring (CBT)
		Mindfulness (DBT)
	Generalized Anxiety Disorder 7-item screening (GAD-7)	Worry time
		Relaxation skills
Negative cognitions	Beck Depression Inventory (BDI)	Cognitive restructuring (CBT)
		Mindfulness (DBT)
		Cognitive Defusion (ACT)
Sleep	Pittsburg Sleep Quality Index (PSQI)	Cognitive-behavioral therapy for insomnia (CBT-I)
		Interpersonal and social rhythm therapy (IPSRT)
Racing thoughts	Focussed clinical interview	Reducing internal and external overstimulation (CBT)
		Organization strategies (PST; CBT)
Interpersonal conflict/strained relationships	Focused clinical interview	Interpersonal Effectiveness (DBT)
Isolation and withdrawal	UCLA Loneliness Scale	Increasing social support and interactions with family/friends (IPT)

solving skills. Stress reframing can be especially valuable for patients with mixed states, many of whom will have developed an enhanced reactivity to stressors.[36,37] Another helpful technique is to identify specific reasons to live, which orients patients to the future. Helping patients to identify or reconnect with social supports, whether family or community groups, is recommended to increase the number of people a patient can rely on for support during times of crisis.

High-Risk Behaviors

Patients who experience increased activation are often at risk of engaging in behaviors endangering themselves and possibly others. High-risk sexual behaviors, excessive spending, and making investments in ventures that are seemingly too good to be true are common behaviors that signal to others a patient is unwell and in need of treatment. Oftentimes, insight is limited regarding the negative consequences of these behaviors in the moment, but may be improved after the fact. A discussion about the short-term versus long-term consequences of the behaviors should be had, emphasizing the benefit of establishing concrete, practical barriers to safeguard the patient from painful and potentially irreversible long-term consequences. Implementation of these boundaries and safeguards should be discussed with relevant family members and legal or financial representatives.

THERAPY PARTICIPATION
Treatment Adherence

Patients and their support network benefit from being educated on the complexities and challenges that come specifically with mixed states. The goal is to move from compliance and adherence to responsible participation.

Practical Barriers

Patients could face significant practical barriers. Challenges to accessing care because of financial, transportation, and scheduling limitations should be addressed to minimize their impact on treatment.

SYMPTOMS AND DIFFICULTIES

A careful assessment of a patient's current symptoms and concerns will inform the selection of evidence-based interventions to improve: coping skills, social and communication skills, symptom recognition, personal strength and resource recognition, functional and adaptive thinking, problem solving skills, sleep–wake cycles, relaxation, and mindfulness skills. As noted, treatment targets may shift. For example, therapy may initially address a combination of depression and overactivation and the associated risk of suicidal behavior. At a later point, interactions between affect or action control and interpersonal communication may be the appropriate focus of treatment and require different interventions. Controlled clinical trials have shown immediate and sustained effects of those modules to improve depression and mania, improve sleep, improve medication adherence,[19,22–26] and to diminish suicidal behaviors[27] and anxiety.[28] Specific interventions should be selected to best suit a patient's clinical profile, his or her circumstances, and a provider's training in delivering the interventions. **Table 1** displays commonly observed symptoms with mixed states, and displays a variety of evidence-based treatments as examples of interventions for those symptoms.

RELAPSE PREVENTION

In BD, the use of behavioral coping mechanisms during a prodromal phase reduced risk of relapse and was associated with fewer mood episodes.[38] Mood charts are used across a variety of disorders. Several good templates are available online. The mood chart should not be too complex, but should be customized based on episode prodromes that the patient and therapist have identified. Mood charts are a vehicle to increase a sense of control, and to facilitate alliance and communication with the therapist.

CASE STUDY

Laura was a 27-year-old, married, accountant who was referred for psychotherapy by her psychiatrist. She began experiencing a lot of "ups and downs" in college. In her senior year, close friends called Laura's parents because she had stopped attending class, was up most of the night, and had expressed a wish to no longer live. She took a medical leave of absence from school, sought treatment, and was diagnosed with MDD with mixed features. Since then, she had been "off and on" prescribed mood stabilizers, more recently "off" since meeting and marrying her husband 1 year ago. She started feeling more irritable and anxious 6 months after they were married. She also started having difficulty focusing at work. About 3 months ago, conflict with coworkers regarding her increasing unreliability resulted in a confrontation with her boss and his suggestion that she resign. Laura's husband and parents were understanding of Laura's difficulties and tried their best to be supportive. However, they were also growing tired and increasingly frustrated by her moodiness, seeming lack of effort to get herself back on track, and not knowing how to help her.

Laura arrived to her first psychotherapy appointment with her husband and mother, wearing wrinkled, casual attire. She appeared tired and ungroomed. She stated that the past few months had been "awful" since losing her job, and that she experienced significant difficulty maintaining basic self-care habits and keeping up with household chores. She described low mood, irritability, racing thoughts, and chronic worry about her marriage and finances. She also noted binge eating, insomnia, and suicidal ideation in the past month. She spent most of the day in bed watching television while her husband was at work. At night, she paced around her house. Her marriage was especially strained since her husband discovered several thousand dollars of credit card debt from online shopping sprees and a withdrawal from her 401K to purchase a lavish all-inclusive vacation for their anniversary. Laura reported abstaining from alcohol and denied engaging in illicit substance use. During the initial phase of treatment, the provider conducted an assessment of safety concerns, factors that posed barriers to engaging in treatment, and current symptoms associated with presenting concerns. **Fig. 1** illustrates the organization of the treatment planning as well as the focal points and interventions used.

Psychoeducation

Psychoeducation was provided to Laura and her family on the expected course, recurrence, and prognosis of MDD with mixed features. Family members were also provided with information regarding the evidence of effectiveness and benefits of psychotherapy. Expectations for therapy were addressed, particularly the recommendation that Laura's family be involved in her treatment. This process included her family helping to establish structure and provide support during periods of greater illness severity, as well as learning to spot emerging prodromal symptoms and helping her to access appropriate levels of care. Laura's reported history of noncompliance with prescribed medications was addressed by providing psychoeducation on the effectiveness of medication. This information was shared with Laura's husband and parents to support compliance during periods when Laura was feeling better and might feel less motivated to take her medication.

Safety Concerns

A safety plan was developed using the crisis response plan model to address suicidal ideation. Laura was guided in a narrative assessment of the most recent crisis and identified thoughts, emotions, behaviors, and bodily sensations to outline possible warning signs of increased risk. Contacts she could reach out to when feeling at increased risk of self-harm were also identified. These people included Laura's husband, parents, and a cousin. Distracting and pleasant activities that were familiar, relaxing, and did not pose risk for overspending were identified, including taking her dog for walk, working on a puzzle, and baking. Laura expressed often feeling overwhelmed by the intensity of her suicidal thoughts. For this reason, distress tolerance skills taken from DBT were introduced and included into her safety plan. Finally, cognitive restructuring techniques were applied to challenge and modify suicidal thoughts.

Targeted Symptom Interventions

The following treatment interventions were applied to target Laura's symptoms and to improve her general coping skills. A variety of evidence based interventions may have been used for these symptoms and were selected based on Laura's receptiveness to the CBT and DBT models:

- *Irritability*: In addition to relaxation skills to decrease irritability, mindfulness skills were introduced to increase emotion awareness, bodily sensations, and the presence of primary and secondary emotions. Emotion regulation skills from DBT were also introduced to address emotional reactivity.
- *Racing thoughts*: To combat Laura's racing thoughts, factors contributing to overstimulation in the environment (noise, clutter, and being in crowds) were identified and removed where possible. She was also educated on the importance of being adherent to medication to manage this symptom. Finally, Laura was taught organizational and time management strategies.
- *Anxiety and worry*: Laura learned cognitive restructuring skills to address thoughts that perpetuated her anxiety and worry. Relaxation techniques such as progressive muscle relaxation and paced breathing were also practiced during and between sessions.
- *Negative cognitions*: Laura engaged in chronic negative thoughts about unemployment, hygiene, and perceived burden on her spouse. Cognitive restructuring techniques were used to identify and modify maladaptive thinking patterns.
- *Isolation and withdrawal*: Since she became ill, Laura significantly decreased time spent outside of her home and with other people. Small goals were made each week to engage in pleasurable, easy-going activities with a friend or a family member outside of the house. It was important when selecting these activities that they felt manageable and were familiar, so as not to induce anxiety.
- *Interpersonal conflict*: Laura's symptoms and history of illness contributed to significant strain on her marriage. They had also made it difficult for Laura to maintain friendships and get along with others. Interpersonal effectiveness skills taken from DBT were introduced to increase her comfort in communicating emotions and needs that increased responsiveness from spouse, parents, and friends.
- *Impulsivity*: Emotional regulation strategies such as (i) chain analysis of the presenting problem and distress tolerance skills taken from DBT were incorporated to increase awareness of impulsive urges, and (ii) mindfulness of possible consequences and alternative behaviors. These coping skills helped Laura to problem solve and identify practical steps to manage her urges to shop online.

Relapse Prevention Interventions

After mapping out Laura's patterns associated with the described symptoms, Laura became more aware of the contributing factors and warning signs that her symptoms were emerging and worsening. **Fig. 2**—drawn from the CBT model—was completed to personalize the relationship between Laura's specific triggers, thoughts, emotions, behaviors, and physical sensations. The figure was shared with her family members to educate them on early warning signs as well. A copy was kept on Laura's phone and posted at home for reference. To decrease risk of relapse, Laura's sleep habits and daily routines were evaluated. Sleep interventions from CBT for insomnia (sleep restriction is contraindicated for Laura),

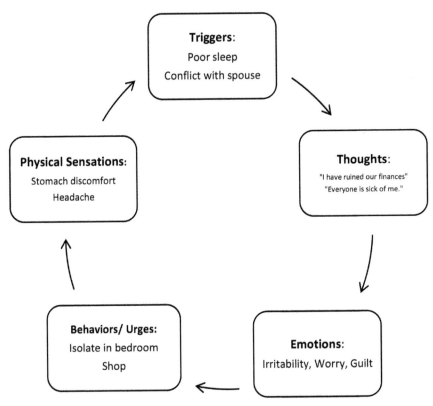

Fig. 2. Laura's personalized illness cycle.

including stimulus control, were applied. Laura was also recommended to regularly exercise. Laura and her provider developed regular daily routines that helped her to plan ahead and balance tasks, chores, and leisure activities to support her mood and relationships. As her symptoms remitted, Laura felt well enough to return to work. She and her provider prepared for changes to her routines and modified daily schedule to ensure she had adequate time to complete scheduled activities during the day and maintain good sleep habits.

SUMMARY

Current treatment guidelines for patients with mixed depression or (hypo)mania focus almost exclusively on psychopharmacological and electroconvulsive therapy interventions,[10] foregoing evidence-based psychosocial treatments. Psychosocial interventions have been proven effective for MDD,[39–41] BD,[19,24] suicidal behaviors,[27] and anxiety.[28] In MDD, psychological and pharmacologic interventions have both similar efficacy, with combined treatment having effects that could be twice as large compared with single interventions.[11,12,39] Adding CBT to treatment as usual in patients with treatment-resistant depression significantly improved depression severity.[42] In addition, there is a lower rate of refusal to start and continue psychological interventions than pharmacologic interventions,[43] which may importantly help to support and enhance medication initiation and compliance, if clinically appropriate. Psychotherapy has been associated with dropout of 19.2% of patients with MDD and 15.2% of individuals with generalized anxiety disorder,[44] with discontinuation possibly signifying a misfit between patient and treatment.

Certain interventions, although effective in the context of major depression or other disorders, may not be optimal for patients with mixed states of depression. For instance, behavioral activation aims to increase the number of daily (enjoyable) activities that a patient engages in to combat low mood[41] and may be less appropriate for mixed states owing to a possible general activating effect. In addition, treatments should also take into account symptoms of psychosis, coexisting substance use disorders and other psychopathological characteristics that can manifest with mixed states[4,5,45] and that have not been the focus of this article. However, the possible combinations of disorders and symptoms associated with mixed depression and mixed mania, well as the case presented in this article, illustrate that interventions must be selected after careful assessment a patient's individual needs. These needs could change across the course of illness, although there is evidence that individuals who experience a pure or mixed manic episode are more likely to experience the same types of episodes in the future.[46] This makes psychological treatment of mixed states defined as MDE or an episode of (hypo)mania with at least 2 symptoms of the opposite pole including irritability and agitation, economically viable, especially when implemented (with medication) at the first appearance of a mixed episode.

DISCLOSURE

The authors have nothing to disclose related to this work. Drs B. O'Brien, A.C. Swann, S.J. Mathew and M. Lijffijt are supported by the use of resources and facilities at the Michael E. Debakey VA Medical Center, Houston, Texas.

REFERENCES

1. Kessler RC, Sampson NA, Berglund P, et al. Anxious and non-anxious major depressive disorder in the World Health Organization World Mental Health Surveys. Epidemiol Psychiatr Sci 2015;24:210–26.
2. Merikangas KR, Jin R, He J-P, et al. Prevalence and correlates of bipolar spectrum disorder in the world mental health survey initiative. Arch Gen Psychiatry 2011;68:241–51.
3. Vázquez GH, Lolich M, Cabrera C, et al. Mixed symptoms in major depressive and bipolar disorders: a systematic review. J Affect Disord 2018;225:756–60.
4. Swann AC, Janicak PL, Calabrese JR, et al. Structure of mania: depressive, irritable, and psychotic clusters with different retrospectively-assessed course patterns of illness in randomized clinical trial participants. J Affect Disord 2001;67:123–32.
5. Swann AC, Steinberg JL, Lijffijt M, et al. Continuum of depressive and manic mixed states in patients with bipolar disorder: quantitative measurement and clinical features. World Psychiatry 2009;8:166–72.
6. Balázs J, Benazzi F, Rihmer Z, et al. The close link between suicide attempts and mixed (bipolar) depression: implications for suicide prevention. J Affect Disord 2006;91:133–8.
7. Azorin J-M, Aubrun E, Bertsch J, et al. Mixed states vs. pure mania in the French sample of the EMBLEM study: results at baseline and 24 months–European mania in bipolar longitudinal evaluation of medication. BMC Psychiatry 2009;9:33.

8. Jha MK, Malchow AL, Grannemann BD, et al. Do baseline sub-threshold hypo-manic symptoms affect acute-phase antidepressant outcome in outpatients with major depressive disorder? Preliminary findings from the randomized CO-MED trial. Neuropsychopharmacology 2018;43:2197–203.

9. Yuen LD, Shah S, Do D, et al. Current irritability associated with hastened depressive recurrence and delayed depressive recovery in bipolar disorder. Int J Bipolar Disord 2016;4(1):15.

10. Verdolini N, Hidalgo-Mazzei D, Murru A, et al. Mixed states in bipolar and major depressive disorders: systematic review and quality appraisal of guidelines. Acta Psychiatr Scand 2018;138:196–222.

11. Cuijpers P, Sijbrandij M, Koole SL, et al. Adding psychotherapy to antidepressant medication in depression and anxiety disorders: a meta-analysis. World Psychiatry 2014;13:56–67.

12. Cuijpers P, Dekker J, Hollon SD, et al. Adding psychotherapy to pharmacotherapy in the treatment of depressive disorders in adults: a meta-analysis. J Clin Psychiatry 2009;70(9):1219–29.

13. APA. Diagnostic and statistical manual of mental disorders. 5th edition. Arlington (VA): American Psychiatric Association; 2013.

14. Sato T, Bottlender R, Schröter A, et al. Frequency of manic symptoms during a depressive episode and unipolar "depressive mixed state" as bipolar spectrum. Acta Psychiatr Scand 2003;107:268–74.

15. Malhi GS, Byrow Y, Outhred T, et al. Exclusion of overlapping symptoms in DSM-5 mixed features specifier: heuristic diagnostic and treatment implications. CNS Spectr 2017;22:126–33.

16. Koukopoulos A, Sani G, Ghaemi SN. Mixed features of depression: why DSM-5 is wrong (and so was DSM-IV). Br J Psychiatry 2013;203:3–5.

17. Sani G, Vöhringer PA, Napoletano F, et al. Koukopoulos' diagnostic criteria for mixed depression: a validation study. J Affect Disord 2014;164:14–8.

18. Akiskal HS, Benazzi F, Perugi G, et al. Agitated "unipolar" depression reconceptualized as a depressive mixed state: implications for the antidepressant-suicide controversy. J Affect Disord 2005;85(3):245–58.

19. Geddes JR, Miklowitz DJ. Treatment of bipolar disorder. Lancet 2013;381:1672–82.

20. Hofmann SG, Asnaani A, Vonk IJJ, et al. The efficacy of cognitive behavioral therapy: a review of meta-analyses. Cognit Ther Res 2012;36:427–40.

21. Leichsenring F, Hiller W, Weissberg M, et al. Cognitive-behavioral therapy and psychodynamic psychotherapy: techniques, efficacy, and indications. Am J Psychother 2006;60:233–59.

22. Chu C-S, Stubbs B, Chen T-Y, et al. The effectiveness of adjunct mindfulness-based intervention in treatment of bipolar disorder: a systematic review and meta-analysis. J Affect Disord 2018;225:234–45.

23. Hofmann SG, Sawyer AT, Witt AA, et al. The effect of mindfulness-based therapy on anxiety and depression: a meta-analytic review. J Consult Clin Psychol 2010;78:169–83.

24. Vallarino M, Henry C, Etain B, et al. An evidence map of psychosocial interventions for the earliest stages of bipolar disorder. Lancet Psychiatry 2015;2:548–63.

25. Eisner L, Eddie D, Harley R, et al. Dialectical behavior therapy group skills training for bipolar disorder. Behav Ther 2017;48:557–66.

26. Lukens EP, McFarlane WR. Psychoeducation as evidence-based practice: considerations for practice, research, and policy. Brief Treat Crisis Interv 2004;4: 205–25.
27. Tarrier N, Taylor K, Gooding P. Cognitive-behavioral interventions to reduce suicide behavior: a systematic review and meta-analysis. Behav Modif 2008;32: 77–108.
28. Carpenter JK, Andrews LA, Witcraft SM, et al. Cognitive behavioral therapy for anxiety and related disorders: a meta-analysis of randomized placebo-controlled trials. Depress Anxiety 2018;35:502–14.
29. Swales MA. Dialectical behaviour therapy: description, research and future directions. Int J Behav Consult Ther 2009;5(2):164–77.
30. DeCou CR, Comtois KA, Landes SJ. Dialectical behavior therapy is effective for the treatment of suicidal behavior: a meta-analysis. Behav Ther 2019;50: 60–72.
31. Panos PT, Jackson JW, Hasan O, et al. Meta-analysis and systematic review assessing the efficacy of Dialectical Behavior Therapy (DBT). Res Soc Work Pract 2014;24:213–23.
32. Endicott J, Spitzer RL. Use of the research diagnostic criteria and the schedule for affective disorders and schizophrenia to study affective disorders. Am J Psychiatry 1979;136:52–6.
33. Endicott J, Spitzer RL. A diagnostic interview: the schedule for affective disorders and schizophrenia. Arch Gen Psychiatry 1978;35:837–44.
34. Endicott J, Cohen J, Nee J, et al. Hamilton depression rating scale. Extracted from regular and change versions of the schedule for affective disorders and schizophrenia. Arch Gen Psychiatry 1981;38(1):98–103.
35. Ellis TE, Green KL, Allen JG, et al. Collaborative assessment and management of suicidality in an inpatient setting: results of a pilot study. Psychotherapy 2012. https://doi.org/10.1037/a0026746.
36. Lijffijt M, Hu K, Swann AC. Stress modulates illness-course of substance use disorders: a translational review. Front Psychiatry 2014;5:83.
37. Lijffijt M. Stress and addiction. In: Swann AC, Moeller FG, Lijffijt M, editors. Neurobiology of addiction. 1st edition. New York: Oxford University Press; 2016. p. 153–75.
38. Lam D, Wong G, Sham P. Prodromes, coping strategies and course of illness in bipolar affective disorder–a naturalistic study. Psychol Med 2001;31: 1397–402.
39. Cuijpers P, Berking M, Andersson G, et al. A meta-analysis of cognitive-behavioural therapy for adult depression, alone and in comparison with other treatments. Can J Psychiatry 2013;58:376–85.
40. Barth J, Munder T, Gerger H, et al. Comparative efficacy of seven psychotherapeutic interventions for patients with depression: a network meta-analysis. PLoS Med 2013;10:e1001454.
41. Ekers D, Webster L, Van Straten A, et al. Behavioural activation for depression; an update of meta-analysis of effectiveness and sub group analysis. PLoS One 2014;9(6):e100100.
42. Ijaz S, Davies P, Williams CJ, et al. Psychological therapies for treatment-resistant depression in adults. Cochrane common mental disorders group. Cochrane Database Syst Rev 2018. https://doi.org/10.1002/14651858.CD010558.pub2.
43. Swift JK, Greenberg RP, Tompkins KA, et al. Treatment refusal and premature termination in psychotherapy, pharmacotherapy, and their combination: a meta-analysis of head-to-head comparisons. Psychotherapy 2017;54:47–57.

44. Swift JK, Greenberg RP. A treatment by disorder meta-analysis of dropout from psychotherapy. J Psychother Integr 2014;24:193–207.

45. Swann AC. The strong relationship between bipolar and substance-use disorder. Ann N Y Acad Sci 2010;1187:276–93.

46. Baldessarini RJ, Salvatore P, Khalsa H-MK, et al. Dissimilar morbidity following initial mania versus mixed-states in type-I bipolar disorder. J Affect Disord 2010;126(1–2):299–302.